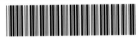

Advances in Endocrine Therapy of Breast Cancer

Advances in
Endocrine Therapy of
Breast Cancer

Proceedings of the 2003 Gleneagles Conference

edited by

James N. Ingle
The Mayo Clinic
Rochester, Minnesota, U.S.A.

Mitchell Dowsett
The Royal Marsden Hospital
London, England

MARCEL

DEKKER

Library of Congress Cataloging-in-Publication Data
A catalog record for this book is available from the Library of Congress.

ISBN: 0-8247-2228-0 (Dekker)
ISBN: 0-932763-01-5 (Summit)

Headquarters:
Marcel Dekker, 270 Madison Avenue, New York, NY 10016, U.S.A.
tel: 212-696-9000, fax: 212-685-4340

Distribution and Customer Service
Marcel Dekker, Cimarron Road, Monticello, New York 12701, U.S.A.
tel: 800-228-1160; fax: 845-1772

Current printing (last digit):

10   9   8   7   6   5   4   3   2   1

PRINTED IN CANADA

Contributors

D. Craig Allred / *Baylor College of Medicine, Houston, Texas, U.S.A.*

Tom J. Anderson / *Edinburgh University, Edinburgh, Scotland*

Denise Barrow / *Welsh School of Pharmacy, Cardiff University, Cardiff, Wales*

Michael Baum / *University College Hospital London and The Portland Hospital, London, England*

Christopher C. Benz / *Buck Institute for Age Research, Novato, California, U.S.A.*

Jonas C. S. Bergh / *Karolinska Institute and Hospital, Stockholm, Sweden*

Ajay S. Bhatnagar / *WWS Group Ltd, Muttenz, Switzerland*

Wayne Bocchinfuso / *Eli Lilly & Co., Research Triangle Park, North Carolina, U.S.A.*

Jacques M. Bonneterre / *Centre Oscar Lambret, Lille, France*

David Britton / *Welsh School of Pharmacy, Cardiff University, Cardiff, Wales*

Ercole Cavalieri / *Eppley Institute, Nebraska Medical Center, Omaha, Nebraska, U.S.A.*

Prabu Devanesan / *PPD Discovery, Morrisville, North Carolina, U.S.A.*

J. Mike Dixon / *Western General Hospital, Edinburgh, Scotland*

Mitchell Dowsett / *The Royal Marsden Hospital, London, England*

Dean P. Edwards / *University of Colorado Health Sciences Center, Denver, Colorado, U.S.A.*

Wolfgang Eiermann / *Frauenklinik von Roten Kreuz, Munich, Germany*

Matthew J. Ellis / *Washington University, St. Louis, Missouri, U.S.A.*

Dean B. Evans / *Novartis Pharma AG, Basel, Switzerland*

Gini F. Fleming / *University of Chicago, Chicago, Illinois, U.S.A.*

Julia Gee / *Welsh School of Pharmacy, Cardiff University, Cardiff, Wales*

Paul E. Goss / *Princess Margaret Hospital, University Health Network, Toronto, Ontario, Canada*

Adrian L. Harris / *Churchill Hospital, Oxford, England*

Maureen Harper / *Welsh School of Pharmacy, Cardiff University, Cardiff, Wales*

I. Craig Henderson / *University of California at San Francisco, San Francisco, California, U.S.A.*

Iain Hutcheson / *Welsh School of Pharmacy, Cardiff University, Cardiff, Wales*

Steven Hiscox / *Welsh School of Pharmacy, Cardiff University, Cardiff, Wales*

James N. Ingle / *The Mayo Clinic, Rochester, Minnesota, U.S.A.*

Raimund Jakesz / *Vienna General Hospital, Vienna, Austria*

Stephen R. D. Johnston / *The Royal Marsden Hospital, London, England*

Walter Jonat / *Universitatsklinikum Frauenklinik, Kiel, Germany*

Nicola Jordan / *Welsh School of Pharmacy, Cardiff University, Cardiff, Wales*

Manfred Kaufmann / *J.W. Goethe Universitat, Frankfurt, Germany*

Fredrika Killander / *Lund University Hospital, Lund, Sweden*

Jan G. Kiljn / *Eramus University, Rotterdam, The Netherlands*

Sara Kinhult / *Lund University Hospital, Lund, Sweden*

Janice Knowlden / *Welsh School of Pharmacy, Cardiff University, Cardiff, Wales*

Kenneth Korach / *National Institute of Environmental Health Services, Research Triangle Park, North Carolina, U.S.A.*

Yubai Li / *University of Virginia Health System, Charlottesville, Virginia, U.S.A.*

Niklas Loman / *Lund University Hospital, Lund, Sweden*

Y. Miki / *Tohoku University School of Medicine, Sendai, Japan*

William R. Miller / *University of Edinburgh and Western General Hospital, Edinburgh, Scotland*

Henning T. Mouridsen / *Rigshospitalet, Copenhagen, Denmark*

Robert I. Nicholson / *Welsh School of Pharmacy, Cardiff University, Cardiff, Wales*

C. Kent Osbourne / *Baylor College of Medicine and The Methodist Hospital, Houston, Texas, U.S.A.*

Trevor J. Powles / *The Royal Marsden Hospital, London, England*

Paul Ramage / *Novartis Pharma AG, Basel, Switerland*

Eleanor G. Rogan / *Eppley Institute, Nebraska Medical Center, Omaha, Nebraska, U.S.A.*

Carsten Rose / *Lund University Hospital, Lund, Sweden*

Jose Russo / *Fox Chase Cancer Center, Philadelphia, Pennsylvania, U.S.A.*

Richard J. Santen / *University of Virginia Health System, Charlottesville, Virginia*

Hironobu Sasano / *Tohoku University School of Medicine, Sendai, Japan*

Rachel Schiff / *Baylor College of Medicine and The Methodist Hospital, Houston, Texas, U.S.A.*

S. G. Silverberg / *University of Maryland, School of Medicine, Baltimore, Maryland, U.S.A.*

E. R. Simpson / *Prince Henry's Institute of Medical Research, Monash Medical Centre, Clayton, Victoria, Australia*

Kathrin Strasser-Weippl / *Princess Margaret Hospital, University Health Network, Toronto, Ontario, Canada*

T. Suzuki / *Tohoku University School of Medicine, Sendai, Japan*

Michael Verderame / *Penn State University, Hershey, Pennsylvania, U.S.A.*

Ji-Pang Wang / *University of Virginia Health System, Charlottesville, Virginia*

Norman Wolmark / *Allegheny General Hospital, Pittsburgh, Pennsylvania, U.S.A.*

Wei Yue / *University of Virginia Health System, Charlottesville, Virginia*

Contents

Contents

Contents

Preface

Endocrine therapy is assuming an increasingly important role in the management of women with breast cancer. This is justified by new evidence from clinical research and new knowledge from the laboratory. The use of endocrine manipulations covers the spectrum from metastatic disease, adjuvant therapy, and neoadjuvant therapy to prevention, the last representing the ultimate goal. The pace of new information is accelerating, particularly from the clinical trials sector with maturation of multiple randomized clinical trials. The appearance of new agents, especially the aromatase inhibitors, has provided the basis for substantial interest and enthusiasm from investigators in the field. Laboratory investigations have also yielded important and potentially exploitable information related to the biology of breast cancer. Because of this rapidly evolving field, 36 leading authorities in clinical, basic, and translational breast cancer research assembled in Gleneagles, Scotland, to review the current state of knowledge and discuss future research directions. This book presents reviews from speakers and the discussions that ensued.

The meeting consisted of five areas of focus. Part I evaluated the clinical pharmacology of the selective estrogen receptor modulators (SERMs), selective estrogen receptor downregulators (SERDs), and aromatase inhibitors (AIs). Part II considered endocrine therapy in postmenopausal women in the metastatic, adjuvant, and neoadjuvant settings. Part III examined endocrine therapy in premenopausal women and addressed its use in the advanced disease in adjuvant settings as well as the role of chemotherapy in women with an estrogen-receptive-positive tumor. Part IV examined chemoprevention and considered the biology of premalignant lesions, estrogen-induced carcinogenesis, and the use of SERMs and AIs in clinical trials. Part V addressed new therapeutic approaches based on emerging knowledge of the biology of breast cancer. The areas examined included the interaction of the estrogen-receptor pathway with other growth factor pathways, surrogate biomarkers, new antibodies for immunohistochemical staining of aromatase, and novel therapeutics for enhancing the efficacy of endocrine therapy.

Over recent years a large number of SERMs have been developed with the primary aim of reducing the agonist activity present in the prototype drug tamoxifen on normal endometrial and malignant breast cells. The rationale for this has been enhanced by an improved understanding of the molecular pharmacology of tamoxifen. However, many of these new SERMs have been tested in comparative clinical trials, yet none have demonstrated superiority over tamoxifen. In contrast, although the pure anti-estrogen, fulvestrant, also has no greater efficacy than tamoxifen in Phase 3 studies, its ability to elicit responses in patients with acquired resistance to tamoxifen (and AIs) provides an opportunity for this drug to find a place in the hormonal treatment cascade. Comprehensive pharmacological characterization of AIs has shown that, unlike earlier inhibitors, the third-generation compounds lead to near obliteration of plasma and tumor estrogens in postmenopausal women with excellent specificity.

The value of endocrine therapy is undisputed in all breast cancer patients whose tumors express the estrogen receptor and/or progesterone receptor. Considering postmenopausal women, further work is needed relating to dose-response relationships with the third-generation AIs. In particular, better means of evaluating impact of AIs on the target organ, specifically the breast, are needed. Laboratory studies have demonstrated that breast cancer cells can adapt to a changing estrogen environment and strategies for dealing with this adaptation are needed. Two classes of AIs, that is, nonsteroidal and steroidal, are available, and research is ongoing to determine if there are meaningful therapeutic differences between these two classes. Both the AIs and tamoxifen have demonstrated efficacy in the adjuvant setting, and multiple clinical trials are addressing the optimal utilization of these agents. When used as adjuvant therapy, the optimal duration of AIs therapy remains to be determined.

In premenopausal women, in the adjuvant setting, the role of chemotherapy and endocrine therapy needs resolution. A major question is whether women who receive adjuvant chemotherapy but do not become amenorrheic should also receive ovarian function suppression. Although ovarian function suppression with LHRH analogues is effective therapy, the optimal duration of such therapy needs to be determined. Evidence exists about the value of the combination of LHRH analogues plus tamoxifen but the value of AIs in place of tamoxifen needs to be resolved. Clinical trials are ongoing to address the value of ovarian function suppression and AIs in adjuvant therapy of premenopausal women, both in the presence and absence of chemotherapy.

Chemoprevention represents a major focus of breast cancer research today. The relationship of estrogens to the risk of developing breast cancer is indisputable. Tamoxifen has been studied in multiple trials and has been demonstrated to produce clear reductions in the incidence of invasive breast cancer. The large randomized trial of tamoxifen versus raloxifene (STAR) will complete accrual of

19,000 patients in 2004. Other studies involving the AIs are both underway and being planned. Cautionary notes were sounded regarding the use of potent AIs in the prevention setting, and measures to monitor patients for adverse events were emphasized. There was agreement that clinical trials of prevention strategies need to continue but that emphasis should be placed on the identification of risk profiles in order to target the most appropriate patients in prevention trials.

The session on biology and novel therapeutics addressed the extensive information forthcoming from the laboratory on signaling pathways in addition to the estrogen-receptor pathway. Multiple interactions between these pathways have been identified. It is clear that there is cross-talk between the estrogen-receptor pathway and other growth-factor-signaling pathways, and this knowledge is leading to hypotheses that can ultimately be tested in the clinic. Major opportunities exist for combining classic endocrine manipulations with growth-factor inhibitors and small molecule signal transduction inhibitors. Characterization of tissues from patients to determine the key factors responsible for de novo and acquired resistance to individual hormonal treatments will be required to deliver rational combinations of the new agents with current endocrine agents, which are likely to remain the bedrock of our therapy in hormone-receptor-positive disease for the foreseeable future. The neoadjuvant setting, whereby specimens can be obtained before, during, and after therapy, is ideal for studying surrogate biomarkers and mechanisms of de novo resistance, but tissue collections will also be required from patients at relapse to allow characterization of mechanisms of acquired resistance.

The quickening pace of discovery related to endocrine therapy was evident in the presentations and discussions from this meeting. Whereas discovery always raises questions and challenges, it is clear that the issues for future study are being articulated. The fact that breast cancer research has become a concerted, collaborative, and global effort is shown in the substance of this meeting. This second Gleneagles colloquium in the homeland of Sir George Thomas Beatson augers well for the quest to eliminate the burden of breast cancer.

James N. Ingle
Mitchell Dowsett

1

Clinical Pharmacology of SERMs and Pure Anti-estrogens

Stephen R. D. Johnston
The Royal Marsden Hospital
London, England

I. OVERVIEW

Estrogens play a predominant role in the growth and development of breast cancer. Hence, efforts at disease treatment and prevention have focused on the blockade of estrogen formation and action. Although tamoxifen, a nonsteroidal estrogen antagonist, is the most widely used therapy for the treatment of breast cancer, its effectiveness is limited by mixed agonist/antagonist activity and by the development of long-term resistance in most patients. This has led to the development of more selective anti-estrogens, as well as so-called pure anti-estrogens with no agonist activity. This chapter reviews data from preclinical and clinical trials on selective estrogen receptor modulators (SERMs) and selective estrogen downregulators (SERDs) in an attempt to understand their current therapeutic role.

II. INTRODUCTION

The anti-estrogen tamoxifen is established as first-line endocrine therapy for women with breast cancer, where it is most effective in estrogen-receptor-positive (ER+) disease. However, most tumors that respond eventually develop acquired resistance and begin to regrow. It has been hypothesized that the partial estrogen receptor (ER) agonist activity of tamoxifen or its metabolites is responsible for the acquisition of tamoxifen-stimulated growth, which can be reversed by tamoxifen withdrawal or inhibited by other anti-estrogens with less agonist activity. Accordingly, attention has focused in recent years on the development of more selective anti-estrogens, such as the benzothiophene selective ER modulators (i.e., raloxifene, arzoxifene), and the so-called pure anti-estrogens (i.e., fulvestrant) that downregulate ER with no agonist activity (also termed selective estrogen receptor downregulators, SERDs). This chapter reviews data from preclinical models and clinical trials on successive generations of selective estrogen receptor modulators (SERMs) and SERDs in an attempt to understand their current therapeutic role, especially in terms of the rapidly evolving use of aromatase inhibitors (AIs) that function by lowering estrogen levels.

III. SELECTIVE ESTROGEN RECEPTOR MODULATORS (SERMs)

As a class, the so-called selective estrogen receptor modulators or SERMs are targeted anti-estrogens that bind ER and alter receptor conformation. They may also differentially activate and/or repress estrogen-regulated genes in different tissues, a mechanism that may be tissue- or gene-dependent. Impetus for the development of SERMs originally derived from the desire to improve on the safety and/or efficacy of tamoxifen. For example, toremifene was developed in the hope that it might prevent genotoxicity, whereas other agents were sought to overcome the endometrial toxicity associated with tamoxifen. In terms of efficacy, some of the prospective SERM compounds displayed greater potency against the receptor, while others had greater binding affinity. Important efficacy criteria included whether SERMs might overcome tamoxifen resistance resulting from its agonist effects or, more importantly, whether they could delay the time to disease progression if the agonist effects of tamoxifen were the cause.

A.   Tamoxifen-like SERMs

The chemical structures for various first generation SERMs in development about a decade ago are shown in Figure 1 (1). Compared to the triphenyl ethylene structure of tamoxifen, there are subtle changes, in some cases yielding beneficial pharmacologic differences. For example, the chlorine atom in toremifene resulted in a compound that did not induce DNA adducts, and the hydroxyl group in position 3 in droloxifene resulted in a molecule with enhanced receptor binding affinity (2,3). Structural alterations in idoxifene included a pyrrolidene ring on the side chain and an iodine atom in position 4 where hydroxylation occurs that, modulated metabolism and enhanced binding affinity respectively (4). Experiments in MCF-7 hormone-sensitive xenografts indicated that idoxifene reduced growth support compared to tamoxifen, although maximum growth suppressive activity still resulted from estrogen deprivation (5). Although both in vitro and in vivo experimental studies often suggested differences in various SERMs compared to tamoxifen, not all studies showed differences (1).

2

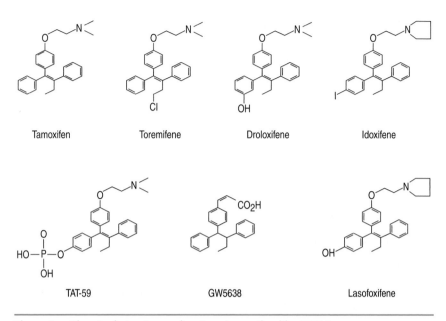

Figure 1 Chemical structures of various tamoxifen-like SERMs.

In view of the reduced agonist activity, a number of Phase II studies were conducted in tamoxifen-resistant patients. However, results were disappointing, showing an objective response (OR) rate of only 5%, and a clinical benefit that included stable disease for at least 6 months of 18% of patients (Table 1) (1). Attempts were then made to see whether, in the first-line setting, the reduced agonist profile of SERMs would result in improved clinical efficacy compared with tamoxifen either in terms of OR or time to progression of disease (TTP). By and large, these clinical studies with toremifene, droloxifene, and idoxifene also yielded disappointing results. Toremifene was probably the best studied, and a meta-analysis of five studies involving 1,421 patients with advanced breast cancer showed no difference in OR or TTP compared to tamoxifen (6). A multicenter Phase III trial comparing tamoxifen (20 mg/day) and idoxifene (40 mg/day) in 220 postmenopausal women with ER+ metastatic breast cancer was stopped early after no clear differences in either efficacy or toxicity emerged. The OR rate was 20% for idoxifene vs. 19% for tamoxifen, with a median duration of OR of 8.1 months for idoxifene and 7.3 months for tamoxifen. Overall, there was no significant difference in TTP or survival (7). A parallel study in the United States showed similar results (8). A summary of results from phase II/III clinical studies with toremifene, droloxifene, and idoxifene, as first-line therapy in hormone-sensitive disease, indicates a median OR rate of about 30% with a median TTP of 7 months, i.e., comparable to tamoxifen (Table 1) (1).

3

Table 1 Efficacy of Tamoxifen-like SERMs in Advanced Breast Cancer

Drug	Tamoxifen-resistant ORR (SD) (%)	1st-line Phase III (*II) ORR (median TTP)
Toremifene	0–14 (16–30)	21–38% (4.9–11.9 mo)
Droloxifene	15 (19)	*30–51% (5.6–8.3 mo)
Idoxifene	9 (9)	20% (6.5 mo)
Median	5 (18)	31% (6.9 mo)

ORR = objective response rate; SD = stable disease; TTP = time to progression.
Source: Adapted from Ref. 1.

B. Second- and Third-Generation SERMs

Chemical structures for second and third generation SERMs, which are based on the benzothiophene structure of raloxifene, are shown in Figure 2. In preclinical studies these drugs appeared especially attractive as they lacked any agonist effects on the endometrium (1). The following drugs will be discussed: 1) raloxifene; 2) arzoxifene, the so-called sister of raloxifene, which had better oral bioavailability and enhanced potency; and 3) EM-652.

1. Raloxifene

Compared with tamoxifen, preclinical data showed that raloxifene had significantly less estrogenic activity on endometrial cells and could inhibit tamoxifen-stimulated endometrial cancer growth in vivo (9). Raloxifene was developed subsequently for osteoporosis, based on clinical studies that showed prevention of bone loss in postmenopausal women (10). Although raloxifene was not developed as an antiestrogen for breast cancer, limited data (albeit disappointing) exist on its activity in patients with advanced breast cancer. An early study by Buzdar et al. evaluated the response of 14 patients with disseminated breast with primary or secondary resistance to tamoxifen. There were no complete or partial responses, and 1 patient showed a minor response, leading to the conclusion that raloxifene had no significant antitumor activity in patients previously treated with tamoxifen (11). Another small phase II study by Gradishar et al. evaluated raloxifene in 21 patients with tamoxifen- sensitive, ER+ disease. Although well tolerated, raloxifene therapy resulted in an OR rate of 19%, with stable disease in 14% of patients (12).

2. Arzoxifene

LY35381 (arzoxifene) is a benzothiophene analogue that is a more potent antiestrogen with an improved SERM profile compared with raloxifene (13). In particular, arzoxifene was a more potent inhibitor of breast cancer cells in vitro than either tamoxifen or raloxifene, and it inhibited growth of mammary tumor

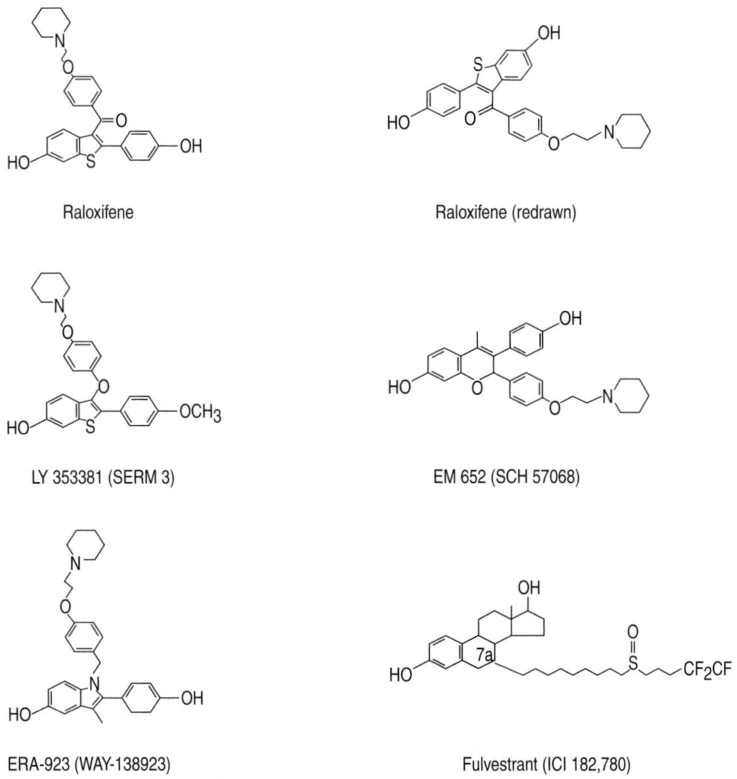

Figure 2 Chemical structures of second- and third-generation SERMs.

xenografts in vivo (14). A study by Detre et al. compared the activity of arzoxifene and tamoxifen, in the setting of continued estrogen, using an MCF-7 xenograft model. At doses of 20 mg/kg, arzoxifene and tamoxifen were equally effective at antagonizing tumor growth over a 4-week period (Fig. 3). Tumors harvested at defined time points (3, 7, 14, and 28 days) and tested for various biomarkers showed equal downregulation of progesterone receptors (PR) and P27 by both compounds. Overall, then, results from this study were unable to differentiate arzoxifene from tamoxifen (15).

Clinically, a randomized, double-blind, Phase II study published recently by Buzdar et al. compared two different doses of arzoxifene (20 mg, 50 mg) in tamoxifen-sensitive ($n = 49$) and tamoxifen-resistant women ($n = 63$) with advanced or metastatic breast cancer. The primary endpoint was OR rate, with TTP included as a secondary endpoint. Among tamoxifen-resistant patients, the OR rate was comparably low (10%) in both treatment groups, with no difference

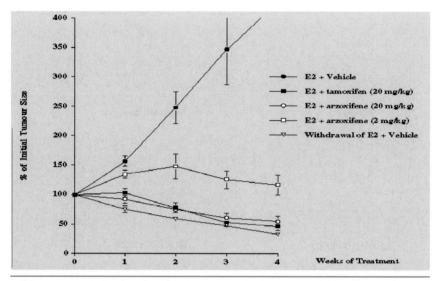

Figure 3 Comparative inhibition of estrogen-stimulated growth of MCF-7 xenografts in oophorectomized athymic mice by either tamoxifen or the SERM arzoxifene. (From Ref. 15)

in TTP (2.7–2.8 months). Interestingly, among tamoxifen-sensitive patients, the OR was numerically higher in the 20-mg arm than the 50-mg arm (26.1% vs. 8.0%) and the TTP was also longer (8.3 months vs. 3.2 months) (16). However, a subsequent Phase III trial was terminated early because results with arzoxifene were apparently no better than tamoxifen.

3. EM-652

EM-652 is a so-called pure anti-estrogen that is nonsteroidal and still basically a benzopyrene in terms of its structure. Johnston et al. have compared the effect of increasing doses (0.01–10 mg/kg) of EM-652, tamoxifen, and raloxifene in an immature rat uterine model, which is perhaps the most sensitive preclinical measure for differentiating the antagonist and agonist effects of these agents. In the absence of estrogen, increasing doses of tamoxifen resulted in a significant increase in uterine weight (a surrogate of agonist effects in this model) with minimal increase seen with raloxifene (Fig. 4). For EM-652, there was no increase in agonist effects over the entire dosage range. On the other hand, EM-652 appeared to be much more potent as an antagonist on a per-dose effect compared to either tamoxifen or raloxifene (17).

To test the hypothesis that a more potent and specific anti-estrogen might show increased clinical efficacy, Labrie et al. administered the prodrug of EM-652

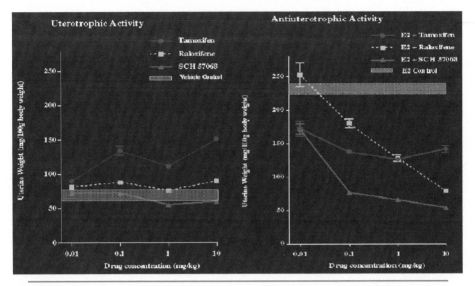

Figure 4 Uterotrophic and antiuterotrophic effects of tamoxifen, and the SERMs raloxifene and EM-652. (From Ref. 17)

(EM-800, 20 mg or 40 mg) to 43 postmenopausal women who had tamoxifen-resistant breast cancer. The OR rate was 14% (1 patient with complete response and 5 patients with partial response), while 10 patients (23%) had stable disease (≥ 6 months) (18). However, a recent large, Phase III multicenter trial comparing EM-800 to anastrozole in patients resistant to tamoxifen was terminated after EM-800 appeared inferior at predefined interim analysis.

Table 2 summarizes the efficacy results for these second- and-third generation SERMs. Although there are less clinical data available than for the first-generation agents, the results are about the same. There is very little activity

Table 2 Efficacy of Second- and Third-Generation SERMs in Advanced Breast Cancer

Drug	Tamoxifen-resistant ORR (SD) (%)	1st-line Phase II ORR (median TTP)
Raloxifene	0	19%
Arzoxifene	3–10 (3–7)	30–36% (8.3–10.4 mo)
EM-800	14 (23)	—
Median	6.5 (7)	30% (9.4 mo)

ORR = objective response rate; SD = stable disease; TTP = time to progression.

Source: Adapted from Ref. 1.

7

against tamoxifen-resistant disease (6.5%) and, because most of the trials were stopped, the limited data on their use as first-line agents show an efficacy rate comparable to tamoxifen (1).

IV. SELECTIVE ESTROGEN RECEPTOR DOWNREGULATORS (SERDs)

A separate class of endocrine agents has recently been recognized with the development of the so-called pure anti-estrogen fulvestrant (ICI 182,780 or Faslodex®). Fulvestrant is a steroidal anti-estrogen that is structurally related to estradiol, but with a long side-chain that results in its potent anti-estrogenic activity (Fig. 5). It is devoid of partial agonist effects, and different in that respect from some of the other nonsteroidal anti-estrogens and the nonsteroidal SERMs. Its defining characteristic involves ER downregulation, which may result in greater efficacy, particularly in tamoxifen-resistant disease. Preclinical studies indicate an absence of agonist effects on the endometrium and possibly a reduced thromboembolic effect compared to tamoxifen.

A. Preclinical Data

Fulvestrant lacks agonist estrogen-like activity both in breast and uterine tissues. When administered alone, fulvestrant showed no uterotrophic activity; when coadministered with estradiol, fulvestrant blocked the uterotrophic activity of estradiol in a dose-dependent manner, with complete antagonism of estrogen action at a dose of 0.5 mg/kg of body weight/day (19). In vitro, fulvestrant's binding affinity for the ER is approximately 100-fold greater than tamoxifen, and in ER+ MCF-7 breast cancer cells, fulvestrant, unlike tamoxifen, is a pure antagonist of estrogen-regulated gene

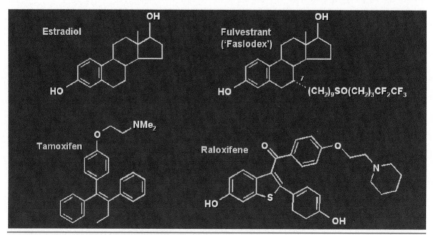

Figure 5 Chemical structures of estradiol, tamoxifen, raloxifene, and fulvestrant.

expression (cathepsin D and pS2) (20). ER expression is suppressed and downregu-lated by fulvestrant, without any concomitant rise in epidermal growth factor recep-tor (EGFR) or transforming growth factor (TGF)-alpha expression (21). In vitro studies have demonstrated that tamoxifen-resistant breast cancer cell lines remained sensitive to growth inhibition by fulvestrant, whereas in vivo studies in oophorec-tomized athymic mice showed that fulvestrant suppressed the growth of established MCF-7 xenografts for twice as long as tamoxifen and significantly delayed the onset of resistant tumor growth (22, 23). Taken collectively, these preclinical data suggest that fulvestrant could be a more effective estrogen antagonist than tamoxifen, and that the lack of adverse agonist effects on breast cancer cells may be advantageous in the endocrine-resistant setting.

B. Clinical Studies

Early clinical data from Robertson et al. that measured the effect of fulvestrant on ER further confirmed its novel mechanism of action compared to tamoxifen and other SERMs. Previously untreated patients with ER+ or ER-unknown tumors were randomized to receive a single IM dose of fulvestrant 50 mg ($n = 31$), ful-vestrant 125 mg ($n = 32$), fulvestrant 250 mg ($n = 32$), oral tamoxifen ($n = 25$), or placebo ($n = 29$) at 14–21 days prior to tumor resection surgery. Fulvestrant decreased ER expression in a dose-dependant manner, with statistically signifi-cant reductions in ER expression at all doses of fulvestrant compared to placebo, and for fulvestrant 250 mg compared to tamoxifen (24).

The clinical efficacy of fulvestrant in women with tamoxifen-refractory advanced breast cancer was shown in a small Phase-II trial in 19 patients who received the monthly IM formulation, starting with 100 mg in the first month and increasing to 250 mg for the second and subsequent months. Seven patients demonstrated a partial response in their tumors, and six patients demonstrated stable disease for at least 6 months. Overall, the median duration of clinical ben-efit for the 13 patients was 25 months. These data clearly confirmed the lack of cross-resistance with tamoxifen that had been suggested in preclinical studies, supporting a mechanism of action distinct from tamoxifen (25). Osborne et al. then compared the efficacy and tolerability of fulvestrant with anastrozole in the treatment of tamoxifen-resistant disease. Postmenopausal women with advanced breast cancer ($n = 400$) received either an IM injection of fulvestrant 250 mg once monthly or a daily oral dose of anastrozole 1 mg. The primary endpoint was TTP, with secondary endpoints including OR rate. After a median follow-up period of 16.8 months, there was no significant difference in TTP (5.4 months for fulvestrant vs. 3.4 months for anastrozole), OR rates (17.5% for both treatments), or clinical benefit rates, indicating an activity level for fulvestrant that is compa-rable to AIs in the setting of tamoxifen failure. On extended follow-up (median 21.3 months), however, there was a significantly greater duration of response

(19 months vs. 10.8 months) in patients who received fulvestrant compared to anastrozole (ratio of average response durations = 1.35; 95% CI = 1.10−1.67; $p < 0.01$) (26). A similar-sized European study that compared fulvestrant with anastrozole in a similar population showed no statistical difference between the efficacies of the two treatments (27).

Another recently reported Phase III trial evaluated the efficacy of fulvestrant as first-line therapy compared to tamoxifen. Patients ($n = 597$) with metastatic or locally advanced breast cancer, previously untreated with endocrine or cytotoxic chemotherapy, received either fulvestrant 250 mg IM once monthly or tamoxifen 20 mg orally per day. The primary endpoint was TTP; secondary endpoints included OR rate and clinical benefit. Given the agonist effects of fulvestrant, one would expect to see a greater duration of response. After a median follow-up of 14.5 months, there were no significant differences between the treatment groups in either TTP or OR rate. Clinical benefit was significantly lower with fulvestrant than with tamoxifen (54.3% vs. 62.0%; $p = 0.03$). In those patients with ER+ and PR+ tumors, however, a retrospective analysis found that the OR rate was significantly higher for fulvestrant vs. tamoxifen (44.3% vs. 29.8%, $p = 0.019$) (28). At first glance, these results may appear disappointing in light of the promising preclinical data that suggested fulvestrant might control hormone-sensitive breast cancer for substantially longer than tamoxifen (23). There have been a number of possible explanations put forward to explain these data, and current studies are exploring a loading dose schedule to achieve higher concentrations of fulvestrant more quickly.

V. ROLE OF SERD IN RELATION TO AIs

Given a scenario in which AIs are likely to become first-line therapy in the adjuvant setting, what might be the role for fulvestrant or other SERDs? Although one might certainly consider tamoxifen or exemestane in a patient who failed AI therapy, data are emerging to suggest that resistance to AIs is associated with enhanced ER signaling, which includes upregulated activation and expression of ER. If the ER pathway indeed plays a central role in the development of resistance in hormone-positive breast cancer, then it may be appropriate to target ER with a downregulator such as fulvestrant, especially insofar as tamoxifen may still function as an agonist in breast cancer cells that become resistant to long-term estrogen deprivation (LTED).

A. Preclinical Models

Emerging laboratory data suggest that endocrine sensitivity may not only be maintained but also enhanced following acquired resistance to LTED with AIs. Hormone-sensitive MCF-7 breast cancer cells treated by LTED eventually adapt and become hypersensitive to the very low levels of estradiol (E2) (29). In part, this is caused by an adaptive increase in ER expression and function (30). There is also evidence for "cross-talk" between various growth factor receptor signaling pathways and ER at the time of relapse, with ER becoming activated and supersensitized by a number of different intracellular kinases, including mitogen-activated protein kinases (MAPK) and the insulin-like growth factor (IGF)/AKT pathway (31–33). Basal estrogen-regulated gene transcription was elevated 7.5-fold in LTED compared with wt MCF-7 cells. LTED resistant cells showed enhanced sensitivity to low levels of estrogen, yet the cells were refractory to the anti-estrogenic effects of tamoxifen. In contrast, fulvestrant fully antagonized estrogen-stimulated transcription in both wt MCF-7 and LTED cells, and it significantly reduced basal gene transcription in the LTED cells (31).

B.   Clinical Studies

To date, response to fulvestrant following disease progression on endocrine therapy with AIs has been evaluated only in small clinical trials. Perey et al. reported on an ongoing trial to assess the efficacy of fulvestrant as third-line therapy in advanced breast cancer patients ($n = 20$) whose disease progressed after treatment with tamoxifen and AIs. After a follow-up of at least 6 months, 2 patients showed a partial response and 5 patients had stable disease ($\geq$ 6 months), which represented 41% of eligible patients (34). More recently, Steger et al. presented data in patients ($n = 48$) with ER+ and/or PR+ metastatic breast cancer who were treated with fulvestrant 250 mg IM once per month following the failure of at least two other hormone therapy modalities. After a median follow-up of 5 months, 3 patients (7%) had a partial response, 17 patients (43%) had stable disease (6 months), and 20 patients (50%) had disease progression, resulting in a clinical benefit rate of 50% (35).

An important finding in the preclinical study by Martin et al. was that, although fulvestrant alone inhibited growth of LTED MCF-7 cells, increasing concentrations of estrogen were able to reverse the inhibitory effects of the drug, essentially resulting in an escape phenomenon (31). This result has played a role in the design of the Study of Fulvestrant With or Without Concomitant Anastrozole vs. Exemestane Following Progression on Non-Steroidal Aromastase Inhibitors (SOFEA) in the United Kingdom. In this large, recently initiated trial, ER+ postmenoupausal women ($n = 750$), with locally advanced/metastatic breast cancer whose disease has progressed on therapy with nonsteroidal AIs, will be randomized to receive either fulvestrant and continued AI (anastrozole) therapy, or fulvestrant and placebo. The control arm will be exemestane. The primary endpoint of the study will be TTP of the disease. A similar study in the United States (EFFECT) will compare fulvestrant with exemestane in patients whose disease has progressed on nonsteroidal AIs.

It is hoped that both of these studies will define the optimal role of fulvestrant in the endocrine treatment sequence for postmenopausal women following prior AI therapy.

VI. SUMMARY

Despite early preclinical promise, SERMs have shown minimal activity in tamoxifen-resistant disease and no superiority over tamoxifen in the first-line setting. Their tolerability profile is similar to tamoxifen, with the only major advantage being a decrease in agonist effects on the endometrium. With the development of the AIs, one might yet question whether there is a role for SERMs in combination with these new agents or in an adjuvant or prevention setting.

As estrogen down-regulators, SERDs have an advantage in terms of mechanism of action, and the lack of agonist effects in preclinical models is very promising. In phase III trials, fulvestrant appears equivalent both to tamoxifen as first-line therapy and to anastrozole in tamoxifen-resistant disease. Preclinical models suggest a potential role for fulvestrant and other SERDs in targeting activated and hypersensitive ER in AI-resistant tumors, and this will now be tested prospectively in clinical trials.

REFERENCES

1. Johnston SRD. Endocrine manipulation in advanced breast cancer—recent advances with SERMs therapies. Clin Cancer Res 2001; 7:4376–4387.
2. Disalle E, Zaccheo T, Ornati G. Antiestrogenic and antitumour properties of the new triphenylethylene derivative toremiphene in the rat. J Steroid Biochem 1990; 36:203–206.
3. Roos WK, Oeze L, Loser R, Eppenberger U, et al. Antiestrogen action of 3-hydroxy tamoxifen in the human breast cancer cell line MCF-7. J Natl Cancer Inst 1983; 71:55–59.
4. Chandler SK, McCague R, Luqmani Y, Newton C, Dowsett M, Jarman M, Coombes RC. Pyrrolidino-4-iodotamoxifen and 4-iodotamoxifen, new analogues of the antiestrogen tamoxifen for the treatment of breast cancer. Cancer Res 1991; 51:5851–5858.
5. Johnston SRD, Riddler S, Haynes BP, Hern RA, Smith IE, Jarman M, Dowsett M. The novel anti-oestrogen idoxifene inhibits the growth of human MCF-7 breast cancer xenografts and reduces the frequency of acquired anti-oestrogen resistance. Br J Cancer 1997; 75:804–809.
6. Pyrhonen S, Ellman J, Vuorinen J, Gershanovich M, Tominaga T, Kaufman M, Hayes DF. Meta-analysis of trials comparing toremiphene with tamoxifen and factors predicting outcome of antiestrogen therapy in postmenopausal women with breast cancer. Breast Cancer Res Treat 1999; 75:804–809.
7. Johnston SR, Gorbunova V, Lichinister M, Manikas G, Koralewski P, Pluznaska A, Garin A, Harvey E, for the International Idoxifene Study Group. A multicentre double-

blind randomised phase-III trial of idoxifene versus tamoxifen as first-line endocrine therapy for metastatic breast cancer. Proc Am Soc Clin Oncol 2001; 20:29a [A113].

8. Arpino G, Krishnan M, Dinesh D, Bardou VJ, Clark GM, Elledge RM. Idoxifene versus tamoxifen: a randomized comparison in postmenopausal patients with metastatic breast cancer. Ann Oncol 2003; 14; 233–241.

9. Gottardis, MM, Ricchio MD, Satyaswaroop PG, Jordan VC. Effect of steroidal and nonsteroidal antiestrogens on the growth of a tamoxifen-stimulated human endometrial carcinoma (EnCa101) in athymic mice. Cancer Res 1990; 50:3189–3192.

10. Delmas PD, Bjarnason NH, Mitlak BH, Ravoux AC, Shah AS, Huster WJ, Draper M, Christiansen C. Effects of raloxifene on bone mineral density, serum cholesterol concentrations, and uterine endometrium in postmenopausal women. N Engl J Med 1997; 337:1641–1647.

11. Buzdar AU, Marcus C, Holmes F, Hug V, Hortobagyi G. Phase II evaluation of Ly156758 in metastatic breast cancer. Oncology 1988; 45:344–345.

12. Gradishar WJ, Glusman JE, Vogel CL, et al. Raloxifene HCL, a new endocrine agent, is active in estrogen receptor positive (ER+) metastatic breast cancer. Breast Cancer Res Treat 1997; 46:53 [A209].

13. Sato M, Turner CH, Wang TY, Adrian MD, Rowley E, Bryant HU. A novel raloxifene analogue with improved SERM potency and efficacy in vivo. J Pharmacol Exp Ther 1998; 287:1–7.

14. Fuchs-Young R, Iversen P, Shelton P, et al. Preclinical demonstration of specific and potent inhibition of mammary tumour growth by new selective estrogen receptor modulators (SERMs). Proc Am Assoc Cancer Res 1997; 38:A3847.

15. Detre S, Riddler S, Salter J, A'Hern R, Haynes BP, Dowsett M, Johnston SRD. Comparison of the selective estrogen receptor modulator arzoxifene (LY353381) with tamoxifen on tumor growth and biomarker expression in an MCF-7 human breast cancer xenograft model. Cancer Res 2003. In press.

16. Buzdar A, O'Shaughnessy JA, Booser DJ, Pippen JE Jr, Jones SE, Munster PN, Peterson P, Melemed AS, Winer E, Hudis C. Phase II, randomized, double-blind study of two dose levels of arzoxifene in patients with locally advanced or metastatic breast cancer. J Clin Oncol 2003; 21:1007–1014.

17. Johnston SRD, Detre S, Riddler S, Dowsett M. SCH 57068 is a selective estrogen receptor modulator (SERM) without uterotrophic effects compared with either tamoxifen or raloxifene. Breast Cancer Res Treat 2000 [A163].

18. Labrie F, Labrie C, Belanger A, Simard J, Gauthier S, Luu-The V, Merand Y, Giguere V, Candas B, Luo S, Martel C, Singh SM, Fournier M, Coquet A, Richard V, Charbonneau R, Charpenet G, Tremblay A, Tremblay G, Cusan L, Veilleux R. EM-652 (SCH 57068), a third generation SERM acting as pure antiestrogen in the mammary gland and endometrium. J Ster Biochem Mol Biol 1999; 69:51–84.

19. Wakeling AE, Dukes M, Bowler J. A potent specific pure antiestrogen with clinical potential. Cancer Res 1991; 51:3867–3873.

20. Rajah TT, Dunn ST, Pento JT. The influence of anti-estrogens on pS2 and cathepsin D mRNA induction in MCF-7 breast cancer cells. Anticancer Res 1996; 16:837–842.

21. McClelland RA, Gee JMW, Francis AB, Robertson JF, Blamey RW, Wakeling AE, Nicholson RI. Short-term effects of pure antiestrogen ICI 182,780 treatment

on oestrogen receptor, epidermal growth factor receptor and transforming growth factor-alpha protein expression in human breast cancer. Eur J Cancer 1996; 32A:413–416.

22. Lykkesfeldt AE, Madsen MW, Briand P. Altered expression of estrogen-regulated genes in a tamoxifen-resistant and ICI-164,384 and ICI-182,780 sensitive human breast cancer cell line, MCF-7/TAMR-1. Cancer Res 1994; 54:1587–1595.

23. Osborne CK, Coronado-Heinsohn EB, Hilsenbeck SG, McCue BL, Wakeling AE, McClelland RA, Manning DL, Nicholson RI. Comparison of the effects of a pure steroidal antiestrogen with those of tamoxifen in a model of human breast cancer. J Natl Cancer Inst 1995; 87:746–750.

24. Robertson JF, Nicholson RI, Bundred NJ, Anderson E, Rayter Z, Dowsett M, Fox JN, Gee JMW, Webster A, Wakeling AE, Morris C, Dixon M. Comparison of the short-term biological effects of 7alpha-[9-(4,4,5,5,5-pentafluoropentylsulfinyl)-nonyl]estra-1,3,5, (10)-triene-3,17beta-diol (Faslodex) versus tamoxifen in post-menopausal women with primary breast cancer. Cancer Res 2001; 61:6739–6746.

25. Howell A, Defriend DJ, Robertson JF, Blamey R, Walton P. Response to a specific antiestrogen (ICI 182,780) in tamoxifen-resistant breast cancer. Lancet 1995; 345:29–30.

26. Osborne CK, Pippen J, Jones SE, Parker LM, Ellis M, Come S, Gertler SZ, May JT, Burton G, Dimery I, Webster A, Morris C, Elledge R, Buzdar A. Double-blind, randomized trial comparing the efficacy and tolerability of fulvestrant versus anastrozole in postmenopausal women with advanced breast cancer progressing on prior endocrine therapy: Results of a North American trial. J Clin Oncol 2002; 20:3386–3395.

27. Howell A, Robertson JRF, Albano J, Aschermannova A, Mauriac L, Kleeberg UR, Vergote I, Erikstein B, Webster A, Morris C. Fulvestrant, formerly ICI 182,780, is as effective as anastrozole in postmenopausal women with advanced breast cancer progressing after prior endocrine treatment. J Clin Oncol 2002; 20:3396–3403.

28. Robertson JFR, Howell A, Abram P, Lichinitser MR, Elledge R. Fulvestrant versus tamoxifen for the first-line treatment of advanced breast cancer (ABC) in postmenopausal women. Ann Oncol 2002; 13(suppl 5):46(A1640).

29. Jeng MH, Shupnik MA, Bender TP, Westin EH, Bandyopadhyay D, Kumar R, Masamura S, Santen RJ. Estrogen receptor expression and function in long-term estrogen-deprived human breast cancer cells. Endocrinology 1998; 139:4164–4174.

30. Chan CM, Martin LA, Johnston SR, Ali S, Dowsett M. Molecular changes associated with acquisition of oestrogen hypersensitivity in MCF-7 breast cancer cells on long-term oestrogen deprivation. J Steroid Biochem Mol Biol 2002; 81:333–341.

31. Martin L-A, Farmer I, Johnston SRD, Simak A, Marshall C, Dowsett M. Enhanced estrogen receptor (ER)alpha, ERBB2, and MAPK signal transduction pathways operate during the adaptation of MCF-7 cells to long term estrogen deprivation. J Biol Chem 2003; 278:30458–30468.

32. Shim WS, Conaway M, Masamura S, Yue W, Wang JP, Kmar R, Santen RJ. Estradiol hypersensitivity and mitogen-activated protein kinase expression in long-term estrogen deprived human breast cancer cells in vivo. Endocrinology 2000; 141:396–405.

33. Stephen RL, Shaw LE, Larsen C, Corcoran D, Darbre PD. Insulin-like growth factor receptor levels are regulated by cell density and by long-term estrogen deprivation in

MCF-7 human breast cancer cells. J Biol Chem 2001; 276: 40080–40086.

34. Perey L, Thurlimann B, Hawle H, Bonnefoi H, Aebi S, Pagani O, Goldhirsch A, Dietrich D. Fulvestrant "faslodex" as hormonal treatment in postmenopausal patients with advanced breast cancer progressing aftrer treatment with tamoxifen and aromatase inhibitors. San Antonio Breast Cancer Symposium, Dec 11–14, 2002, A249.

35. Steger GG, Bartsch R, Wenzel C, Pluschnig U, Locker G, Mader RM, Zielinski CC. Fulvestrant beyond the second hormonal treatment line in metastatic breast cancer. Proc Am Soc Clin Oncol 2003; A78.

2

Aromatase Inhibitors: The Third Generation

William R. Miller
University of Edinburgh and Western General Hospital
Edinburgh, Scotland

I. OVERVIEW

As a result of rational drug development, a third generation of breast cancer drugs that are able to inhibit the aromatase enzyme (which is responsible for estrogen biosynthesis) with immense potency and great specificity have been developed. In comparison with anti-estrogens, such as tamoxifen, which block signaling through the estrogen receptor (ER), aromatase inhibitors (AIs) have the advantage of being devoid of estrogen agonistic action and antagonizing non-ER mediated events, but they will not influence the effect of exogenous estrogens or estrogen mimetics. Among the newly developed inhibitors, anastrozole, letrozole, and exemestane are currently being used to treat postmenopausal women with breast cancer. All are a magnitude of order more potent than the prototype, first-generation drug aminoglutethemide, when given to postmenopausal women in daily milligram doses, often reduce circulating estrogens to undetectable levels without evident effects on other circulating hormones. However, differences exist between the AIs in terms of structure and mechanism of action. Thus, exemestane is steroidal, its mechanism of action competing with natural androgen at the enzyme's active site where it binds irreversibly. In contrast, letrozole and anastrozole are triazoles, which interact with the cytochrome p450 prosthetic group of the enzyme; their action is reversible. Among the inhibitors, letrozole appears most potent, having the lowest IC_{50} for aromatase and reducing estrogen levels to the greatest extent. Optimal use of AIs requires: 1) accurate prediction of which breast cancer is most likely to respond to which inhibitor, and 2) identification of markers of primary and acquired resistance and the means of bypassing such resistance. Tumor estrogen receptor status is currently the best single marker of response to treatment. In terms of resistance, mechanisms may be shared with other forms of endocrine treatment, but it is becoming clear that certain forms of resistance may be particular to AIs; conversely, they may not show cross-resistance with other endocrine agents such as tamoxifen.

II. TARGETING ESTROGEN

Many breast cancers appear to require estrogens for their continued growth and will regress if deprived of these trophic hormones. In postmenopausal women, there are two major strategies by which to produce estrogen blockade (Fig. 1), either: 1) to use agents (SERMs) that interfere with estrogen signaling at the level of ERs within tumor cells, or 2) to block the synthesis of estrogen, which, in patients with breast cancer, occurs both in peripheral tissues (fat and muscle) and the tumor itself. This is most specifically achieved by inhibiting the last step in the biosynthetic sequence of the conversion of androgens to estrogens by the aromatase enzyme using AI.

Although both SERMs and AIs have the potential to reduce the trophic effects of estrogen and cause regression of hormone-dependent cancers in common, there are differences in their mechanism of action, which may have important biological and clinical implications (Table 1).

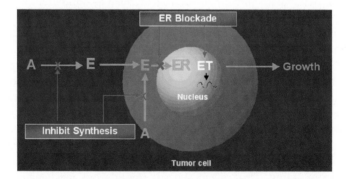

Figure 1 Two major strategies by which to effect estrogen deprivation by: 1) ER block using drugs that block estrogen (E) signaling at the level of the estrogen receptor (ER), thus interfering with estrogen signal transduction (ET); 2) using drugs that reduce the synthesis of estrogen by directly inhibiting the transformation of androgens (A) into estrogen catalyzed by the aromatase enzyme (peripherally/intratumorally).

Table 1 Differences Between Anti-estrogens and AIs

	Aromatase inhibitor	SERM
Endogenous estrogens	Reduced	Unchanged
Exogenous estrogens	Unaffected	Blocked
Agonist activity	No	Yes

For example, there are differences in effects on endogenous estrogens. AIs reduce endogenously synthesized estrogens, but, in contrast, agents that block the effects of estrogen at the level of the receptors generally do not inhibit synthesis; estrogen levels remained unaltered or may even increase (1). This difference may be important because metabolites of natural estrogens can have influences independent of receptor-induced mechanisms (2). Although specific aromatase inhibitors reduce levels of classical estrogen synthesized endogenously, they will not affect the activity of exogenous estrogens or estrogen mimics. Thus, environmental pollutants, plant-derived phyto-estrogens, and adrenal androgens may all interact with the estrogen receptor (3–6) and induce estrogenic activity, including stimulation of estrogen-dependent growth of breast cancer cells (7). In contrast, anti-estrogens, such as tamoxifen, will interfere with ER signaling regardless of ligand. It is, however, interesting that the third-generation AIs appear more effective as anti-endocrine agents than tamoxifen (8–13), which would not support the hypothesis that environmental disruptors are responsible for breast cancer growth (14).

Finally, in contrast to the most widely used anti-estrogen—tamoxifen—AIs are without estrogen agonist activity. This can most readily be illustrated by the effects of treatment on the expression of classical markers of estrogenic activity such as progesterone receptors (PRs). Thus, although AIs reduce the tumor expression, the most common effect of tamoxifen is to increase expression (15).

III. AROMATASE INHIBITORS

AIs represent several generations of development, each generation reflecting a reduced spectrum of inhibition (increased specificity) and greater potency (Table 2). The latest AIs (letrozole, anastrozole, and exemestane) are third-generation drugs. All reduce aromatase activity, reduce estrogen levels, and can cause the regression of hormone-dependent breast cancers in postmenopausal women. However, the drugs differ in their structure, potency, and interaction with the enzyme.

Table 2 AIs by Generation and Type

Generation	Type I	Type II
First	Testolactone	Aminoglutethimide
Second	Formestane	Fadrozole
Third	Exemestane	Anastrozole
		Letrozole

A. Structure

Inhibitors have been divided into two subtypes. Type I inhibitors consist of molecules that compete directly with the natural androgen substrate for the substrate binding site of the enzyme. These agents, such as exemestane, are invariably steroidal, because they are androgen analogues (Fig. 2). The second subtype comprises Type II inhibitors, which interact with the haem moiety of the cytochrome P_{450} prosthetic group in the aromatase molecule, inhibiting electron transfer. Type II inhibitors (anastrozole and letrozole) are nonsteroidal because they are azoles.

These structural differences may have implications for long-term treatment, whereby the steroidal agents may result in androgenic effects. For example, increasing doses of the steroidal agent exemestane (including those used clinically) appear to suppress sex hormone-binding globulin (SHBG) progressively (16). Similar changes in SHBG and other hormone plasma concentrations—including follicle-stimulating hormone and luteinizing hormone—have been seen with another steroidal AI, formestane (17, 18). The effects are only rarely associated with overt androgenic side effects. Indeed, steroidal influences may be beneficial in normal tissues subject to long-term estrogen deprivation. In this respect, results have been presented suggesting that exemestane can protect against bone mineral density loss in ovariectomized mice, whereas the non-steroidal inhibitor, letrozole, does not (19). Whether these differences observed in an animal model are relevant to postmenopausal women treated with AIs remains to be established.

B. Potency

The potency of AIs has been tested in a variety of model systems including placental microsomes, particulate tumor fractions, and whole-cell systems (20). The latest generations of agents are magnitudes of order more potent than the prototype drug, aminoglutethimide. Thus, whereas micromolar concentrations were required for aminoglutethimide, only nanomolar concentrations are needed with letrozole, anastrozole, exemestane, and formestane. Typical IC_{50} values (50% inhibitory concentration) derived from placental microsomes, breast cancer homogenates, and cultured fibroblasts of breast adipose tissue as the test system are summarized as shown in Table 3. Relative potency compared with

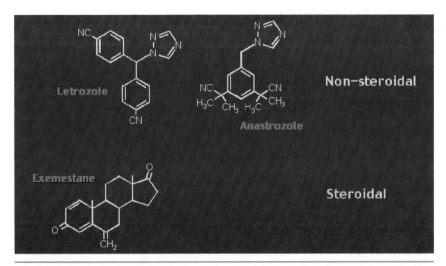

Figure 2   Structure of different AIs.

aminoglutethimide in the fibroblasts ranged from 10,000 times greater for letrozole, to 1,600 times for exemestane and 570 times for anastrozole.

Interestingly, letrozole appears to be more active in whole-cell cultures than in disrupted-cell preparations (Table 3). More detailed comparisons of the two third-generation Type II AIs, letrozole and anastrozole, have been made across several cell systems and reported by Bhatnagar et al. (21). These comparisons confirmed that letrozole was more potent than anastrozole, but in disrupted cell preparations, the difference was only two-fold as compared with 12- to 30-fold in whole cell systems. This increase in potency may reflect differences between the two drugs in pharmacokinetics or drug uptake (22).

In vivo effects of AIs have been assessed on peripheral aromatase activity and circulating estrogens in postmenopausal women. At clinically used doses, anastrozole, letrozole, and exemestane all markedly suppress in vivo aromatization (letrozole: 98.9%; exemestane: 97.9%; anastrozole: 96.7%) (23–25). As a consequence, circulating estrogens in postmenopausal women fall to levels that are often below the detection limit of current assays. However, differences between AIs have also been reported. Geisler et al. conducted a cross-over experiment comparing the effects of therapy in patients given letrozole first followed by anastrozole, or vice versa (26). Each group of patients was treated for 6 weeks. Following crossover from anastrozole to letrozole, whole body estrogen inhibition increased significantly from 97.3% to > 99.1% (the detection limit of the assays) in all six patients studied ($p = .0022$) (Fig. 3). In the reverse direction—switching from letrozole to anastrozole—the suppressive effects of letrozole to below the level of detection were lost on transfer to anastrozole, with aromatase activity becoming detectable in

Table 3 Inhibition of Aromatase Activity in Whole-Cell and Disrupted-Cell Preparation

	Placental microsomes		Breast cancer homogenates		Mammary fibroblast cultures	
	IC_{50} (nM)	Relative potency	IC_{50} (nM)	Relative potency	IC_{50} (nM)	Relative potency
Aminoglutethimide	3000	1	4500	1	8000	1
Anastrozole	12	250	10	450	14	570
Letrozole	12	250	2.5	1800	0.8	10,000
Formestane	50	60	30	150	45	180
Exemestane	50	60	15	300	5	1600

five of six cases. Data from the same study showed that these differences also applied to levels of circulating estrogen. Thus, letrozole produced greater suppression of plasma estrone (84.3 vs 81.0%), estrone sulfate (98.0 vs 93.5%), and estradiol (values) than anastrozole. Differences reached significance for estrone ($p = 0.019$) and estrone sulfate ($p = 0.0037$), but that for estradiol did not reach significance, most likely because many measurements were below the assay's level of detection. It still remains to be determined if these differences in suppression of aromatase translate into differences in clinical benefit.

C.   Inhibitor-Enzyme Interaction

Differences exist between the mechanisms by which AIs bind and interact with the aromatase enzyme. Inhibitors, such as formestane and exemestane, bind irre-

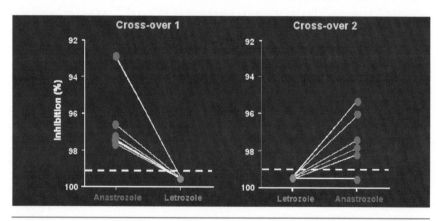

Figure 3   Patients switching to letrozole consistently achieved greater inhibition of whole body aromatization than with anastrozole. In contrast, patients switching to anastrozole lost the level of inhibition achieved by letrozole.

versibly to the aromatase enzyme and, as such, have been termed aromatase inactivators. Indeed, it may be that the parent compound is metabolized by the enzyme into reactive intermediates which results in irreversible binding. This type of inhibition is mechanism-based (27) and, because the enzyme is inactivated as a result of its own metabolism, the drugs have been termed "suicide inhibitors" (27). A further consequence of such inactivation is that the inhibition is generally specific and long term, and continued presence of the drugs is not required for inhibition (28). Conversely, Type II inhibitors, which include letrozole and anastrozole, bind reversibly by associating with the moiety of the cytochrome P_{450} of the aromatase enzyme, and continued presence of the drug is required for effective inhibition.

These differences may be illustrated in an experimental system (29). Thus, if cultured fibroblasts are incubated with either Type I or II AIs prior to an assay of aromatase when inhibitors are removed, irreversible Type I agents—exemestane and formestane—are associated with decreased aromatase activity, whereas the reversible properties of Type II inhibitors, such as aminoglutethimide, anastrozole, fadrozole, and letrozole, mean that inhibition is not apparent without their continued presence during assay. Interestingly, in this experiment design, increased levels of aromatase activity may be observed with Type II nonsteroidal inhibitors upon discontinuation of the drug. This is because the azoles may both induce aromatase mRNA and stabilize the enzyme protein (30, 31). Confirmation of these effects may be seen in surgical specimens derived from patients given AIs. Thus, in a study in which breast fat was collected before and after 3 months of therapy and assayed in vitro for aromatase, an increase in activity was seen following treatment with aminoglutethimide-hydrocortisone (Fig. 4) (29); similar but lesser effects were seen with both anastrozole and letrozole, particularly when there were low levels of aromatase activity in the fat, but the irreversible Type I inhibitor, exemestane, was always associated with decreased activity. Thus, it is possible that, although reversible, Type II agents may be highly potent in the short term, but they may be less effective in the long term if effects lead to the induction and stabilization of the aromatase enzyme. More research is needed in this area because it is not yet clear whether the effect is clinically relevant.

D. Predictors of Response

Although AIs produce strong estrogen deprivation and are effective endocrine agents in postmenopausal women with breast cancer, not all tumors respond to therapy. Currently, the single most useful predictive marker for response to AIs is ER status. This can be most clearly illustrated by observations from neoadjuvant studies in which ERs are measured in pretreatment biopsies and response is monitored by volume changes in the same primary tumor. Thus, in

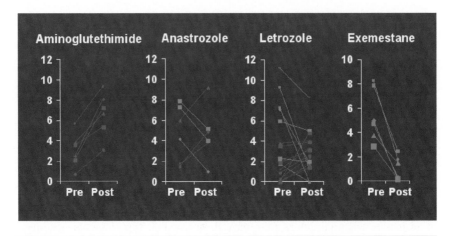

Figure 4 Reduction of breast fat aromatase activity following the administration of different AIs (pre = baseline; post = after 3 months of therapy).

a study from a single center (Table 4), no ER-poor (< 20 fmol/mg cytosol protein) tumor responded to either aminoglutethimide or formestane. Patients with such tumors should not be candidates for treatment with AIs. Although the responses came from the ER-rich tumor cohort, the presence of ER did not guarantee benefit. The problem that still remains is how to differentiate those ER-rich patients who will respond to therapy and those who will not. The PR has been investigated in this respect. However, although patients who have ER+/PR+ tumors tend to have higher response rates than those with ER+/PR− tumors (32), benefits of aromatase inhibition may occur in PgR− tumors (Table 4).

Although ER and PR are predictive for all forms of endocrine therapy, it is possible that some markers may be predictive for individual forms of therapy. In this respect, overexpression of the human epidermal growth factor receptors (HERs) appear to be associated with a low likelihood of response to tamoxifen, whereas tumors that overexpressed HER genes B-1 and B-2 were more likely to respond to letrozole compared with those that were negative for these markers (33).

However, additional markers are required so that management with AIs may be more completely optimized. Studies have been initiated to identify such markers in the neoadjuvant setting. Serial biopsies are taken before treatment and between 10 and 14 days of therapy with aromatase inhibition. Following 3 months of treatment, the patients undergo surgery, and samples are taken from the excised

Table 4 Estrogen/Progesterone (ER/PR) Receptor
Status and Response to AIs

	Response	Nonresponse
ER rich	6 (43%)	8
ER poor	0 (0%)	8
PR+	46 (88%)	6
PR–	4 (57%)	3

breast tumor. This protocol allows the identification of molecular change that occurs before any clinical response is seen. It is hoped that candidate genes will be found by micro-array of the tissue samples. These candidate genes will then be used as markers to dictate therapy.

E. Resistance Mechanisms

Substantial numbers of patients with breast cancer benefit from endocrine therapy, but most still die of disease that appears resistant to treatment. Thus, it is essential to understand the mechanism(s) by which both primary and acquired resistance can occur. Resistance to therapy can be either as de novo or acquired. Underlying mechanisms may also be common to all forms of estrogen deprivation whereas others may be specific to particular forms of therapy, such as AIs (34–36).

1. General Mechanisms

These mechanisms include: 1) the absence of a functional estrogen signaling system; 2) inefficient hormone deprivation; 3) hormone compensation; 4) clonal outgrowth of insensitive cells; 5) estrogen hypersensitivity; and 6) dependence on other signaling systems. The detailed evidence for these mechanisms has been reviewed elsewhere (37) and, although it is clear that all are theoretically possible and may be detected in model systems, clinical experience may be summarized as follows.

Breast cancers that have no (or low) ERs, do not appear to require estrogen for their continued growth (38). These tumors are, therefore, unlikely to respond to measures that are specifically designed to block synthesis or action of estrogen. This mechanism is a major reason for de novo resistance to therapy. Patients with ER– tumors should not be candidates for endocrine treatment.

Therapies that do not adequately suppress estrogen signaling may be associated with apparent hormone insensitivity; however, these tumors may respond to more efficient hormone deprivation. Clinical experience suggests that responses to second-line therapies are not infrequent. Hormone compensation can occur and lead to resistance. This is the underlying reason for the reluctance to use AIs in premenopausal women, because first-generation inhibitors, such as aminoglutethimide, are largely ineffective at reducing circulating estrogens and producing clinical benefit (39–41) as a result of compensatory feedback loops in the hypothalamus/pituitary (42). These raise levels of gonadotrophins, which stimulate the ovary, resulting in increased androgen substrate and aromatase. Although the latest generation of more potent inhibitors may produce effective blocks, they have yet to be used routinely in premenopausal women.

Hormone-insensitive clones of tumor cells that were present at initiation of therapy may emerge under the selective pressure of treatment. However, although cellular heterogeneity related to hormone receptors and sensitivity has been documented (43, 44), clinical observations are not compatible with differential destruction of cell clones being uniquely (or even generally) associated with acquired resistance. Thus, if successful endocrine treatment selectively kills ER+ cells so ER– clones emerge at relapse, tumor receptor content should fall progressively with therapy. This can occur (45), but tumors relapsing after endocrine treatment are very often ER+ (46).

Breast cancers may have a hormone-resistant phenotype if tumors are/become hypersensitive to estrogen (47). One of the mechanisms by which this may occur is by ligand-independent phosphorylation of ERs. The consequence is that signal transduction can occur even in an environment of low estrogen (48). Therefore, it is pertinent that high expression of either EGF-receptor (49, 50), protein kinase A (51) or insulin-like growth factor receptor (50) confers hormone resistance clinically (52).

2. Specific Resistance to AIs

There are several possible mechanisms by which tumors may have the phenotype of selective resistance to AIs. These include: 1) high/over-expression of aromatase, 2) mutant aromatase, and 3) tumor stimulation by nonclassical and/or exogenous estrogens.

High or over-expression of aromatase may mean that effective inhibition of aromatase is not achieved by the clinical dose of drugs. For example, in premenopausal women, high aromatase activity in the ovary is difficult to block, and AIs have not been effective in this setting (40). Although levels of aromatase activity in peripheral tissues of postmenopausal women are substantially lower than those in the premenopausal ovary, it is possible to induce activity. Thus, breast cancers from patients treated with aminoglutethimide display paradoxically high levels of aromatase as assessed ex vivo. These effects are consistent with aminoglutethimide's ability to induce microsomal cytochrome P_{450} hydroxylases (53). Similar effects have been observed with other nonsteroidal inhibitors, such as anastrozole and letrozole (28). The phenomenon might reduce the long-term efficacy of this class of drug. Interestingly, response to steroidal Type I inhibitors (which are not known to induce aromatase) have been reported in patients relapsing on nonsteroidal agents (54–56).

Structure-function studies of aromatase suggest that selective resistance to inhibitors may occur as a result of gene mutation. For example, one particular point mutation, induced experimentally in cDNA coding for the active site of the aromatase enzyme, decreased sensitivity to 4-hydroxyandrostenedione without changing either sensitivity to aminoglutethimide or inherent aromatase activity (57). This phenotype has also been observed in about 15% of breast cancers that display aromatase activity sensitive to nonsteroidal inhibitors, such as amino-glutethimide and fadrozole, but relatively resistant to 4-hydroxyandrostenedione (58). Studies in which aromatase activity has been measured in breast cancer before and during treatment with 4-hydroxyandrostenedione also support the concept that certain tumors may be resistant to 4-hydroxyandrostenedione (59, 58). Interestingly, these resistant tumors also do not show the reduction in DNA synthesis or proliferative activity that is usually observed in tumors that respond to 4-hydroxyandrostenedione (Fig. 5) (59).

AIs block the synthesis of classical estrogens, but they do not affect other sources of estrogenic activity including: 1) Δ^5androgens, which are produced in large amounts by the adrenal cortex, and 2) exogenously derived estrogens, which include synthetic estrogens (60), industrial pollutants (5), and phyto-estrogens (6). If these sources make a substantial contribution to the tumor environment, these par-

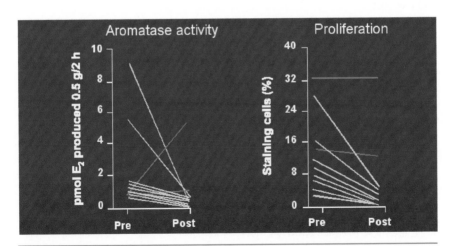

Figure 5 Change in tumor aromatase activity and proliferation following the administration of formestane. These changes are usually observed in tumors that respond to 4-hydroxyandrostenedione.

27

ticular cancers will appear resistant to AIs, but they could still be estrogen-dependent and respond to other forms of endocrine blockage, e.g., anti-estrogens. However, it is interesting that recent trials indicate that AIs are at least equivalent to tamoxifen, if not superior (10–15, 20, 61, 62), suggesting that endogenously synthesized estrogens (rather than exogenous agents) drive growth in the majority of breast cancers.

IV. CONCLUSIONS

In conclusion, a new generation of potent and specific AIs have been developed that can suppress aromatase activity and levels of endogenous estrogens in postmenopausal women more effectively than ever before. All these agents, which include letrozole, anastrozole, and exemestane, offer significant advantages over earlier AIs and other endocrine modalities for breast cancer patients with respect to efficacy and tolerability. However, the drugs differ in structure, potency, and interaction with the aromatase enzyme, such that individual inhibitors may be optimal in different breast cancers and management settings. This offers the opportunity for more tailored therapy in individual cancers based on specific tumor genotypes to particular inhibitors.

In order to aid this identification, it will be important to have good, reliable markers that will accurately predict response to therapy. Finally, the methods by which tumors develop resistance to aromatase therapy need to be identified.

REFERENCES

1. Santen RJ, Manni A, Harvey H, Redmond C. Endocrine treatment of breast cancer in women. Endocr Rev 1990; 11:1–45.
2. Liehr JG. Breast carcinogenesis and its prevention by inhibition of estrogen genotoxicity. In: Miller WR, Ingle JN, eds. Endocrine Therapy in Breast Cancer. New York: Marcel Dekker, 2002; pp. 287–301.
3. Sharpe RM. Could environmental oestrogenic chemicals be responsible for some disorders of human male reproductive development? Curr Opin Urol 1994; 4:295–301.
4. Setchell KDP, Borriello SP, Hulme P, Kirk DN, Axelson M. Nonsteroidal estrogens of dietary origin: possible roles in hormone-dependent disease. Am J Clin Nutr 1984; 40:569–578.
5. McLachlan JA, Newbold RR. Estrogens and development. Environ Health Perspect 1987; 75:25–27.
6. Adams JB, Garcia M, Rochefort H. Estrogenic effects of physiological concentrations of 5-androstene 3β17β diol and its metabolism in MCF-7 human breast cancer cells. Cancer Res 1981; 42:470–4726.
7. Boccuzzi G, Brignardello E, di Monaco M, Forte C, Leonardi L, Pizzini A. Influence of dehydropiandrosterone and 5-en-androstene-3-beta,17-beta-diol on the growth of

MCF-7 human breast cancer cells induced by 17-beta estradiol. Anticancer Res 1992; 12:799–803.

8. Mouridsen H, Gershanovich M, Sun Y, Perez-Carrion R, Boni C, Monnier A, Apffelstaedt J, Smith R, Sleeboom HP, Janicke F, Pluzanska A, Dank M, Becquart D, Bapsy PP, Salminen E, Snyder R, Lassus M, Verbeek JA, Staffler B, Chaudri-Ross HA, Dugan M. Superior efficacy of letrozole versus tamoxifen as first-line therapy for post-menopausal women with advanced breast cancer: results of a Phase III study of the International Letrozole Breast Cancer Group. J Clin Oncol 2001; 19(10):2596–2606.

9. Mouridsen H, Sun Y, Gershanovich M, et al. Final survival analysis of the double-blind, randomized, multinational Phase III trial of letrozole (Femara®) compared to tamoxifen as first-line hormonal therapy for advanced breast cancer. Breast Cancer Res Treat 2001; 69:211.

10. Nabholtz JM, Buzdar A, Pollak M, Harwin W, Burton G, Mangalik A, Steinberg M, Webster A, von Euler M. Anastrozole is superior to tamoxifen as first-line therapy for advanced breast cancer in postmenopausal women: results of a North American multicenter randomized trial. Arimidex Study Group. J Clin Oncol 2000; 18:3758–3767.

11. Dixon JM, Love CD, Bellamy CO, Cameron DA, Leonard RC, Smith H, Miller WR. Letrozole as primary medical therapy for locally advanced and large operable breast cancer. Breast Cancer Res Treat 2001; 66:191–199.

12. Eiermann W, Paepke S, Appfelstaedt J. Letrozole Neoadjuvant Breast Cancer Study Group. Preoperative treatment of postmenopausal breast cancer patients with letrozole. A randomized double-blind multicenter study. Ann Oncol 2001; 12:1527–1532.

13. The ATAC Trialist's Group. Anastrozole alone or in combination with tamoxifen versus tamoxifen alone for adjuvant treatment of postmenopausal women with early breast cancer: first results of the ATAC randomised trial. Lancet 2002; 359:2131–2139.

14. Miller WR, Sharpe RM. Environmental oestrogens and human reproductive cancers. Endocr Relat Cancer 1998; 5:69–96.

15. Miller WR, Dixon JM, Macfarlane L, Cameron D, Anderson TJ. Pathological features of breast cancer response following neoadjuvant treatment with either letrozole or tamoxifen. Eur J Cancer 2002; 39:462–468.

16. Johannessen DC, Engan T, di Salle E, Zurio MG, Paolini J, Ornati G, Piscitelli G, Kvinnsland S, Lonning PE. Endocrine and clinical effects of exemestane (PNU 155971), a novel steroidal aromatase inhibitor, in postmenopausal breast cancer patients: a Phase I study. Clin Cancer Res 1997; 3:1101–1108.

17. Boeddinghaus IM, Dowsett M. Comparative clinical pharmacology and pharmaco-kinetic interactions of aromatase inhibitors. J Steroid Biochem Mol Biol 2001; 79:85–91.

18. Bajetta E, Zilembo N, Bichisao E, Pozzi P, Toffolatti L. Steroidal aromatase inhibitors in elderly patients. Crit Rev Oncol Hematol 2000; 33:137–142.

19. Goss P, Cheung AM, Lowery C, Hu H, Qi S. Comparison of the effects of exemestane, 17-hydroexemestane and letrozole on bone and lipid metabolism in the ovariectomized rat [abstr 415]. Breast Cancer Res Treat 2002; 76 (Suppl 1).

20. Miller WR, Jackson J. The therapeutic potential of aromatase inhibitors. Expert Opin Investig Drugs 2003; 12:1–15.

21. Bhatnagar AS, Brodie AM, Long BJ, Evans DB, Miller WR. Intracellular aromatase and its relevance to the pharmacological efficacy of aromatase inhibitors. J Steroid Biochem Mol Biol 2001; 76:199–202.

22. Bhatnagar AS, Miller WR. Pharmacology of inhibitors of estrogen biosynthesis. In: Oettel M, Schillinger E, eds. Handbook of Experimental Pharmacology: Estrogens and Antiestrogens. Berlin: Springer-Verlag, 1999; pp. 223–230.

23. Miller WR, Dixon JM. Local endocrine effects of aromatase inhibitors within the breast. J Steroid Biochem Mol Biol 2001; 79:93–102.

24. Dowsett M, Jones A, Johnston SR, Jacobs S, Trunet P, Smith IE. In vivo measurement of aromatase inhibition by letrozole (CGS 20267) in postmenopausal patients with breast cancer. Clin Cancer Res 1995; 1:1511–1515.

25. Geisler J, King N, Dowsett M, Ottestad L, Lundgren S, Walton P, Kormeset PO, Lonning PE. Influence of anastrozole (Arimidex), a selective non-steroidal aromatase inhibitor, on in vivo aromatisation and plasma oestrogen levels in postmenopausal women with breast cancer. Br J Cancer 1996; 74:1286–1291.

26. Geisler J, Haynes B, Anker G, Dowsett M, Lonning PE. Influence of letrozole and anastrozole on total body aromatization and plasma estrogen levels in postmenopausal breast cancer patients evaluated in a randomized, cross-over study. J Clin Oncol 2002; 20:751–757.

27. Johnston JO, Metcalf BW. Aromatase: a target enzyme in breast cancer. In: Sunkara PS, eds. Novel Approaches to Cancer Chemotherapy. London: Academic Press, 1984; pp. 307–328.

28. Miller WR, Vidya R, Mullen P, Dixon JM. Induction and suppression of aromatase by inhibitors. In: Miller WR, Santen RJ, eds. Aromatase Inhibition and Breast Cancer. New York: Marcel Dekker, 2001; pp. 213–225.

29. Miller WR, Dixon JM. Antiaromatase agents: preclinical data and neoadjuvant therapy. Clin Breast Cancer 2000; 1(Suppl 1):S9–S14.

30. Harada N, Nonda SI, Hatano O. Aromatase inhibitors and enzyme stability. Endocr Relat Cancer 1999; 6:211–218.

31. Chen S, Zhou D, Okubo T, Kao YC, Yang C. Breast tumor aromatase: functional role and transcriptional regulation. Endocr Relat Cancer 1999; 6:149–156.

32. Dowsett M, Ellis MJ. Role of biologic markers in patient selection and application to disease prevention. Am J Clin Oncol 2003; 26:S34–S39.

33. Ellis MJ, Coop A, Singh B, Mauriac L, Llombert-Cussac A, Janicke F, Miller WR, Evans DB, Dugan M, Brady C, Quebe-Fehling E, Borgs M. Letrozole is more effective neoadjuvant endocrine therapy than tamoxifen for ErbB-1- and/or ErbB-2-positive, estrogen receptor-positive primary breast cancer: evidence from a phase III randomized trial. J Clin Oncol 2001; 19:3808–3816.

34. Miller WR. Oestrogen and breast cancer: biological considerations. Br Med Bull 1991; 49:470–483.

35. Miller WR, Langdon SP. Steroid hormones and cancer: (III) observations from human subjects. Eur J Surg Oncol 1997; 23:163–183.

36. Geisler J, Lonning PE. Resistance to endocrine therapy of breast cancer: recent advances and tomorrow's challenges. Clin Breast Cancer 2001; 1:297–308.

37. Miller WR. Biological rationale for endocrine therapy in breast cancer. Best Prac Res Clin Endo Metab 2004; 18:1–32.

38. Miller WR. Prediction of estrogen sensitivity/dependence. Estrogen and Breast Cancer. Austin, Texas: RG Landes Co, 1996; pp. 151–169.

39. Santen RJ, Samojlik E, Wells SA. Resistance of the ovary to blockade of aromatization with aminoglutethimide. J Clin Endocrinol Metab 1980; 51:473–477.

40. Harris AL, Dowsett M, Jeffcoate SL, McKinna JA, Morgan M, Smith IE. Endocrine and therapeutic effects of aminoglutethimide in premenopausal patients with breast cancer. J Clin Endocrinol Metab 1982; 55:718–720.

41. Wander HE, Blossey HC, Nagel GA. Aminoglutethimide in the treatment of premenopausal patients with metastatic breast cancer. Eur J Cancer Clin Oncol 1986; 22:1371–1374.

42. Miller WR. Aromatase inhibitors in the treatment of advanced breast cancer. Cancer Treat Rev 1989; 16:83–93.

43. Hamon TJ, Allegra JC. Loss of hormonal responsiveness in cancer. In: Stoll BA, ed. Endocrine Management of Cancer: Biological Basis. Basel: Karger, 1988; pp. 61–71.

44. Isaacs JT. Clinical heterogeneity in relation to response. In: Stoll BA, ed. Endocrine Management of Cancer: Biological Basis. Basel: Karger, 1988; pp. 125–145.

45. Taylor RE, Powles TJ, Humphreys J, Bettelheim R, Dowsett M, Casey AJ, Neville AM, Coombes RC. Effects of endocrine therapy on steroid receptor content of breast cancer. Brit J Cancer 1982; 45:80–85.

46. Robertson JF. Oestrogen receptor: a stable phenotype in breast cancer. Br J Cancer 1996; 73:5–12.

47. Masamura S, Santner SJ, Heitjan DF, Santen RJ. Estrogen deprivation causes estradiol hypersensitivity in human breast cancer cells. J Clin Endocrinol Metab 1995; 80:2918–2925.

48. Katzenellenbogen BS. Estrogen receptors: bioactivities and interaction with cell signalling pathways. Biol Reprod 1996; 54:287–293.

49. Nicholson RJ, Hutcheson IR, Harper ME, Knowlden JM, Barrow D, McClelland RA, Jones HE, Wakeling AE, Gee JM. Modulation of epidermal growth factor receptor in endocrine resistant, oestrogen receptor-positive breast cancer. Endocr Relat Cancer 2001; 8:175–182.

50. Ellis MJ. The insulin-like growth factor network and breast cancer. In: Bowcock AM, ed. Breast Cancer: Molecular Genetics, Pathogenesis and Therapeutics. Totowa, New Jersey: Humana Press, 1999; pp. 121–142.

51. Miller WR. Regulatory subunits of PKA and breast cancer. Ann N Y Acad Sci 2002; 968:37–48.

52. Nicholson RI, Madden TA, Bryant S, Gee JMW. Cellular and molecular actions of estrogens and antiestrogens in breast cancer. In: Robertson JF, Nicholson RI, Hayes DF, eds. Endocrine Therapy of Breast Cancer. London: Martin Dunitz Ltd, 2002; pp. 127–153.

53. Santen RJ, Misbin RI. Aminoglutethimide: review of pharmacology and clinical use. Pharmacology 1981; 1:95–120.

54. Thurlimann B, Paridaens R, Serin D, Bonneterre J, Roche H, Murray R, di Salle E, Lanzalone S, Zurlo MG, Piscitelli G. Third-line hormonal treatment with exemestane in postmenopausal patients with advanced breast cancer progressing on aminoglutethimde: a phase II multicentre multi-national trial. Eur J Cancer 1997; 33:1767–1773.

55. Carlini P, Frassoldati A, De Marco S, Casali A, Ruggeri EM, Nardi M, Papaldo P, Fabi A, Paoloni F, Cognetti F. Formestane, a steroidal aromatase inhibitor after fail-

ure of non-steroidal aromatase inhibitors (anastrozole and letrozole): is a clinical benefit still available? Ann Oncol 2001; 12:1539–1543.

56. Coombes RC, Goss P, Dowsett M, Gazet JC, Brodie A. 4-hydroxyandrostenedione in treatment of postmenopausal patients with advanced breast cancer. Lancet 1984; ii:1237–1239.

57. Kadohama N, Yarborough C, Zhou D, Chen S, Osawa Y. Kinetic properties of aromatase mutants Pro308Phe, Asp309Asn and Asp309Ala and their interactions with aromatase inhibitors. J Steroid Biochem Mol Biol 1992; 43:693–701.

58. Miller WR. In vitro and in vivo effects of 4-hydroxyandrostenedione on steroid and tumour metabolism. In: Coombes RC, Dowsett, M, eds. 4-Hydroxyandrostenedione: A New Approach to Hormone-dependent Cancer. International Congress and Symposium Series. London: Royal Society of Medicine Services, 1991; pp. 45–50.

59. James VHT, Reed MJ, Adams EF, Ghilchick M, Lai LC, Coldham NG, Newton CJ, Purohit A, Owen AM, Singh A, Islam S. Oestrogen uptake and metabolism in vivo. In: Beck JS, ed. Oestrogen and the Human Breast. Edinburgh: The Royal Society of Edinburgh, 1989, Vol 95B; pp.185–193.

60. Ginsburg E. Environmental oestrogens. Lancet 1994; 343:284–285.

61. Bonneterre J, Thurlimann B, Robertson JF, Krzakowski M, Mauriac L, Koralewski P, Vergote I, Webster A, Steinberg M, von Euler M. Anastrozole versus tamoxifen as first-line therapy for advanced breast cancer in 668 postmenopausal women: results of the Tamoxifen or Arimidex Randomized Group Efficacy and Tolerability study. J Clin Oncol 2000; 18:3748–3757.

62. Goss PE, Strasser K. Aromatase inhibitors in the treatment and prevention of breast cancer. J Clin Oncol 2001; 19:881–894.

3

Systemic Therapy of Metastatic Breast Cancer in Postmenopausal Patients

Carsten Rose, Niklas Loman, Fredrika Killander, and Sara Kinhult

Lund University Hospital
Lund, Sweden

I. OVERVIEW

Since the 1980s, tamoxifen has been the preferred therapy for postmenopausal patients with metastatic breast cancer. This attribute stems from tamoxifen achieving response rates of 35% and its relative safety compared to cytotoxic chemotherapy. Therefore, it is worthwhile to discuss whether any other endocrine treatment has significant advantages over cytotoxic chemotherapy as first-line therapy for this devastating disease. Recent research has added to the armamentarium of endocrine therapies. One of the characteristics of endocrine therapy is that new remissions can be achieved using subsequent treatments. Hence, it is important to evaluate their optimal sequence. This brief review addresses two basic questions: Should we initiate treatment in metastatic breast cancer with cytotoxic or endocrine therapy? What currently is the optimal sequence of endocrine therapy?

II. INTRODUCTION

It is well established that both endocrine and cytotoxic therapy improve survival in early breast cancer (1, 2). In contrast, treatment of metastatic breast cancer is palliative with survival in the range from a few months to several years. Optimally, efficacy of cytotoxic therapy has been reached by achieving response rates of 60–70% and medium times of progression of 8–12 months and corresponding median survival figures in the order of 18–24 months. This has resulted in a renewed interest in the various endocrine therapies due to their efficacy in patients with steroid receptor positive (SR+) tumors, lower treatment-related acute toxicity, lower long-term morbidity, and lower costs than cytotoxic approaches.

This review of systemic therapy of metastatic breast cancer discusses: 1) treatment with initial chemotherapy compared to treatment with initial endocrine therapy, and 2) the optimal sequence of endocrine therapy in post-menopausal patients with the first recurrence of breast cancer.

III. CYTOTOXIC CHEMOTHERAPY VERSUS ENDOCRINE THERAPY

When approaching this question there is, of course, the possible approach of making a decision based upon personal experience and personal preference. In contrast, the methodology behind evidence-based decision making is to scour all available literature thoroughly and as systematically as possible (3). The gold standard in terms of literature analysis are those performed and critiqued by the Cochrane Collaboration (4).

One such systematic review compared the evidence of effectiveness of chemotherapy alone to endocrine therapy alone for metastatic breast cancer in randomized controlled trials (RCTs) (5). The authors of this systematic review searched through more than 5,000 RCTs in breast cancer in the Cochrane database in order to identify eligible studies. Fifty trials concerning chemotherapy and endocrine therapy predominantly in the metastatic disease setting were initially reviewed according to predefined protocol criteria. After a thorough examination of the method section independently performed by two investigators with a blinded review of the whole manuscript, nine randomized control trials were included in the analysis. All nine studies were published before 1995 and they included in general only a small number of patients (range, $n = 50$–226). Also, the cytotoxic treatment regimens among these trials varied, as did the endocrine therapies, and tamoxifen was used in only three out of the nine trials. The largest single body of data in this respect comes from the Australian/New Zealand Breast Cancer Trial Group (ANZBCTG) of adriamycin and cyclophosphamide (AC) in combination, versus endocrine therapy with tamoxifen (6). The response rate to chemotherapy was 45% for AC versus the response rate to tamoxifen of 22%. Overall, six of these nine randomized control trials showed a higher response rate for cytotoxic agents, while three of the studies showed a response rate that favored endocrine therapy.

However, the situation is different if the data from seven out of the nine studies are analyzed in terms of overall survival, defined as time from date of randomization to date of death. In this outcome, there is a trend toward prolongation of overall survival in favor of those patients starting out on endocrine therapies (Fig. 1). This trend becomes more pronounced by omitting the survival

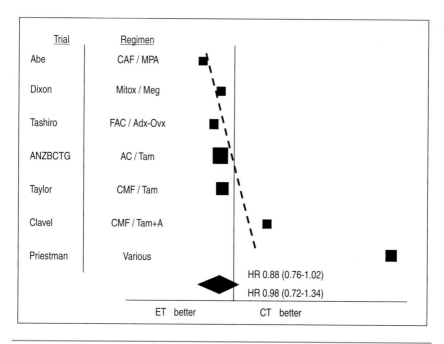

Figure 1 Cytotoxic chemotherapy (CT) versus endocrine therapy (ET) for first-line treatment on overall survival as hazard ratios (HR). HR = 0.98 refer to all seven studies. HR = 0.88 correspond to survival data after exclusion of the study by Priestman et al. (7). A: drostanolone; AC: doxorubicin plus cyclophosphamide; Adx: adrenalectomy; C: cyclophosphamide; CAF: cyclophosphamide, adriamycin, and fluorouracil; CMF: cyclophosphamide, methotrexate and fluorouracil; FAC: fluorouracil, doxorubicin and cyclophosphamide; MPA: medroxyprogesterone acetate; Meg: megesterol; Mitox: mitoxantrone; Ovx: ovariectomy; Tam: tamoxifen. (Adapted from Ref. 5)

figures—a distinct outlier—from the oldest trial performed by Priestman and colleagues (7). This particular trial included both pre- and postmenopausal patients and five different forms of endocrine therapy.

Of course there are limitations with extrapolating the outcomes on the basis of evidence from this systematic review. The studies pooled included: patients with tumors both positive and negative for estrogen receptors (ER); the endocrine therapy varied from study to study; the comparative treatment arm did not always include tamoxifen; and modern aromatase inhibitors of the third generation (AIs) were not used. Looking at the chemotherapy regimens used: chemotherapy was relatively conventional; taxanes were not used at all; modern supportive therapies were not available, nor were oral combination or weekly low-toxicity chemotherapies. Hence, when these pooled studies are aligned against current

35

standards of therapy, overall survival was probably biased against endocrine therapy, and toxicity was biased against chemotherapy.

One of the characteristics of endocrine therapy is that the response can be predicted by the presence of estrogen and/or progesterone receptors in a patient's tumor tissue. Moreover, one of the most intriguing characteristics of endocrine therapy is that subsequent remissions can be obtained with successive endocrine therapies. The various forms of endocrine therapies have different mechanisms of resistance, and it is universally accepted that, in comparison with cytotoxic therapy, endocrine therapy is relatively nontoxic. It is, therefore, pertinent, on the strength of the best available evidence, to suggest that the established systemic therapy of metastatic breast cancer in SR+ patients should be various trials of endocrine therapy in sequence. In steroid-receptor-negative (SR–) patients and nonresponders to endocrine therapy, combination chemotherapy is by all means appropriate (Fig. 2).

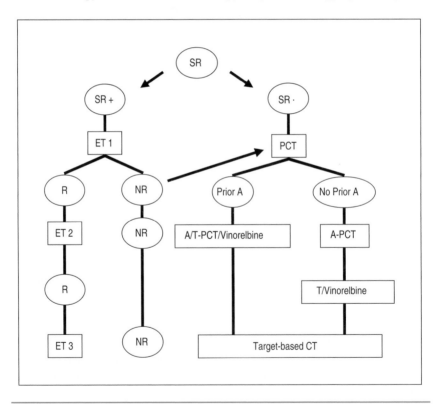

Figure 2 Systemic therapy routes for metastatic breast cancer. A: anthracycline; ET1: first-line endocrine therapy; ET2: second-line endocrine therapy; ET3: third-line endocrine therapy; NR: non-responders; PCT: polychemotherapy; R: responders; SR–: steroid-receptor negative; SR+: steroid-receptor positive; T: taxanes.

Table 1 Response Rates in Clinical Studies Comparing Cytotoxic Versus Endocrine Therapy in Metastatic Breast Cancer

Trial (Ref.)	Therapy	N	RR–CT	RR–ET	RR:ratio
Abe (25)	CAF:MPA	50	36	24	1.5
Dixon (26)	Mitox:Meg	60	23	13	1.77
Tashiro (27)	FAC:Adx/Ovx	56	54	33	1.64
ANZBCTG (6)	AC:Tam	226	45	22	2.05
Taylor (28)	CMF:Tam	181	38	45	0.84
Clavel (29)	CMF:Tam/A	64	13	29	0.44
Priestman (7)	FACV:Various	92	49	21	2.33
Rosner (30)	A/FCP:Adx	57	44	33	1.33
Newsome (31)	C:DES/A	68	13	17	0.76

A: drostanolone; AC: doxorubicin plus cyclophosphamide; Adx: adrenalectomy; A/FCP: adriamycin/5FU-cylophosphamide-prednisone; C: cyclophosphamide; CAF: cyclophosphamide, adriamycin, and fluorouracil; CMF: cyclophosphamide, methotrexate, and fluorouracil; DES/A: diethylstilbestrol/androgen; FAC: fluorouracil, doxorubicin, and cyclophosphamide; MPA: medroxyprogesterone acetate; Meg: megesterol; Mitox: mitoxantrone; Ovx: ovariectomy; Tam: tamoxifen.

Source: Adapted from Ref. 5.

IV. PROPER SEQUENCE OF ENDOCRINE THERAPY

A. Diethylstilbestrol as First-Line Treatment

By analyzing the available literature, Henderson investigated the optimal sequence of endocrine therapies and proposed a treatment outline in 1981 (8). In the 1970s, diethylstilbestrol was the first-line treatment. Responders were either withdrawn from diethylstilbestrol, given adrenalectomy, or given third-line treatment with progestins or androgens. This treatment outline was based upon a nonsystematic review of the literature.

B. Tamoxifen as First-Line Endocrine Therapy

Therapy sequences devised using post-1981 literature have to look at additional factors besides efficacy, such as side effects, quality of life, and cost. In the case of side effects, endocrine therapy is widely regarded as relatively nontoxic. Cost-benefit analyses have major implications but will not be dealt with here. Quality of life was not measured in the listed studies; therefore, for the purposes of outlining optimal-treatment sequences in the context of this review, it is appropriate to concentrate on efficacy data.

Efficacy of endocrine therapies can be established and compared through time-event measurements, response rate, predictive factors such as steroid receptors, and site of the disease, and efficacy. Efficacy analysis can be taken further by looking at crossover data from RCTs. Ideally, optimal sequence should be evaluated from RCTs with full crossover of all patients accrued for first-line therapy. However, such studies have not been performed. The closest was the ANZBCTG, where around 70% of the patients were actually crossed over after a trial of either chemotherapy or tamoxifen. However, in most of the studies, only minor fractions of patients are crossed over and we are, therefore, left with the only alternative of analyzing studies with a partial crossover.

In an analysis of the literature (9), it could be demonstrated how diethylstilbestrol, the drug of choice for first-line endocrine therapy in the 1970s, was replaced by tamoxifen. Tamoxifen and diethylstilbestrol were compared in six RCTs. In all of these studies, endpoints were overall response rate (RR). Time to a first response (TFR) was not given in any of these studies, and duration of response (DoR) was given only in two-thirds of the studies. Basic time events such as time to failure (TTF) or time to progression (TTP) were only mentioned in a third of these trials, and only half of these studies mentioned survival data. However, response rate for diethylstilbestrol was similar to the response rate for tamoxifen in these six studies (28% versus 27%; total $n = 497$ patients). But despite this and regardless of the lack of investigative rigor by today's standard, diethylstilbestrol was replaced by tamoxifen mainly due to side effects. It is, however, noteworthy that Peethambaram et al. in an update of their trial comparing diethylstilbestrol versus tamoxifen, could show a significant survival advantage for diethylstilbestrol over tamoxifen, with 5-year survival figures at 35% for the diethylstilbestrol arm and 16% for the tamoxifen arm (10).

This literature search conducted in the late 1980s comparing tamoxifen to other forms of endocrine therapy (oophorectomy, adrenalectomy, aminoglutethimide, progestins, and androgens) yielded 26 RCTs. Again, RRs were given in all, but TFRs only in one of the studies. Duration of remission was only covered in 81% of these papers. What is now considered the primary endpoint, TTFs/TTPs were only given in 42% of the 26 studies, with only 62% of these studies showing overall survival data. By today's standards this seems to be very weak evidence by which to establish tamoxifen as the treatment of choice for first-line metastatic disease.

Comparing the percentage RR of tamoxifen with other endocrine therapies did not show a marked clinical advantage for tamoxifen. The RR to tamoxifen in a heterogeneous population of both ER+ and ER− patients varied from mid-20% to a little above 30%. In these trials, patient populations were small, so it cannot be said with confidence that the RR of tamoxifen differs from the rates of the other forms of endocrine therapy.

SR data coming from these RCTs do not securely establish the precision of tamoxifen either. Again, the patient numbers are very small. On the basis of response rate in patients who are ER+, ranging from 25–56%, the predictive power of steroid-receptors is questionable. The assay of the time was basically the ligand-binding assay performed on the primary tumor. Also, the order of magnitude achieved was not in the 60% range expected by today's standards. The situation is entirely the same for the other endocrine therapies in question.

The change in paradigm from using diethylstilbestrol or progestins to tamoxifen for metastatic breast cancer was rooted in these 26 trials published in the 1980s (9). However, only three of these trials met the tyranny of N and had sufficent power (1 − Beta = > 80%) to demonstrate a true benefit in a RR of 50% (e.g., an increase from 20–30% in RR). Such a demonstrable difference was not achieved in any of these 26 trials, and with a few notable exceptions, this has never been achieved in any trial of endocrine therapy. Nevertheless, by 1980 tamoxifen had become the gold standard. At that time, the best treatment sequence for postmenopausal ER+ or unknown women was to start out with a trial of tamoxifen. Responders were then taken further with a progestin or a first-generation AI. For responders to second-line endocrine therapy, diethylstilbestrol or androgen therapy was the third-line treatment option.

C.   Third-Generation AIs Versus Tamoxifen in First-Line Therapy

In a recent commentary, "A rose is no longer a rose" (11), Craig Hendersen alluded to the indications of higher efficacy for third-generation AIs over tamoxifen as first-line endocrine therapy for metastatic disease. Overall, the results of these large, well-conducted RCTs comparing letrozole (12), anastrozole in two trials (13, 14), and exemestane—preliminary data (15), versus tamoxifen gave indications of significant differences for some of the efficacy endpoints like RR, clinical benefit rate (CBR), TTF, TTP, and toxicity, but none of the studies gave indications of overall survival.

In a combined analysis of the two anastrozole trials, anastrozole could only demonstrate superiority to tamoxifen for TTP in a retrospective analysis of the subgroup of patients known to be SR+ (13). For letrozole, all subsets of patients analyzed showed that those on letrozole fared better in terms of TTP than those on tamoxifen (12). In the predominantly SR+ group, letrozole had a RR of 32% versus 21% for tamoxifen. However, it was nowhere near the erstwhile 60% expected RR for first-line endocrine therapy in this group of patients. In this study, the TTP on letrozole was 9.4 months, significantly better ($p < 0.001$) than the 6 months on tamoxifen. This study was not designed to demonstrate differences in overall survival. Letrozole patients survived a median of 34 months versus 30 months on tamoxifen ($p = 0.5303$), although the first 30 months showed a superior survival rate for letrozole treated patients (Fig. 3) (16).

In terms of TTP by hormone-receptor status, both patients positive for ER and/or PR and receptor-unknown women did better than the tamoxifen-treated

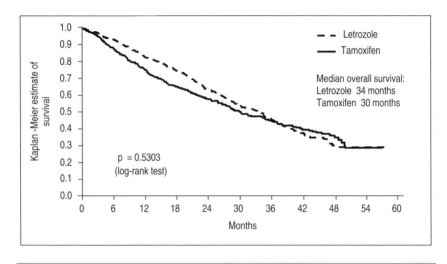

Figure 3 Overall survival analysis of letrozole versus tamoxifen as first-line therapy. (From Ref. 16)

patients. Median TTP by site of metastasis revealed significant differences between letrozole and tamoxifen in patients with visceral and nonvisceral disease; and even in patients with liver metastases there was a small but statistically significant difference in favor of letrozole (Table 2) (17). By applying 95% confidence limits, the RR in the viscera goes from 20% to 33% for letrozole and from 12% to 22% for tamoxifen.

In light of this new evidence, the sequence of endocrine therapy for SR+ postmenopausal patients is as follows: First choice, a third-generation AI, although the use of tamoxifen here is still arguable. Some patients will already have been exposed to an AI in the adjuvant setting. For these patients, the use of tamoxifen is justified. For second-line therapy, third-generation AIs have been

Table 2 Median Time to Progression According to Site of Metastases for Letrozole Versus Tamoxifen

Type of metastasis	Letrozole (mo)	Tamoxifen (mo)	HR (95% CI)	p
All	9.4	6	0.72 (0.62–0.83)	<0.0001
Nonvisceral	10.9	6.3	0.75 (0.62–0.91)	0.0038
Visceral, nonliver	11.9	6.1	0.66 (0.51–0.86)	0.0017
Liver	3.8	3.0	0.72 (0.43–0.94)	0.0232

Source: Ref. 17.

compared to megestrol acetate in very large, well conducted RCTs. The results of these trials showed some differences in favor of third-generation AIs, particularly in terms of TTF and toxicity. However, these differences in efficacy are not overwhelmingly important in clinical terms.

In terms of toxicity data, studies comparing third-generation AIs to megestrol acetate, with the exception of the Buzdar et al. study with letrozole versus megestrol (18), the third-generation AIs were better tolerated than the progestin megestrol acetate.

Second-line comparisons of the various forms of AIs have been conducted in a number of large randomized trials. Letrozole and vorozol have been compared to aminoglutethimide. Letrozole has been compared favorably to fadrozole and anastrozole (19). For some study endpoints, the third-generation AIs are more effective than the older ones. Two studies of anastrozole versus fulvestrant for second-line endocrine therapy showed that these approaches were equivalent (20, 21).

In the case of liver metastasis, a comparison of the response rates between letrozole, aminoglutethimide, and megestrol acetate, with the application of 95% confidence limits, shows a trend in favor of the AIs as a second-line endocrine approach. This implies that there may be important clinical differences between these third-generation AIs and megestrol acetate.

However, only in a few of the studies, comparing AIs with either megestrol acetate or tamoxifen as second- or first-line endocrine therapy, have response data been related to SR− status. All these studies include patients with SR+, unknown, and SR− tumors. Therefore, the RR in patients known to be SR+ should theoretically be higher than the overall RR. To exemplify this, Table 3A and B give the overall RR compared to the RR in patients with SR+ status, SR− status, or unknown (?) status in relation to therapy with either AIs or other forms of endocrine therapy. It can be seen from Table 3A that the RR overall and the RR in SR+ patients are in the same order of magnitude regardless of endocrine therapy. Likewise, there is not much of a difference between the overall RR and the RR in patients known to be SR− or unknown (Table 3B). The compiled data from these large randomized studies do not support our general belief that SR status, predominantly coming from the primary tumors, is of substantial predictive value.

Crossover data define cross-sensitivity and non–cross-resistance. The traditionally expected response rates for sequential therapy in SR+ patients used to be 60% for first-line therapy and 30% for second-line therapy in responders to previous endocrine therapy (22). Cross-sensitivity of tamoxifen versus other endocrine therapies in the 26 "old" RCTs shows that, if treatment is initiated with tamoxifen followed by other endocrine therapies, there will be a higher total rate of response for first- and second-line therapy than vice versa (9). In terms of efficacy, this observation (based upon small numbers) jus-

Table 3

A Response Rates (%), Overall and in Patients with Positive Steroid-Receptor Status (%) to AIs and Other Endocrine Therapy (MA or Tam)

AI	SR+*	RR	RR SR+	ET	SR+*	RR	RR SR+
AG (32)	66	34	38	MA	77	31	28
Fadr (33)	76	27	20	Tam	81	20	30
Form (34)	76	17	16	MA	70	17	17
Ana (35)	62	10	11	MA	58	10	13
Let (36)	65	32	30	Tam	67	21	20

B Response Rates (%) Overall and in Patients with Negative or Unknown Steroid-Receptor Status (%) to AIs and Other Endocrine Therapy (MA or Tam)

AI	SR–/?**	RR	RR– SR–/?	ET	SR–/?*	RR	RR– SR–/?
AG (32)	34	34	—	MA	23	31	—
Fadr (33)	24	27	19	Tam	19	20	17
Form (34)	24	17	—	MA	30	17	—
Ana (35)	34	10	10	MA	38	10	8
Let (36)	34	32	28	Tam	33	21	19

*Percent of patients with SR+ tumors.

**Percent of patients with SR– or unknown tumors

Data from five randomized studies in second- and first-line endocrine therapy comparing aromatase inhibitors with other forms of endocrine therapy.

SR: steroid receptor; AI: aromatase inhibitor; AG: aminoglutethimide; Ana: anastrozole; ET: other endocrine therapy; Fad: fadroxole; Form: formestane; Let: letrozole; MA: megestrol acetate; Tam: tamoxifen; RR: overall response rate; RR SR+: Response rate in SR+ patients; RR SR–/?: Response rate in SR–/? patients; SR+: SR positive; SR–/?: SR negative or unknown.

tified the use of tamoxifen as first-line choice for endocrine therapy—it was fair to start out with tamoxifen.

In more recent trials, there is a large variation in cross sensitivity between either tamoxifen, aminoglutethimide, or medroxyprogesterone acetate as first-line therapy and second-line therapy given with progestins, AIs, or tamoxifen. The RR to second-line endocrine therapy in responders to first-line endocrine therapy varies from 0 to 42%. However, the number of patients with sufficient data to analyze the cross sensitivity is very small. In terms of non–cross-resistance, there is more of a uniform picture. Non–cross-resistance in recent studies is depicted by a RR to second-line endocrine therapy in the neighborhood of 10–15% in nonresponders to tamoxifen or aminoglutethimide.

The steroidal third-generation AI, exemestane, still needs to show that it is as good as tamoxifen for first-line therapy. However, a low RR to exemestane (5–8%) has been demonstrated after prior AI therapy with either aminoglutethimide, or another nonsteroidal AI (23).

For second- and third-line endocrine therapy, progestins can still play a role. In many patients, tamoxifen can still be of use, and fulvestrant still has to be defined better in clinical terms. However, the recent data from the comparison with anastrazole tell us it might be a useful drug in a sequence of endocrine therapies. The third-tier agents could include high doses of estrogens. In a small study of postmenopausal breast cancer patients heavily exposed to endocrine therapy, some response was seen with high doses of estrogens (24).

V. CONCLUSION

To assess where we currently stand, a series of questions can be asked. First, is first-line endocrine therapy equally effective as cytotoxic chemotherapy in SR+ patients? At present, there is no definite answer to that question because larger trials will be necessary to answer it properly. Second, are nonsteroidal AIs really first-line endocrine therapy in metastatic breast cancer? In view of the present data, where anastrozole has shown equivalence to tamoxifen and letrozole has shown superiority, the answer to this is yes. Third, concerning the current role of steroidal AIs like exemestane, are we awaiting confirmative data? Fourth, what is the role of pharmacological doses of estrogens? Because these are very inexpensive therapies, they warrant further investigation. Finally, what will be the future role of fulvestrant? Its place in the treatment paradigm needs to be investigated further, as indeed do the benefits and limitations of the other endocrine therapies.

As Gertrude Stein said, "[A] Rose is a rose is a rose." And in terms of endocrine therapy for metastatic disease, it now seems that we have a whole bouquet of roses, with different bloom, fragrance, and hue.

REFERENCES

1. Early Breast Cancer Trialists' Collaborative Group. Polychemotherapy for early breast cancer: an overview of the randomised trials. Lancet 1998; 352:930–942.
2. Early Breast Cancer Trialists' Collaborative Group. Tamoxifen for early breast cancer: an overview of the randomised trials. Lancet 1998; 351:1451–1467.
3. Sackett DL, Rosenberg WM. The need for evidence-based medicine. J R Soc Med 1995; 88:620–624.
4. Sackett DL. Cochrane Collaboration. Br Med J 1994; 309:1514–1515.
5. Wilcken N, Hornbuckle J, Ghersi D. Chemotherapy alone versus endocrine therapy alone for metastatic breast cancer. Cochrane Database Syst Rev 2003;CD002747.

6. The Australian and New Zealand Breast Cancer Trials Group, Clinical Oncological Society of Australia. A randomized trial in postmenopausal patients with advanced breast cancer comparing endocrine and cytotoxic therapy given sequentially or in combination. J Clin Oncol 1986; 4:186–193.

7. Priestman T, Baum M, Jones V, Forbes J. Comparative trial of endocrine versus cytotoxic treatment in advanced breast cancer. Br Med J 1977; 1:1248–1250.

8. Henderson IC. Less toxic treatment for advanced breast cancer. N Engl J Med 1981; 305:575–576.

9. Rose C. Endocrine therapy of advanced breast cancer. In: Kaufmann M, Henderson IC, Enghofer E, eds. Therapeutic management of metastatic breast cancer. De Gruyter, New York, 1989; pp. 3–17.

10. Peethambaram PP, Ingle JN, Suman VJ, Hartmann LC, Loprinzi CL. Randomized trial of diethylstilbestrol vs. tamoxifen in postmenopausal women with metastatic breast cancer. An updated analysis. Breast Cancer Res Treat 1999; 54:117–122.

11. Henderson IC. A rose is no longer a rose. J Clin Oncol 2002; 20:3365–3368.

12. Mouridsen H, Gershanovich M, Sun Y, Perez-Carrion R, Boni C, Monnier A, Apffelstaedt J, Smith R, Sleeboom HP, Jaenicke F, Pluzanska A, Dank M, Becquart D, Bapsy PP, Salminen E, Snyder R, Chaudri-Ross H, Lang R, Wyld P, Bhatnagar A. Phase III study of letrozole versus tamoxifen as first-line therapy of advanced breast cancer in postmenopausal women: analysis of survival and update of efficacy from the International Letrozole Breast Cancer Group. J Clin Oncol 2003; 21:2101–2109.

13. Bonneterre J, Buzdar A, Nabholtz JM, Robertson JF, Thurlimann B, von Euler M, Sahmoud T, Webster A, Steinberg M; Arimidex Writing Committee; Investigators Committee Members. Anastrozole is superior to tamoxifen as first-line therapy in hormone receptor positive advanced breast carcinoma. Cancer 2001; 92:2247–2258.

14. Nabholtz JM, Buzdar A, Pollak M, Harwin W, Burton G, Mangalik A, Steinberg M, Webster A, von Euler M. Anastrozole is superior to tamoxifen as first-line therapy for advanced breast cancer in postmenopausal women: results of a North American multicenter randomized trial. Arimidex Study Group. J Clin Oncol 2000; 18:3758–3767.

15. Paridaens R, Dirix L, Lohrisch C, Beex L, Nooij M, Cameron D, Biganzoli L, Cufer T, Duchateau L, Hamilton A, Lobelle JP, Piccart M. Mature results of a randomized phase II multicenter study of exemestane versus tamoxifen as first-line hormone therapy for postmenopausal women with metastatic breast cancer. Ann Oncol 2003; 14:1391–1398.

16. Mouridsen H, Sun Y, Gershanovich M. Final survival analysis of the double-blind, randomized multinational phase III trial of letrozole (Femara®) compared to tamoxifen as first-line hormonal therapy for advanced breast cancer [abstr]. 24th Annual San Antonio Breast Cancer Symposium, San Antonio, TX, USA. Dec 10–13, 2001. Breast Cancer Res Treat 2001; 69.

17. Mouridsen H, Chaudri-Ross H. Oncologist 2003. In press.

18. Buzdar A, Douma J, Davidson N, Elledge R, Morgan M, Smith R, Porter L, Nabholtz J, Xiang X, Brady C. Phase III, multicenter, double-blind, randomized study of letrozole, an aromatase inhibitor, for advanced breast cancer versus megestrol acetate. J Clin Oncol 2001; 19:3357–3366.

19. Rose C, Vtoraya O, Pluzanska A, Davidson N, Gershanovich M, Thomas R, Johnson S, Caicedo JJ, Gervasio H, Manikhas G, Ben Ayed F, Burdette-Radoux S, Chaudri-

Ross HA, Lang R. An open randomised trial of second-line endocrine therapy in advanced breast cancer. Comparison of the aromatase inhibitors letrozole and anastrozole. Eur J Cancer 2003; 39:2318–2327.

20. Howell A, Robertson JF, Quaresma AJ, Aschermannova A, Mauriac L, Kleeberg UR, Vergote I, Erikstein B, Webster A, Morris C. Fulvestrant, formerly ICI 182,780, is as effective as anastrozole in postmenopausal women with advanced breast cancer progressing after prior endocrine treatment. J Clin Oncol 2002; 20:3396–3403.

21. Osborne CK, Pippen J, Jones SE, Parker LM, Ellis M, Come S, Gertler SZ, May JT, Burton G, Dimery I, Webster A, Morris C, Elledge R, Buzdar A. Double-blind, randomized trial comparing the efficacy and tolerability of fulvestrant versus anastrozole in postmenopausal women with advanced breast cancer progressing on prior endocrine therapy: results of a North American trial. J Clin Oncol 2002; 20:3386–3395.

22. Ellis MJ, Hayes DF, Lippman ME. In: Harris JR, Lippman ME, Morrow M, Osborne CK, eds. Diseases of the Breast 2nd ed. Philadelphia: Lippincott Williams and Wilkins, 2000; pp. 749–797.

23. Lonning PE, Bajetta E, Murray R, Tubiana-Hulin M, Eisenberg PD, Mickiewicz E, Celio L, Pitt P, Mita M, Aaronson NK, Fowst C, Arkhipov A, di Salle E, Polli A, Massimini G. Activity of exemestane in metastatic breast cancer after failure of nonsteroidal aromatase inhibitors: a phase II trial. J Clin Oncol 2000; 18:2234–2244.

24. Lonning PE, Taylor PD, Anker G, Iddon J, Wie L, Jorgensen LM, Mella O, Howell A. High-dose estrogen treatment in postmenopausal breast cancer patients heavily exposed to endocrine therapy. Breast Cancer Res Treat 2001; 67:111–116.

25. Abe O, Asaishi K, Izuo M, Enomoto K, Koyama H, Tominaga T, Nomura Y, Ohshima A, Aoki N, Tsukada T. Effects of medroxyprogesterone acetate therapy on advanced or recurrent breast cancer and its influences on blood coagulation and the fibrinolytic system. Surg Today 1995; 25:701–710.

26. Dixon AR, Jackson L, Chan S, Haybittle J, Blamey RW. A randomised trial of second-line hormone vs single agent chemotherapy in tamoxifen resistant advanced breast cancer. Br J Cancer 1992; 66:402–404.

27. Tashiro H, Nomura Y, Hisamatsu K. A randomized trial of endocrine therapy, chemotherapy, and chemo-endocrine therapy in advanced breast cancer. Gan To Kagaku Ryoho 1990; 17:2369–2373.

28. Taylor SG, Gelman RS, Falkson G, Cummings FJ. Combination chemotherapy compared to tamoxifen as initial therapy for stage-IV breast cancer in elderly women. Ann Intern Med 1986; 104:455–461.

29. Clavel B, Cappelaere JP, Guerin J, Klein T, Pommatau E, Berlie J. Management of advanced breast cancer in post-menopausal women. A comparative trial of hormonal therapy, chemotherapy, and a combination of both. Sem Hop 1982; 58:1919–1923.

30. Rosner D, Dao TL, Horton J, et al. Randomized study of adriamycin (ADM) vs. combined therapy (FCP) vs. adrenalectomy (ADX) in breast cancer. Proceedings of the American Association of Cancer Research 1974; 15(252).

31. Newsome JF, Powers JA. The comparative results of combined cytotoxic and hormonal agent in the treatment of disseminated breast cancer. Proceedings of the American Association for Cancer Research 1963; 4(12):48.

32. Lundgren S, Gundersen S, Klepp R, Lonning PE, Lund E, Kvinnsland S. Megestrol acetate versus aminoglutethimide for metastatic breast cancer. Breast Cancer Res Treat 1989; 14:201–206.

33. Thürlimann B, Beretta K, Bacchi M, Castiglione-Gertsch M Goldhirsch A, Jungi WF, Cavalli F, Senn HJ, Fey M, Löhnert T for the Swiss Group for Clinical Cancer Research (SAKK). First-line fadrozole HCI (CGS 16949A) versus tamoxifen in postmenopausal women with advanced breast cancer. Prospective randomised trial of the Swiss Group for Clinical Cancer Rsearch SAKK 20/88. Ann Oncol 1996; 7:471–479.

34. Thürlimann B, Castiglione M, Hsu-Schmitz SF, Cavalli F, Bonnefoi H, Fey MF, Morant R, Löhnert T, Goldhirsch A for the Swiss Group for Clinical Cancer Research (SAKK). Formestane versus megestrol acetate in postmenopausal breast cancer patients after failure of tamoxifen: a phase III prospective randomised cross over trial of second-line hormonal treatment (SAKK 20/90). Eur J Cancer 1997; 33(7):1017–1024.

35. Jonat W, Howell A, Blomqvist C, Eiermann W, Winblad G, Tyrrell C, Mauriac L, Roche H, Lundgren S, Hellmund R, Azab M on behalf of the Arimidex Study Group. A randomised trial comparing two doses of the new selective aromatase inhibitor anastrozole (Arimidex) with megestrol acetate in postmenopausal patients with advanced breast cancer. Eur J Cancer 1996; 32A(3): 404–412.

36. Mouridsen H, Gershanovich M, Sun Y, Pérez-Carrion R, Boni C, Monnier A, Apffelstaedt J, Smith R, Sleebom HP, Jönicke F, Pluzanska A, Dank M, Becquart D, Bapsy PP, Salminen E, Snyder R, Lassus M, Verbeek JA, Staffler B, Chaudri-Ross HA, Dugan M. Superior efficacy of letrozole versus tamoxifen as first-line therapy for postmenopausal women with advanced breast cancer: results of a phase III study of the International Letrozole Breast Cancer Group. J Clin Oncol 2001; 19(10): 2596–2606.

4

ATAC: Early Breast Cancer

Michael Baum
University College London and
The Portland Hospital
London, England

I. OVERVIEW

In the adjuvant treatment of postmenopausal women with early breast cancer, tamoxifen is the standard first-choice agent. However, prolonged use of tamoxifen can be associated with an increased risk of endometrial carcinomas and venous thromboembolic disorders. Recent trials on the use of different aromatase inhibitors (AIs), in early breast cancer may provide the alternative answer to these problems. First results have been reported for the Anastrozole, Tamoxifen Alone or in Combination (ATAC) trial, which was designed to examine the efficacy and tolerability of these two agents, as first-line adjuvant therapies in postmenopausal women with early breast cancer. In this large, international, double-blind trial, 9,366 postmenopausal women with early breast cancer were randomized to receive either anastrozole alone, tamoxifen alone, or a combination of both, for 5 years. The primary endpoints were disease-free survival and occurrence of adverse events, with the data analyzed on an intention-to-treat basis. Hormone receptor (HR) status and nodal status of the patients were identified. Patients taking anastrozole alone experienced significantly better disease-free survival compared with tamoxifen alone: Hazard ratio = 0.83; 95% confidence interval (CI) = 0.71–0.96; $p = 0.0129$. This benefit was seen especially in patients with hormone-receptor-positive (HR+) tumors. Similar rates for disease-free survival were observed between the combination therapy arm and the tamoxifen alone arm (hazard ratio = 1.02; 95% CI = 0.88–1.18; p = 0.7718). Patients on anastrozole reported fewer cases of hot flashes, vaginal bleeding and discharge, and endometrial cancer compared with tamoxifen. However, a greater number of cases of musculoskeletal disorders and bone fractures were reported in patients on anastrozole. Overall, the ATAC trial demonstrated the efficacy of anastrozole, and that it is a well-tolerated endocrine agent, for use as adjuvant therapy in postmenopausal women with HR early breast cancer.

II. INTRODUCTION

Breast cancer is one of the leading causes of death in women in developed countries, with only cardiovascular diseases and lung cancer causing higher numbers of death (1,2). Although incidence of breast cancer in women has increased, mortality rates have declined steadily (3). This can be largely attributed to advances in breast cancer treatment over the last 15 years. As breast cancer progression is dependent on estrogens for growth, endocrine blockade has played a large role in improving prognosis. Hence, a large contribution to the reduction in mortality is due to endocrine manipulation, such as ovarian suppression and the antiestrogen, tamoxifen. For early breast cancer in postmenopausal women, tamoxifen is the standard first-choice treatment for adjuvant therapy (4). However, despite its efficacy, prolonged use of tamoxifen is associated with an increased risk of endometrial carcinomas and venous thromboembolic disorders. In addition, recent developments on AIs may demonstrate greater efficacy, competing with tamoxifen as first-line adjuvant treatment.

III. ATAC TRIAL DESIGN

This was the first trial to report results of an AI versus tamoxifen in a head-on comparison, and to examine their efficacy and safety as first-line adjuvant therapies in postmenopausal women (5). The ATAC trial, an international, multicenter, randomized, double-blind study, recruited 9,366 postmenopausal breast cancer patients postoperatively, following radiotherapy or chemotherapy or both. Patients were randomized to anastrozole alone (1 mg OD), tamoxifen alone (20 mg OD) or a combination of both, for 5 years.

The primary endpoints were disease-free survival (which included local, regional, and distant recurrence; new primary breast cancer; and death from any cause), and occurrence of adverse events. The data were analyzed on an intention-to-treat basis. All the treatment groups were well-balanced with one-third patients node-positive and 84% patients with HR+ status. Receptor status was negative in 8% of patients and unknown for the remaining 8% of the study population.

IV. ATAC RESULTS

The total number of events needed to trigger the first protocol analysis and to detect significance was predicted to be 1,056. However, in the main analysis, 1,079 first events were recorded, of which 766 were in receptor-positive patients. Patients taking anastrozole alone experienced significantly better disease-free survival compared with tamoxifen alone (hazard ratio = 0.83; 95% CI = 0.71–0.96; p = 0.0129), and the combination arm (hazard ratio = 0.81; 95% CI = 0.70–0.94; p = 0.006) (6). Similar rates for disease-free survival were observed between the combination therapy arm and the tamoxifen alone arm (hazard ratio = 1.02; 95% CI = 0.88–1.18; p = 0.7718).

In the receptor-positive patients, anastrozole alone also demonstrated higher recurrence-free survival compared with tamoxifen alone (hazard ratio = 0.73; 95% CI = 0.59–0.9; p = 0.003) with no significant difference observed between the combination arm and tamoxifen (hazard ratio = 1.09; 95% CI = 0.90–1.34; p = 0.4). At present, the reason for the combination arm being significantly less effective than anastrozole alone is unclear. A hypothesis for this may be that tamoxifen acts as a weak agonist when endogenous levels of estrogen are low, as is seen in the existing situation of postmenopausal women taking an AI.

Comparing the first events between the monotherapy arms, fewer breast cancer events, such as local recurrence and distant recurrence, occurred in the anastrozole arm. This is also demonstrated in a Kaplan Meier analysis in which the probability of first event in the overall population showed significant advantage in favor of anastrozole (hazard ratio = 0.86; 95% CI = 0.76–0.99; p = 0.03) (Fig. 1).

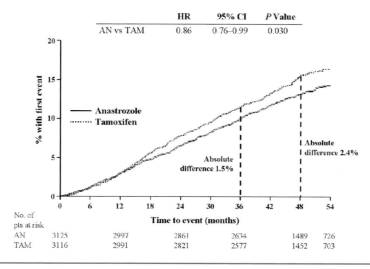

Figure 1   Probability of a first event in the overall population.

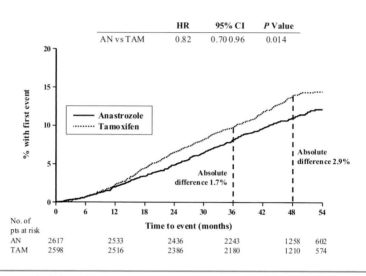

Figure 2   Probability of a first event in HR+ population.

This translates into an absolute difference of 2.4% at 4 years. A similar finding was also seen for probability of recurrence in the overall population, with an absolute difference of 2.3% at 4 years.

The greater efficacy of anastrozole compared with tamoxifen is validated even more in the receptor-positive population. In this group, the probability of first event again favors anastrozole (hazard ratio = 0.82; 95% CI = 0.7–0.96; p = 0.014) (Fig. 2) with a relative risk reduction approaching 20% and an absolute difference of 2.9% at 4 years. These results were also mirrored for the probability of recurrence in the receptor-positive population, as for the overall population.

Further benefit was seen in the anastrozole arm compared with the tamoxifen-arm: Significantly fewer cases of new primary breast cancers in the contralateral breast occurred in the anastrozole arm: Odds ratio (OR) = 0.62; 95% CI = 0.38–1.02; p = 0.0062. This suggests that anastrozole may have a preventive element in breast cancer development, especially in hormone-responsive tumors where the impact on contralateral disease was even greater (OR = 0.56; 95% CI = 0.32–0.94; p = 0.042). As a result of this, anastrozole was incorporated into the design of the second International Breast Cancer Intervention Study (IBIS-II) prevention trial (7).

V.   PROGNOSTIC FACTORS

HR status is a predictive factor in which patients who have receptor-negative breast cancer do not obtain the benefit of hormone-blocking drugs, such as tamoxifen and anastrozole. Therefore, it can be deduced from ATAC trial results, in which the point estimate of comparison for receptor-negative patients is at one

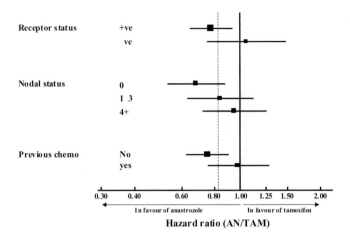

Figure 3 Breast cancer events for prognostic factors.

(Fig. 3), that tamoxifen and anastrozole were equally ineffective in preventing breast cancer events.

With respect to nodal status, anastrozole is clearly more effective than tamoxifen in node-negative patients, but it has less clear-cut superiority in node-positive patients as the confidence intervals overlap 1.0 (Fig. 3). Node-positive patients are more likely to have received chemotherapy, hence a confounding issue: In patients who previously had chemotherapy, anastrozole appears to be similar to tamoxifen. This can readily be misinterpreted to suggest that anastrozole is ineffective after chemotherapy. However, the odds ratio of the tamoxifen versus anastrozole is close to one, and, because it is known that tamoxifen is effective in combination with chemotherapy, it can be suggested that both drugs are equally effective in this setting, but anastrozole is more effective in the chemo-naïve patients. The reason for this is open to speculation.

VI. ADVERSE EVENTS AND TOLERABILITY

In the initial analysis of the ATAC trial, significantly fewer patients on anastrozole experienced hot flashes compared with patients in the tamoxifen-alone arm ($p < 0.0001$) (5). A similar finding was also demonstrated in the final updated analysis (6). However, this should not be used to market the drug considering hot flashes still occurred in one-third of patients in the anastrozole group.

Significantly fewer patients on anastrozole experienced vaginal bleeding or discharge compared with patients on tamoxifen (4.8% vs. 8.7% and 3.0% vs. 12.2%, respectively). This is an advantage for both patients and gynecologists, because this limits the number of invasive investigations required to exclude endometrial car-

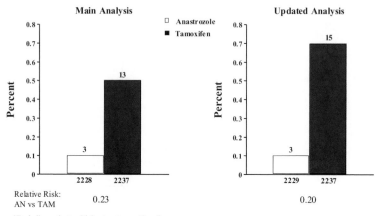

Figure 4 Rates of endometrial cancer, recorded as an adverse event.

cinoma when such symptoms occur. These reductions in vaginal symptoms may eventually translate into a protective element by anastrozole against endometrial cancer. Significantly fewer patients in the anastrozole group developed endometrial carcinoma compared with tamoxifen (0.1% vs. 0.7%; $p = 0.02$) (Fig. 4).

Fewer ischemic cerebrovascular and venous thromboembolic events occurred in the anastrozole-treated group compared with patients on tamoxifen. However, compared with tamoxifen, more musculoskeletal complaints, such as arthralgia, occurred in the anastrozole arm, as well as a higher incidence of bone fractures (30.3% vs. 23.7% and 7.1% vs. 4.4%, respectively). This marked correlation to bone fractures may be due to the acceleration in loss of bone-mineral density through the reduction in estrogen levels. Tamoxifen may confer some advantage over anastrozole in producing a partial agonistic effect at ERs. However, this should not deter the use of anastrozole because osteopenia can be counteracted by the addition of a bisphosphonate. Consequently, baseline and serial measurements of bone-mineral density are recommended prior to starting a breast cancer patient on anastrozole, or indeed when any other hormone-blocking agents are used.

Overall tolerability among the three treatment regimens was similar and of a high degree, with fewer withdrawals due to drug-related adverse events in the anastrozole arm compared with the tamoxifen arm.

VII. CONCLUSION

The results of the ATAC trial demonstrate the significant benefit of anastrozole over tamoxifen in disease-free survival and time-to-recurrence in postmenopausal

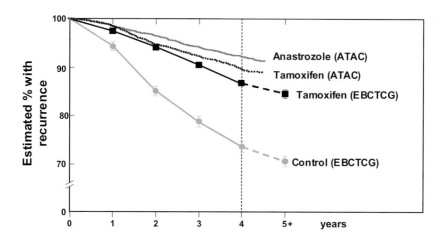

Figure 5 Comparison of ATAC data with EBCTCG 1995 overview—HR+ patients > 50 years of age.

early breast cancer patients, and especially in patients with HR+ tumors. In addition, the overall incidence of contralateral breast cancer was lower in HR+ patients treated with anastrozole alone (OR = 0.56; 95% CI = 0.32–0.94; p = 0.042) compared with tamoxifen.

When these ATAC trial results are compared with the overview by the Early Breast Cancer Trialists' Collaborative Group (4), advances in adjuvant treatment clearly can be seen to have been made (Fig. 5). Over the last 15 years, there has been an improvement in the 4-year recurrence-free rate from 70.5% in control patients, to 92.2% with anastrozole treatment. This marked improvement in efficacy and tolerability for anastrozole over tamoxifen suggests it should be considered as a choice for postmenopausal women with hormone-responsive early breast cancer. At present, there are no restrictions to the licensing of anastrozole as an adjuvant treatment for breast cancer in Japan and North America. However, its current license in Europe is limited to patients in whom tamoxifen is contraindicated.

Although the ATAC trial results introduce the concept of anastrozole being an equivalently effective adjuvant agent to tamoxifen, many additional aspects should be considered. The precise, optimal duration of therapy has yet to be determined. In the ATAC trial, the choice of 5-years' duration of treatment was arbitrary. The most effective sequence regimen is also in question, with other trials presently studying the different situations in which aromatase inhibitors might be used, e.g., in place of tamoxifen or after 5 years of tamoxifen.

It has been suggested that the HER-2/neu status of a tumor may be predictive of a preferential response for an AI over tamoxifen; therefore, an analysis of

HER-2/neu status in the patients from the ATAC trial is presently being conducted retrospectively to determine the predictive role of this marker. With the differences between the classes of AIs (for example, steroidal versus nonsteroidal), there is a need to ascertain whether these differences confer any additional advantages in efficacy and tolerability. Within the Type II group of AIs, letrozole, another third-generation agent, may prove to be more potent than anastrozole, and hence it should pave the way for more comparative trials in the future to determine which is the better drug.

Although cytotoxic chemotherapeutic regimens were believed to be the most effective antitumor treatments for breast cancer 20 years ago, endocrine therapies have emerged to provide better prognosis and tolerability. AIs, especially the third-generation group, have further enhanced the superiority of endocrine therapies as adjuvant agents. The updated results of the ATAC trial have shown evidence of superior therapeutic index for anastrozole compared with tamoxifen. Hence, anastrozole should be considered as a first treatment of choice as an adjuvant agent, for postmenopausal women with hormone-sensitive early breast cancer. However, when selecting this therapy, close monitoring of bone-mineral density is recommended, with the introduction of a bisphosphonate if the patient should become osteopenic.

REFERENCES

1. The World Health Report Archives 1995–2000. World Health Organization 2001.
2. Jemal A, Thomas A, Murray T, Thun M. Cancer Statistics, 2002. CA Cancer J Clin 2002; 52:23–47.
3. Botha JL, Bray F, Sankila R, Parkin DM. Breast cancer incidence and mortality trends in 16 European countries. Eur J Cancer 2003; 39:1718–1729.
4. Early Breast Cancer Trialists' Collaborative Group. Tamoxifen for early breast cancer: an overview of the randomised trials. Lancet 1998; 351:1451–1467.
5. The ATAC Trialists Group. Anastrozole alone or in combination with tamoxifen versus tamoxifen alone for adjuvant treatment of postmenopausal woman with early breast cancer: first results of the ATAC randomized trial. Lancet 2002; 359:2131–2139.
6. The ATAC (Arimidex, Tamoxifen Alone or in Combination) Trialists' Group. Anastrozole alone or in combination with tamoxifen versus tamoxifen alone for adjuvant treatment of postmenopausal woman with early breast cancer: results of the ATAC Trial efficacy and safety update analysis. Cancer 2003; 98:1802–1810
7. Cuzick J. Aromatase inhibitors in prevention—data from the ATAC (Arimidex, Tamoxifen Alone or in Combination) trial and the design of IBIS-II (the second International Breast Cancer Intervention Study). Recent Results Cancer Res 2003; 163:96–103.

5

Aromatase Inhibitors and Other Agents in Early-Stage Breast Cancer

Paul E. Goss and Kathrin Strasser-Weippl
Princess Margaret Hospital
University Health Network
Toronto, Ontario, Canada

I. OVERVIEW

Aromatase inhibitors (AIs) provide a novel approach to the management of breast cancer in postmenopausal women. AIs are superior to megestrol acetate as second-line therapy and to tamoxifen as initial therapy of metastatic disease. The available third-generation AIs include the steroidal exemestane, and the non-steroidals anastrozole and letrozole. Although both types of inhibitors act on the aromatase enzyme, they do so by different mechanisms and have different effects on cellular aromatase activity. In cultures of human breast fibroblasts, non-steroidal agents increase aromatase enzyme content, whereas steroidal agents decrease the levels. The increase seen with nonsteroidals may, in part, explain the development of drug resistance to these agents and the ability of the steroidal inhibitor exemestane to still induce a response when non-steroidal agents have failed. Because AIs almost completely eliminate endogenous estrogen production, they not only affect breast cancers, but may also alter the function of other estrogen-responsive tissues. The steroidal inhibitor exemestane has positive effects on both bone and lipid metabolism in a preclinical rat model, and neutral effects in short-term human volunteer studies. In addition, no increase in clinical fracture rate has been noted in women treated with exemestane in metastatic trials, but the fracture risk has not yet been studied following prolonged exposure in healthy women. The beneficial effects associated with exemestane on these end organs may be due to the steroidal nature of both the parent compound and its principal metabolite, 17-hydroexemestane.

Based on their excellent activity in metastatic disease, AIs are now being evaluated in the adjuvant setting and in pilot studies for chemoprevention. These studies will provide data on the long-term safety of the agents in healthy women and will help to differentiate the AIs from each other, both in terms of efficacy and toxicities. This chapter reviews some of the problems associated with tamoxifen and presents preclinical and clinical data showing the value AIs demonstrate in the treatment of metastatic breast cancer. The new adjuvant trials that are ongoing or in planning that employ AIs are also be discussed.

II. INTRODUCTION

Breast cancer is a complicated disease, and although enormous progress has been made over the last decade, many challenges lie ahead. An important area is post-menopausal adjuvant therapy. Estrogen and progesterone stimulate the growth of normal breast cells and have also been implicated in the development or progression of tumors in the breast. Cancers that are estrogen-receptor positive (ER+) grow in response to estrogen that is synthesized from conversion of androgens ubiquitously in the body. The enzyme catalyzing the final and rate-limiting step in estrogen biosynthesis is aromatase, which is present in fat, muscle, ovaries, breast cells and adrenal glands. When estrogen binds to the estrogen receptors in ER+ cancer cells, the cells divide and tumor growth is promoted. Estrogen-receptor negative (ER−) tumors are unaffected by systemic estrogens or progesterone (1, 2).

To circumvent these deleterious tumor promoting effects of estrogen, selective estrogen receptor modulators (SERMs) were developed, of which tamoxifen was the first to be approved as an adjuvant endocrine treatment. Tamoxifen is indicated for the treatment of metastatic breast cancer, as adjuvant and neoadjuvant therapy, and as chemoprevention in women at elevated risk of breast cancer. It functions as an estrogen antagonist in most ER+ breast tumors, but displays a paradoxical estrogen-like activity on lipid metabolism, bone, and on the endometrium (3, 4).

Tamoxifen has dominated endocrine treatment of breast cancer for over two decades. It is associated with a 26% decrease in the risk of death independent of age or menopausal status, but is only effective in ER+ tumors. The benefits of tamoxifen must also be considered in light of the side effects and risks associated with treatment. The most common side effects include hot flashes, irregular menstrual periods, and vaginal discharge or bleeding. More serious side effects include an increased risk of thromboembolic events, endometrial cancer, and possibly cerebrovascular disease.

Despite this, tamoxifen remains the most successful anticancer drug ever. It has been the standard first-line adjuvant endocrine treatment for breast cancer for several decades. Accumulated data comparing tamoxifen treatment versus placebo over 5 years in ER+ patients for outcomes of recurrences and breast cancer deaths suggest that 5 years of adjuvant tamoxifen confer a beneficial effect lasting beyond the treatment period for at least 15 years and possibly beyond (5, 6). However, breast cancer can become refractory to tamoxifen or develop resistance to it with ongoing treatment. This resistance involves several complex mechanisms, a review of which is beyond the scope of this chapter. Suffice it to say that receptor mutation, recruitment of co-activators and co-suppressors, as well as possible receptor mutation causing estrogen hypersensitivity have been noted (7).

One of the current and future goals of breast cancer therapy is to increase the efficacy of endocrine therapy without increasing toxicity. AIs hold promise in this area. Another future direction is to find new predictive markers that are able to identify subgroups of patients who are more or less likely to respond to a certain treatment. For example, women with one or more positive axillary nodes have an increased risk of breast cancer recurrence, and the number of positive axillary nodes has been linked to disease-free and overall survival (8). However, there are currently no data to suggest that the number of involved axillary nodes is correlated with response to chemotherapy or to endocrine treatment. One of the important goals is to increase survival of patients that have receptor positive breast cancer and that are node positive by tailoring treatment according to the biological characteristics of the tumor. Tumors that are ER− remain a challenge. One way to approach this issue may be to try to prevent ER− breast cancer.

Another important issue is that some patients are currently being treated who may not benefit from therapy. Thus, if predictive factors could help to identify patients who are at very low risk for developing a recurrence, those patients could be spared the treatment. A recent meeting of the National Cancer Institute Clinical Trials Information Project (NCI CTIP) group addressed this issue and a novel trial design was set up for ER+ premenopausal node-negative women. The trial's objective will be to stratify patients into good-risk versus poor-risk populations based on tumor gene profiling, thereby attempting to avoid unnecessary chemotherapy in certain groups of patients.

III. AIs

Apart from tamoxifen, another way of depriving hormone-dependent breast cancer of estrogen is to prevent its synthesis. Aromatase (estrogen synthase) is the enzyme complex responsible for the final step in estrogen synthesis—the conversion of androstenedione and testosterone to estrone and estradiol, respectively. Inhibitors of this enzyme have been shown to be clinically effective in the treatment of advanced breast cancer in postmenopausal women, in whom estrogen is produced in peripheral tissues by aromatization of adrenal androgens. AIs are logical alternatives to SERMs, not only in the treatment of breast cancer, but also in prevention of the disease. To date, SERMs have shown efficacy only in the prevention of ER+ and progesterone-receptor-positive (PR+) breast cancers, without a reduction in ER–/PR– tumors. By both inhibiting the parent estrogens and their carcinogenic catechol metabolites, true prevention of cancer initiation with AIs might be possible, not only for receptor-positive but also for receptor-negative tumors (9, 10).

The first widely used AI was aminoglutethimide. However, being nonselective, it also inhibits adrenocorticosteroid synthesis, necessitating hydrocortisone supplementation. Therefore, aminoglutethimide is associated with frequent and troublesome side effects (10). The second-generation AI formestane, which was also the first selective inhibitor to be developed, has an improved safety profile over aminoglutethimide. However, its use has been somewhat limited by its inconvenient administration via intramuscular injection (10). Newer, orally administered, third-generation AIs include the nonsteroidals anastrozole (Arimidex®) and letrozole (Femara®), and the steroidal exemestane (Aromasin®). These compounds are highly specific at clinical doses, and have little or no effect on basal levels of cortisol or aldosterone (11). They are able to reduce circulating plasma estrogen concentrations in postmenopausal women to below detectable limits, and significantly inhibit aromatase in normal breast tissue and breast tumors. Significant gains in clinical efficacy with these agents over tamoxifen and the older AIs have led to their evaluation as adjuvant therapy (10).

The third-generation AIs are very well tolerated with a low incidence of short-term adverse effects. The nonspecific side effects associated with AIs include headache, nausea, peripheral edema, fatigue, vomiting, and dyspepsia. In addition, certain endocrinological side effects in postmenopausal women have been noted, namely, hot flashes and vaginal dryness. In advanced breast cancer, these side effects result in treatment withdrawal in few (4%) women. Of concern, however, are the potential long-term endocrinological side effects in women receiving treatment as first-line adjuvant therapy or in sequence or combination with tamoxifen or other SERMs.

Current studies of adjuvant treatment for breast cancer in healthy women are carefully evaluating the effects of AIs on bone, lipid metabolism, cardiovascular risk, quality of life, and menopausal symptoms, in addition to general toxicities. Careful evaluation of all-cause morbidity and mortality is necessary to plan trials and justify long-term use of AIs in the treatment or prevention of breast cancer in healthy women (6).

Ongoing adjuvant breast cancer trials are exploring AIs as alternatives to tamoxifen, as well as in sequence or in combination with tamoxifen. The rationale for these adjuvant trials are clinical trials in the metastatic setting and several preclinical models. Brodie et al. for example, (12, 13), have demonstrated that

AIs are superior to tamoxifen in a preclinical model. In the clinical arena, AIs have shown superiority over tamoxifen as first- and second-line endocrine therapy in women with hormone-responsive metastatic breast cancer (14–18). In the neoadjuvant setting, it has been demonstrated that letrozole is more effective than tamoxifen (19). Apart from their superior efficacy, another important advantage of AIs is that they have no agonist effects and thus an improved profile relating to the endometrium compared to tamoxifen. In particular, AIs eliminate the possibility of estrogen operating through non-ER pathways (20). Therefore, current data suggest that AIs will replace tamoxifen as the gold standard in earlier stages of disease, as they have in the advanced disease setting.

IV. ADJUVANT TRIALS WITH AIs

As discussed earlier, the use of AIs in adjuvant therapy is currently being explored (6). Several major ongoing clinical trials with a variety of treatment regimens are comparing the relative efficacy of tamoxifen with the steroidal and nonsteroidal AIs in the adjuvant setting. These are summarized in Figure 1.

The first strategy compares an AI against tamoxifen directly. Among these are the ATAC (Arimidex, Tamoxifen Alone or in Combination) trial, the BIG FEMTA (Femara-Tamoxifen Breast International Group) study, and the EXEM and TEAM trials (exemestane). The ATAC trial was a randomized, double-blind, multicenter trial that compared tamoxifen with anastrozole, alone and in combination with

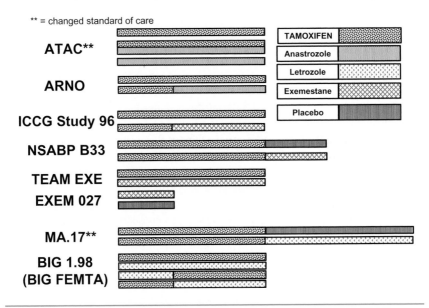

Figure 1   Summary of ongoing first-generation adjuvant trials with AIs.

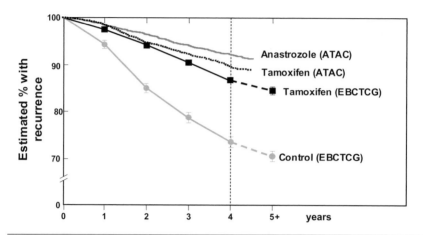

Figure 2 Comparison of ATAC data with EBCTCG receptor-positive patients >50 years old. (Adapted from the EBCTCG overview with ATAC data superimposed. Lancet 1998; 351:1451–1467.)

tamoxifen, as adjuvant endocrine treatment for postmenopausal patients with invasive, early stage breast cancer (21). The results of the ATAC trial show anastrozole to be more effective and better tolerated than tamoxifen in this group of patients (Fig. 2). Anastrozole is now emerging as a new standard for the adjuvant treatment of postmenopausal women with hormone-sensitive early-stage breast cancer. Based on the published results from ATAC, the American Society of Clinical Oncology technology assessment included the option of giving anastrozole to postmenopausal women in the adjuvant breast cancer setting, although tamoxifen is still seen as the standard of care (22). At least one ongoing new adjuvant trial is using anastrozole in the control arm of the study (23).

The adverse events in the ATAC trial showed an increased risk of long-bone fractures in patients receiving anastrozole (Figs. 3 and 4) (21). It is difficult, however, to determine from the ATAC trial whether this was a protective effect of tamoxifen or a detrimental effect of anastrozole, as there was no placebo arm. Figure 4 demonstrates that there is a stable difference in bone fractures over time in the ATAC study. There are several possible explanations for these findings. It has been hypothesized, for example, that women treated with AIs suffer from cognitive dysfunction, and thus, may fall more frequently and fracture their bones. The importance of increased bone turnover induced by AIs has therefore yet to be definitively determined.

In the ATAC study, Baum et al. (21) reported on the side effects as determined by study protocol. In contrast to these data, which favored anastrozole, Fallowfield (24) reported on a quality of life substudy with 1,000 patients. In this study, patients reported their side effects themselves, with somewhat unexpected findings.

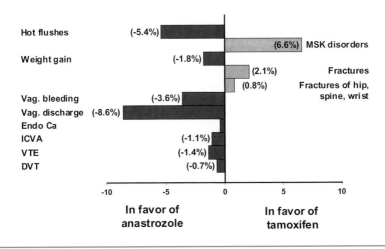

Figure 3 Adverse events in the ATAC.

The patients significantly favored tamoxifen over AIs because of significant differences in categories such as vaginal dryness, pain with intercourse, loss of interest in sex, vomiting, and diarrhea. Whether this type of reporting is more reliable or more accurate than the usual reporting by the trial investigators remains to be determined.

A second set of trials is evaluating the use of an AI as an extension after the initial 5 years of tamoxifen. Examples of this trial design are the MA.17 (letrozole) and

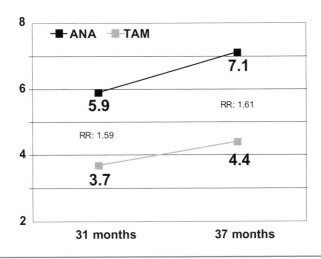

Figure 4 Percentage of bone fractures in the ATAC trial.

the National Surgical Adjuvant Breast and Bowel Project (NSABP B-33, exemestane) trials. Recently, the results of the MA.17 adjuvant study, comparing 5 years of letrozole versus placebo following 5 years of adjuvant tamoxifen were published (25). The women in this study had their study medication unblinded at the first interim analysis because of a highly significant reduction in breast cancer recurrences in the letrozole arm. After a median follow-up of 2.4 years, the hazard ratio for local and distant recurrence or new contralateral breast cancer in the letrozole group as compared with the placebo group was 0.57 (95% CI = 0.43–0.75; p = .00008). Low-grade hot flashes, arthritis, arthralgia, and myalgia were more frequent in the letrozole group, but vaginal bleeding was less frequent. Similar to the ATAC trial, there were more new diagnoses of osteoporosis in women in the AI group, but this was not statistically significant (25).

A third approach of introducing AIs into the adjuvant setting is their use in sequence with tamoxifen as therapy within the initial 5 postoperative years. Examples of this approach are the International Collaboration Cancer Group trial (tamoxifen for 2 to 3 years followed by either tamoxifen or exemestane for the remainder of the 5-year period), the BIG FEMTA trial (patients are crossed over from tamoxifen to letrozole or letrozole to tamoxifen), and the Arimidex-Nolvadex (ARNO) trial (patients receiving tamoxifen are randomized either to continue with tamoxifen or to switch to anastrozole).

The MA.17 trial is one of three adjuvant studies that will collect placebo-controlled data about toxicity. Several companion trials to MA.17 are designed to study end organ effects. Among them, MA.17B specifically addresses bone metabolism with the study endpoints being bone metabolism markers and bone density. MA.17L assesses lipid metabolism and quality of life using tools specific for menopausal women. The results from these trials will be reported shortly (5, 6).

As indicated by the results of the ATAC and the MA.17 trials, the AIs seem to be very promising from an efficacy point of view. A crucial point, however, which cannot be answered at present, is whether AIs have the long-term protective effects on cancer recurrence similar to tamoxifen. In addition, menopausal symptomatology or deleterious effects on bone and lipid metabolism and other end organs may be potentially exacerbated by AIs (10).

V. EXEMESTANE

The third orally active third-generation AI, exemestane, has demonstrated excellent selectivity, tolerability, and efficacy in the treatment of postmenopausal breast cancer. The chemical structures of both exemestane and its major metabolite, 17-hydroexemestane, have the potential to exert minimal steroidal activity, which may counterbalance the effects of estrogen deprivation in some tissues (26). At clinical doses, exemestane causes a dose-dependent reduction in sex hormone-binding globulin (SHBG), indicating that it has an androgenic effect. When exemestane was tested in the castrated immature male rat, a standard model for androgenicity, it produced an increase in ventral prostate weight and hypertrophy of the levator ani muscle mass. It is not clear whether these androgenic effects are due to exemestane or to 17-hydroxymetabolite, which is present both in rats and humans. Labrie et al. demonstrated that when exemestane is added to hormone-sensitive MCF-7 cells under a steady-state milieu of estrogen, it has an antiproliferative effect, which is in contrast to other AIs.* This effect can be reversed by flutamide, which blocks the androgen receptor.

The effects of exemestane on bone and lipid metabolism were investigated in comparison to letrozole and ovariectomy in 10-month-old Sprague-Dawley rats (Fig. 5). The animals were sorted into three groups: intact control (sham operated); ovariectomized control; ovariectomized and treated with exemestane 100 mg/kg weekly. Exemestane completely protected against the adverse changes in lipid and bone metabolism associated with ovariectomy (27). These data demonstrate that exemestane has a distinct effect on bone metabolism. As the castrated animal is devoid of estrogen, it is only the androgenicity of this compound that can explain its protective effect on bone mineral density. In this rat model, the changes in cholesterol levels are similar to those in bone metabolism. In the group of animals treated with ovariectomy, a prompt rise in serum cholesterol was noted, whereas in the group treated with exemestane no rise in serum cholesterol levels was seen (Fig. 6).

In a Phase-II study there was no difference in the incidence of pathologic fractures in postmenopausal women with metastatic breast cancer treated with exemestane versus megestrol acetate (5). In another Phase-II trial in women with metastatic breast cancer, there were also no negative effects on lipid profile after 24 weeks of treatment with exemestane as initial therapy (28, 29). A 3-month human volunteer study investigated the effects of placebo, exemestane, and letrozole on bone biomarkers (30). The effects of exemestane were similar to placebo in this study, showing no increase in bone turnover in postmenopausal women. Letrozole was substantially worse, demonstrating a steep reduction in bone formation. An ongoing, 6-month follow-up study with anastrozole, letrozole, exemestane, and placebo will provide additional information on this important finding.

The protective effects on bone zoledronic acid (Zometa®), a bisphosphonate approved for the treatment of hypercalcaemia of malignancy, will be evaluated in a new study in the adjuvant setting. Postmenopausal women with ER+ tumors will receive letrozole 2.5 mg daily in this trial. Zoledronic acid will either be given concurrently with letrozole from the start of the study or it will be started at a later stage as "salvage therapy," if signs and symptoms of bone demineralization are reported.

---

*Labrie F, personal communication, 2002.

A

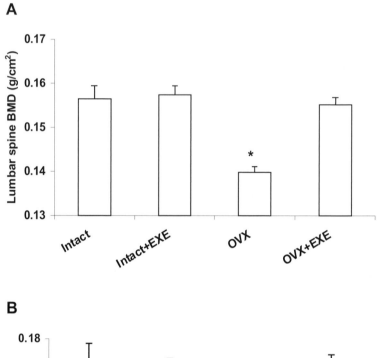

B

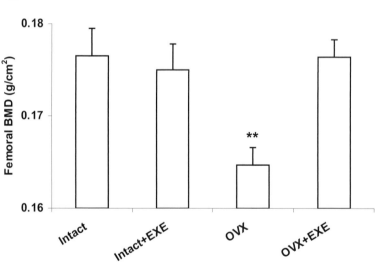

Figure 5 Bone mineral density of the lumbar vertebrae (A) and whole femora (B). Bars represent the mean ± SEM (n = 13–16). * = Significant difference among all other groups ($p < 0.0001$); ** = significant difference among all other groups ($p < 0.001$).

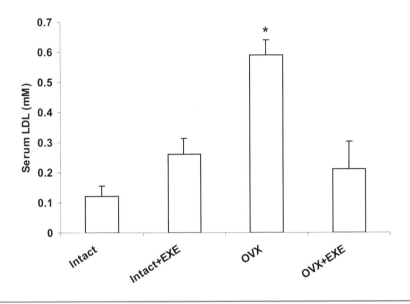

Figure 6   Effect of EXE serum LDL levels. Bars represent the mean ± SEM (*n* = 13−16). * = Significant difference among all other groups (*p* < 0.0001).

VI.   DURATION OF TREATMENT WITH AIs

In the adjuvant setting, the optimal duration of tamoxifen therapy has not yet been fully determined. Two ongoing clinical trials, Adjuvant Tamoxifen Offer More (ATOM) and Adjuvant Tamoxifen Longer Against Shorter (ATLAS), are attempting to resolve this issue. The results from these trials should appear in 2010 or somewhat earlier. The ATAC trial may support the use of anastrozole in the first 5 years of therapy, whereas MA.17 may support the use of letrozole for 5 years after tamoxifen, but neither trial answers the question of how long patients should receive AI therapy. One consideration of duration is being made via rerandomizing the patients coming off the MA.17 trial or other adjuvant trials to another 5 years of therapy versus placebo.

Another important issue in endocrine treatment is that of timing, particularly in relation to chemotherapy. The data from Albain et al. (31) have demonstrated that regarding chemotherapy, tamoxifen is probably best given after and not concurrent with chemotherapy. This question also has to be answered for AIs. The same issue applies to radiation therapy, where there is some evidence to suggest that concurrent irradiation with endocrine therapy is more toxic and less effective (32). Therefore, it might be possible that completing radiation therapy before initiating hormone therapy may be clinically superior.

VII. COMBINATION THERAPY WITH AIs AND COX-2 INHIBITORS

The COX-2 pathway is activated by tissue injury, chemotherapy, radiation, and cancer. Its activation leads to cancer growth promotion by pleiotropic mechanisms in many solid tumor types. Among the COX-2-dependent targets in breast cancer are angiogenesis, cell growth and invasion, tumor-associated inflammation, anti-apoptotic effects, and association with c-erbB-2 (33).

The diagrammatic representation in Figure 7 shows COX-2 in a central role, in which tumor cells invoke the inflammatory mechanism that is in turn driven by the inducible COX-2 enzyme. Once COX-2 has been induced, prostaglandin levels are increased, having a vasoactive endothelial growth factor (VEGF) effect and increasing ligand binding through human epidermal growth factor receptor 2 (HER-2). This mechanism of action has been shown for both ductal carcinoma in-situ (DCIS) as well as invasive cancers. Other COX-2 inducible effects are activation of the MAP kinase and PI3 kinase pathways, leading to an anti-apoptotic effect, and induction of P_{450}. There is evidence that a positive feedback mechanism from some of these loops back to COX-2 exists. Importantly, the aromatase gene is stimulated by the overexpressed COX-2 to produce more estrogen. Estrogen then feeds back, further driving COX-2 stimulation. Aromatase and COX-2 may thus work in concert

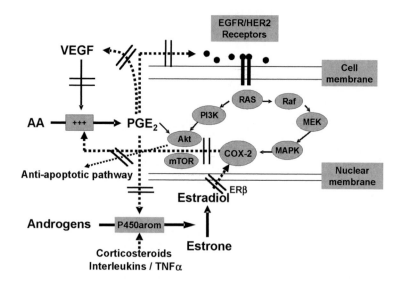

Figure 7 Schematic description of the interactions between COX-2 and AIs.

to increase the growth of premalignant, preinvasive, and invasive tumors, resulting in a vicious circle that could be broken by treatment with an AI or COX-2 inhibitor.

The rationale for combining AIs with COX-2 inhibitors is partly driven by these pleiotropic anticancer effects of COX-2 inhibitors and partly by the fact that the Women's Health Initiative (WHI) reported a 43% reduction in new breast cancers from the use of over-the-counter nonsteroidal anti-inflammatories. There is also a substantial amount of preclinical evidence suggesting that inhibition of the COX-2 pathway may prevent breast cancer.

The DMBA-induced ER+ breast cancer model is reliable for predicting the clinical efficacy of hormone therapies. In this model, exemestane and celecoxib inhibit tumor growth when administered alone, and produce an additive effect when co-administered (34). Interestingly, celecoxib alone also has a dose-dependent inhibiting effect on cell proliferation in ER− breast cancer cell lines in vitro (35).

The combination of an AI and a COX-2 inhibitor is evaluated in a second generation adjuvant trial (NCIC CTG MA.27), which has recently opened to accrual. It is a 6,800-patient study, and the first trial to randomize to one of two AIs without tamoxifen in the control arm. The first question investigated in this study is whether exemestane is superior to anastrozole, both in terms of efficacy and in terms of bone, lipid, and other end-organ toxicities. The second important point to be evaluated is whether the addition of a COX-2 inhibitor provides additional benefit to patients already receiving an AI. For companion studies, a prospective serum and DNA repository, as well as a fresh-frozen and paraffin-embedded tumor bank are being established. In addition to bone and lipid metabolism, quality of life and breast density substudies are being undertaken.

VIII. UNANSWERED ISSUES

In an animal model of ovariectomized nude mice, Long et al. (36) have demonstrated that combining letrozole with tamoxifen, and anastrozole with tamoxifen was not superior to the inhibitors alone. In the case of exemestane, however, the combination with tamoxifen appears to be superior to the inhibitor alone, at least in a preclinical model (37). The reason or mechanism for this finding are unclear to date. These interesting data have prompted a revisiting of the debate about combining AIs with SERMs, called "total estrogen blockade," a strategy that the ATAC trial was initially aiming for. A trial combining exemestane with tamoxifen has, therefore, been proposed in metastatic breast cancer.

Although there is a strong preclinical rationale for this combination, the combination of an AI with SERMs other than tamoxifen might even be superior to this strategy. Toremifene, for example, has a much lower agonistic activity than tamoxifen in an estrogen-depleted environment, although both drugs are equivalent clinically. Thus, combining an AI with a less agonistic SERM may be a more viable treatment combination and a possible way of achieving total estrogen blockade in the way that the combination arm in the ATAC trial failed to do.

When combining AIs with nonendocrine agents, biological pathway inhibitors other than the COX-2 inhibitors have also been used. Among the studies in this field, results from the NCIC CTG MA.14 study will be reported soon. This adjuvant trial investigates whether tamoxifen plus the IGF-1 inhibitor octreotide are superior to tamoxifen alone, a hypothesis that is supported by preclinical data. In the United States, the NSABP trial asking the same question was stopped because of a higher incidence of gall stones in the investigational octreotide arm.

IX. CONCLUSIONS

AIs are a step forward in the treatment of endocrine responsive breast cancer, not only because of their enhanced efficacy, but also because of improved toxicity and possibly fewer resistance mechanisms. In addition, they offer the chance of better chemoprevention in women that are at risk for developing breast cancer.

Further data from the ATAC trial are keenly awaited with regard to disease recurrence, overall survival, and duration of benefit. The optimal regimen for AI therapy in early breast cancer, both in terms of efficacy and toxicity, needs to be carefully evaluated. The ongoing MA.27 trial will address this issue. The NCIC CTG MA.17 trial has provided definitive evidence of the value of letrozole after 5 years of tamoxifen in early-stage breast cancer, and an extension of this trial will help to answer questions about the optimal ongoing duration of therapy. Timing of the AIs in relation to chemo- and radiation therapy has not been prospectively studied yet.

The next generation of studies in this field will address the combination of aromatase inhibitors with other targeted therapies in an attempt to overcome either de novo or acquired resistance to the aromatase inhibitors. Phase-2 and -3 trials are being conducted to explore these possibilities in the advanced disease setting already. Examples include combining aromatase inhibitors with COX-2 inhibitors, iressa, herceptin, and other promising cell signaling pathway inhibitors.

Editorial Note in Reference to the MA.17 Trial
The results of this trial became available after the Gleneagles meeting but have been cited in this chapter to provide a comprehensive overview of this area.

REFERENCES

1. MacGregor JI, Jordan VC. Basic guide to the mechanisms of antiestrogen action. Pharmacol Rev 1998; 50:151–196.

2. Ali S, Coombes RC. Endocrine-responsive breast cancer and strategies for combating resistance. Nat Rev Cancer 2002; 2:101–112.

3. Furr BJ, Jordan VC. The pharmacology and clinical uses of tamoxifen. Pharmacol Ther 1984; 25:127–205.

4. Goss PE, Strasser K. Tamoxifen resistant and refractory breast cancer: the value of aromatase inhibitors. Drugs 2002; 62:957–966.

5. Goss P. Anti-aromatase agents in the treatment and prevention of breast cancer. Cancer Control 2002; 9:2–8.

6. Goss PE. Emerging role of aromatase inhibitors in the adjuvant setting. Am J Clin Oncol 2003; 26:S27–S33.

7. Bentrem DJ, Jordan VC. Antiestrogens: the past and the future. Zentralbl Gynakol 2002; 124:551–558.

8. Nemoto T, Vana J, Bedwani RN, Baker HW, McGregor FH, Murphy GP. Management and survival of female breast cancer: results of a national survey by the American College of Surgeons. Cancer 1980; 45:2917–2924.

9. Miller WR, Jackson J. The therapeutic potential of aromatase inhibitors. Expert Opin Investig Drugs 2003; 12:337–351.

10. Smith IE, Dowsett M. Aromatase inhibitors in breast cancer. N Engl J Med 2003; 348:2431–2442.

11. Bajetta E, Zilembo N, Bichisao E, Martinetti A, Buzzoni R, Pozzi P, Bidoli P, Ferrari L, Celio L. Tumor response and estrogen suppression in breast cancer patients treated with aromatase inhibitors. Ann Oncol 2000; 11:1017–1022.

12. Brodie A, Lu Q, Liu Y, Long B. Aromatase inhibitors and their antitumor effects in model systems. Endocr Relat Cancer 1999; 6:205–210.

13. Brodie A, Jelovac D, Long BJ. Predictions from a preclinical model: studies of aromatase inhibitors and antiestrogens. Clin Cancer Res 2003; 9:455S–459S.

14. Goss PE, Strasser K. Aromatase inhibitors in the treatment and prevention of breast cancer. J Clin Oncol 2001;19:881–894.

15. Nabholtz JM, Buzdar A, Pollak M. Anastrozole is superior to tamoxifen as first-line therapy for advanced breast cancer in postmenopausal women: results of a North American multicenter randomized trial. Arimidex Study Group. J Clin Oncol 2000;18:3758–3767.

16. Bonneterre J, Buzdar A, Nabholtz JM, Robertson JF, Thurlimann B, von Euler M, Sahmoud T, Webster A, Steinberg M; Arimidex Writing Committee; Investigators Committee Members. Anastrozole is superior to tamoxifen as first-line therapy in hormone receptor positive advanced breast carcinoma. Cancer 2001; 92:2247–2258.

17. Mouridsen H, Gershanovich M, Sun Y, Perez-Carrion R, Boni C, Monnier A, Apffelstaedt J, Smith R, Sleeboom HP, Janicke F, Pluzanska A, Dank M, Becquart D, Bapsy PP, Salminen E, Snyder R, Lassus M, Verbeek JA, Staffler B, Chaudri-Ross HA, Dugan M. Superior efficacy of letrozole versus tamoxifen as first-line therapy for postmenopausal women with advanced breast cancer: results of a phase III study of the International Letrozole Breast Cancer Group. J Clin Oncol 2001; 19:2596–2606.

18. Dirix L, Piccart MJ, Lohrisch C, et al. Efficacy of and tolerance to exemestane versus tamoxifen in first line hormone therapy of postmenopausal metastatic breast cancer patients: a European Organisation for the Research and Treatment of Cancer (EORTC Breast Group) Phase II trial with Pharmacia and Upjohn [abstr 114]. Proc Am Soc Clin Oncol 2001; 20.

19. Ellis MJ, Coop A, Singh B, Tao Y, Llombart-Cussac A, Janicke F, Mauriac L, Quebe-Fehling E, Chaudri-Ross HA, Evans DB, Miller WR. Letrozole inhibits tumor proliferation more effectively than tamoxifen independent of HER1/2 expression status. Cancer Res. 2003 Oct 1; 63:6523–31.

20. Miller WR, Dixon JM. Antiaromatase agents: preclinical data and neoadjuvant therapy. Clin Breast Cancer 2000; 1(suppl 1):S9–S14.

21. Baum M, Budzar AU, Cuzick J, Forbes J, Houghton JH, Klijn JG, Sahmoud T. Anastrozole alone or in combination with tamoxifen versus tamoxifen alone for adjuvant treatment of postmenopausal women with early breast cancer: first results of the ATAC randomised trial. Lancet 2002; 359:2131–2139.

22. Winer EP, Hudis C, Burstein HJ, Chlebowski RT, Ingle JN, Edge SB, Edge SB, Mamounas EP, Gralow J, Goldstein LJ, Pritchard KI, Braun S, Cobleig MA, Langer AS, Perotti J, Powles TJ, Browman GP. American Society of Clinical Oncology technology assessment on the use of aromatase inhibitors as adjuvant therapy for women with hormone receptor-positive breast cancer: status report 2002. J Clin Oncol 2002; 20:3317–3327.

23. Buzdar A. Anastrozole as adjuvant therapy for early-stage breast cancer: implications of the ATAC Trial. Clin Breast Cancer 2003; 4(suppl 1):S42–S48.

24. Fallowfield L. Quality of life: a new perspective for cancer patients. Nat Rev Cancer 2002; 2:873–879.

25. Goss PE, Ingle JN, Martino S, Robert NJ, Muss HB, Piccart MJ, Castiglione M, Tu D, Shepherd LE, Pritchard KI, Livingston RB, Davidson NE, Norton L, Perez E A, Abrams JS, Therasse P, Palmer MJ, Pater JL. A randomized trial of letrozole in postmenopausal women after five years of tamoxifen therapy for early-stage breast cancer. New Engl J Med 2003; 349:1793–1802.

26. Lohrisch C, Paridaens R, Dirix LY, Beex L, Nooij M, Cameron D, Biganzoli L, Cufer T, Yague C, Duchateau L, Lobelle JP, Piccart M. No adverse impact on serum lipids of the irreversible aromatase inactivator Aromasin (exemestane [E]) in first line treatment of metastatic breast cancer (MBC): companion study to a European Organization of Research and Treatment of Cancer (Breast Group) trial with Pharmacias' Upjohn [abstr]. Proc Ann Meet Am Soc Clin Oncol 2001; 20:167a.

27. Goss PE, Qi S, Josse RG, Pritzker KPH, Mendes M, Hu H, Waldman SD, Grynpas MD. The steroidal aromatase inhibitor exemestane prevents bone loss in ovariectomized rats. Bone 2003. In press.

28. Paridaens R, Dirix L, Beex L, Nooij MN, Cufer T, Lohrisch C, Biganzoli L, Van H, I, Duchateau L, Lobelle JP, Piccart M. Promising results with exemestane in the first-line treatment of metastatic breast cancer: a randomized Phase II EORTC trial with a tamoxifen control. Clin Breast Cancer 2000; 1(suppl 1):S19–S21.

29. Paridaens R, Dirix L, Lohrisch C, Beex L, Nooij M, Cameron D, Biganzoli L, Cufer T, Duchateau L, Hamilton A, Lobelle JP, Piccart M. Mature results of a randomized phase II multicenter study of exemestane versus tamoxifen as first-line hormone ther-

apy for postmenopausal women with metastatic breast cancer. Ann Oncol 2003; 14:1391–1398.

30. Goss PE, Thomsen T, Banke-Bochita J, et al. A randomized, placebo-controlled, explorative study to investigate the effect of low estrogen plasma levels on markers of bone turnover in healthy postmenopausal women during the 12-week treatment with exemestane or letrozole [abstr 267]. Breast Cancer Res Treat 2002; 69.

31. Albain KS, Green SJ, Ravdin PM, Cobau CD, Levine EG, Ingle JN, Pritchard KI, Schneider DJ, Abeloff MD, Norton L, Henderson IC, Lew D, Livingston RB, Martino S, Osborne CK. Adjuvant chemohormonal therapy for primary breast cancer should be sequential instead of concurrent: initial results from intergroup trial 0100 (SWOG-8814) [abstr 143]. Proc Am Soc Clin Oncol 2003.

32. Pierce LJ, Lew D, Hutchins L, Davidson N, Albain K, Fetting J, Solin L. Patterns of recurrence by sequence of chemotherapy and radiotherapy in early stage breast cancer. Int J Radiat Oncol Biol Phys 2003; 57:S127.

33. Brodie AM, Lu Q, Long BJ, Fulton A, Chen T, Macpherson N, De Jong PC, Blankenstein MA, Nortier JW, Slee PH, van de Ven J, van Gorp JM, Elbers JR, Schipper ME, Blijham GH, Thijssen JH. Aromatase and COX-2 expression in human breast cancers. J Steroid Biochem Mol Biol 2001; 79:41–47.

34. Pesenti E, Masferrer JL, di Salle E. Effect of exemestane and celecoxib alone or in combination on DMBA-induced mammary carcinoma in rats [abstr 445]. San Antonio Breast Cancer Symposium, San Antonio, TX, USA, Dec 10–13, 2001.

35. Arun B, Anthony M, Dunn B. The search for the ideal SERM. Expert Opin Pharmacother 2002; 3:681–691.

36. Long BJ, Jelovac D, Thiantanawat A, Brodie AM. The effect of second-line antiestrogen therapy on breast tumor growth after first-line treatment with the aromatase inhibitor letrozole: long-term studies using the intratumoral aromatase postmenopausal breast cancer model. Clin Cancer Res 2002; 8:2378–2388.

37. Zaccheo T, Giudici D, Di Salle E. Inhibitory effect of combined treatment with the aromatase inhibitor exemestane and tamoxifen on DMBA-induced mammary tumors in rats. J Steroid Biochem Mol Biol 1993; 44:677–680.

6

Neoadjuvant Therapy in Postmenopausal Women

J. M. Dixon
Western General Hospital
Edinburgh, Scotland

I. INTRODUCTION

There are several potential advantages and disadvantages of primary systemic or neoadjuvant therapy in patients with breast cancer (1). The advantages include the presence of a measurable breast mass to allow a direct in vivo assessment of the sensitivity of tumor cells to a particular drug or drugs used. Detection of resistance to treatment allows discontinuation of worthless treatments, which avoids unnecessary toxicity and also allows change to a potentially more effective treatment regimen. Theoretically the earlier the breast cancer is treated, the less likely there is for resistant tumor clones to emerge, and this should ensure that there is only a short delay between diagnosis and treatment of any systemic disease thereby potentially improving outcome. Furthermore neoadjuvant therapy can shrink large primary tumors to allow less extensive surgery, and it can make locally advanced breast cancers operable.

There are some potential disadvantages, however. Diagnosis in the past has relied on fine needle aspiration cytology and this cannot differentiate between invasive and in situ cancer. It is currently routine practice to base diagnosis on a core biopsy, so the danger of treating noninvasive disease with primary systemic therapy should be small. Systemic therapy is usually based on recognized prognostic factors and, in particular, axillary-node status. With neoadjuvant therapy many of the standard prognostic factors including axillary-node status are unknown at the time drug treatment is started. These prognostic factors help to provide crucial information when planning both the length and intensity of chemotherapy regimen.

Although initially neoadjuvant therapy was used only in locally inoperable or locally advanced breast cancer to reduce tumor size and to facilitate mastectomy or radiotherapy, more recently neoadjuvant chemotherapy and hormonal therapy have been used in patients with large, operable breast cancer to produce tumor shrinkage and allow less extensive surgery (2). Clinical experience with both neoadjuvant chemotherapy and hormonal therapy in postmenopausal women is reviewed in the sections that follow.

II. NEOADJUVANT CHEMOTHERAPY IN LARGE OPERABLE BREAST CANCER

A. Nonrandomized Studies of Neoadjuvant Chemotherapy

The first studies of neoadjuvant chemotherapy were conducted in Milan. Between January 1988 and October 1990, 226 women younger than 65-years-old with large operable cancers (greater than 3 cm on mammography) were enrolled (3). Only 34% of these women were over 50 years of age, and the median age of the whole group was 49. The response rate (RR) did not differ between different chemotherapy regimens. The RRs were high with 10.2% having a complete regression, 24.3% a partial response, and 58.9% a minor response; of the remainder, 6.2% showed no change, 3.1% progressed with 1.3% not being evaluable. Of the 226, 203 (90%) were eventually treated with breast-conserving surgery. In eight cases there was no histological disease remaining, and in another five, only in situ disease remained. Of the patients, 60% had axillary node metastasis following chemotherapy. There is no breakdown given in this study of the benefits of therapy in pre- and postmenopausal women. Local recurrence rates were acceptable, with 12 of 203 treated by breast-conserving surgery (5%) developing local recurrence at a mean follow-up of 36 months (4).

B. Randomized Trials of Neoadjuvant Chemotherapy

The first randomized trial of neoadjuvant therapy was conducted between January 1985 and April 1989 in France. It accrued 272 women with large, operable breast cancers (5), with 54% of women in this study postmenopausal. In the 138 patients randomized to standard treatment, all had a modified radical mastectomy and 76 had adjuvant chemotherapy. The remainder received no adjuvant treatment because they had no poor prognostic factors. In the 134 patients randomized to neoadjuvant chemotherapy, breast conservation was possible in 63.1% with 33% ($n = 44$) having radiation alone and 30% ($n = 40$) having breast-conserving surgery followed by radiation. In the patients treated by radiation alone, there were 15 local relapses. In the 44 patients treated by tumorectomy and radiotherapy, there were nine local relapses. This is a high rate of local recurrence in both groups. Overall survival was identical in the two treatment groups after 124 months of follow-up. Looking at the prognostic factors, age did not appear to have any impact on response to therapy or outcome.

The largest randomized studies of neoadjuvant chemotherapy have been performed by the National Surgical Adjuvant Breast Project group (NSABP) (6). In 1988 the NSABP initiated a randomized trial in patients with larger operable breast cancers to compare the preoperative and postoperative administration of chemotherapy. Patients were randomized to receive four cycles of doxorubicin combined with cyclophosphamide given every 21 days for 4 cycles either before or after surgery (6, 7). There were 1,523 patients recruited to this study. Of those patients 36% obtained a complete clinical response to the chemotherapy, and 43% of patients had a clinical partial response giving an overall response rate of 79% following neoadjuvant chemotherapy. Only 3% of women had progressive disease. Of the patients who achieved a complete clinical response, 25% of those who received neoadjuvant chemotherapy (or 9% of the total group) were found to have no tumor present on pathological examination in the lumpectomy or mastectomy specimen. A further 10% of patients with a complete clinical response (4% of the total group) had only noninvasive cancer present in the surgical excision specimen. In total, therefore, 13% of all patients who received chemotherapy had no invasive cancer following chemotherapy (6, 7). There was clear evidence that administration of chemotherapy improved pathological lymph nodes status: 58% of the patients who were randomized to surgery followed by adjuvant chemotherapy had involved nodes histologically whereas only 40% of the group who received neoadjuvant chemotherapy had nodal metastasis. This difference was statistically significant. Overall survival was not different between the two groups and age had no impact on outcome. There was a marginally significant effect of age on outcome in this study. Just less than half the women in both groups were 50 years of age or older (8). Younger women (< 49 years of age) had a better overall 9-year survival with preoperative chemotherapy, 71% vs. 65%, whereas older women had the opposite: 67% for preoperative chemotherapy vs.75% for postoperative chemotherapy (8). This interaction with age was significant ($p = 0.04$). Local recurrence after breast-conserving surgery at 9 years was also less for older women, 13.1% for women < 50 compared with 5.2% for women > 49 ($p = 0.003$). There were more local recurrences in women converted from mastectomy to breast-conserving surgery 11/69 (15.9%) than in the group eligible for breast-conserving surgery at the outset 43/434 (9.9%) ($p = 0.04$). However, this difference is explained by age, with a greater percentage of younger women in the converted group, and after adjustment for age, local recurrence rates were statistically similar in both converted patients and those initially eligible who had breast-conserving surgery (9).

III. NEOADJUVANT ENDOCRINE THERAPY IN LARGE OPERABLE BREAST CANCER

Endocrine treatment is an attractive alternative to chemotherapy in hormone-receptor-positive (HR+) patients, particularly postmenopausal women who may not tolerate the toxicities of chemotherapy. There have been few studies of neoadjuvant endocrine therapy. Initially tamoxifen was used as primary treatment for elderly women regardless of their estrogen-receptor (ER) status (8). These studies showed that prolonged treatment with tamoxifen does not provide long-term control for the majority of women, although one study did suggest that for some women tamoxifen did provide an alternative option for operable breast cancer in selected elderly patients (8).

Two trials compared tamoxifen alone with surgery (9, 10) and two further trials compared tamoxifen alone with surgery and tamoxifen combined (11, 12). Time to local relapse was significantly shorter in the tamoxifen-alone arm of all trials. Surprisingly, in three or four trials the numbers of patients with distant relapse were slightly lower in a group who had no immediate surgery. However, an overview analysis did indicate a significant reduction in deaths from breast cancer in patients who were treated surgically (13).

In Edinburgh, a number of studies have been performed with tamoxifen and the third-generation aromatase inhibitors (AIs). In these studies, postmenopausal women with large operable or locally advanced estrogen-receptor-positive (ER+) breast cancer were treated with either letrozole (36 patients), anastrozole (23 patients) or exemestane (12 patients) (14). The response rates to these new AIs were high (Table 1)—in the region of 80% with few patients progressing on treatment. Furthermore, there was a high rate of conversion from mastectomy to

Table 1 Median-Tumor Volume Reduction in Series of Patients with Locally Advanced Breast Cancer Who Received Neoadjuvant Endocrine Therapy in the Edinburgh Breast Unit*

Agent	No. of patients	Patients with > 50% reduction, n (%)	Patients with < 50% reduction or < 25% increase, n (%)	Patients with > 25% increase, n (%)
Tamoxifen	65	30 (46)	34 (52)	1 (2)
Letrozole	36	32 (89)	3 (8)	1 (3)
Anastrozole	23	18 (78)	5 (13)	0
Exemestane	12	10 (83)	2 (17)	0

*Tumor volume changes (reduction or increase) were assessed by ultrasound measurements during the 3-month treatment period.

Table 2 Patients with Locally Advanced Breast Cancer Requiring Mastectomy Before and After Neoadjuvant Endocrine Therapy in Studies at the Edinburgh Breast Unit

Agent	No. of patients	No. initially requiring mastectomy	No. requiring mastectomy after treatment	Conversion rate, %*
Tamoxifen	65	41	15	63
Letrozole	36	24	2	93
Anastrozole	24**	19	2	89
Exemestane	12	10	2	80

*Percentage of patients initially considered only for mastectomy who underwent breast-conserving surgery following treatment.
**Includes one patient who did not complete full treatment.

breast-conserving surgery (Table 2), with between 63% with tamoxifen and 89% for the AIs (15).

A. Randomized Studies of Neoadjuvant Endocrine Therapy

There have been no large studies comparing neoadjuvant endocrine therapy with standard treatment (16). There has been one small study, called the Edinburgh Randomised Large Tumour study, which randomized 171 patients with large operable breast cancers measuring more than 3 cm between January 1990 and October 1995: 86 patients were randomized to receive standard therapy, which was surgery, mastectomy, or breast-conserving surgery followed by adjuvant chemotherapy or endocrine chemotherapy. The standard at that time in premenopausal node-positive women was chemotherapy, but in all other women (that is, premenopausal node-negative and all postmenopausal women) regardless of ER status, it was tamoxifen. There were 85 patients randomized to the experimental or neoadjuvant arm. Thirty-eight patients, who were ER-poor on an initial biopsy, received neoadjuvant chemotherapy, whereas the 47 patients who had ER-rich breast cancers were treated with either goserelin (17 patients) or tamoxifen (30 patients). There were ten patients who did not respond to their primary endocrine therapy, and they went on to have four cycles of neoadjuvant endocrine therapy. These data were presented at San Antonio last year and showed no detriment to metastatic-free survival by giving neoadjuvant therapy, and there was the suggestion that the preoperative systemic-therapy group had a better outcome (16). Overall survival was no worse for the primary systemic-therapy group with a trend to improved survival for patients receiving neoadjuvant therapy. In the ER+/rich patients, survival was identical in both groups.

Overall, patients who had ER+ cancers had an improved survival compared to those who had (ER–) disease. Metastatic disease-free survival was best in patients who had a partial response. There was a significant relationship between the number of involved nodes after the end of the primary neoadjuvant treatment and survival.

The conclusions from this study are that there is no disadvantage to using ER-directed neoadjuvant therapy, and that axillary-node status at the end of neoadjuvant therapy gives the best guide to outcome in patients treated with neoadjuvant therapy.

A second study randomized 210 patients with T1-4 N0-2 M0 cancer to receive neoadjuvant chemoendocrine therapy or postoperative chemoendocrine therapy (17). Systemic therapy was again based on the ER content of the tumor. ER– patients received chemotherapy, and ER+ patients who were premenopausal received goserelin while postmenopausal women got formestane. At 5 years there was no difference in outcomes between the two groups. There was a reduction in the incidence of metastases in patients responding to primary therapy 4/51 vs.17/49 ($p < 0.01$), and there was a reduction in the extent of surgery in patients receiving neoadjuvant therapy (17).

IV. COMPARISON BETWEEN DIFFERENT ENDOCRINE AGENTS IN THE NEOADJUVANT SETTING

Two randomized trials have compared different endocrine agents in the neoadjuvant setting—one of which has not yet been published. The published trial (P024), the largest of its kind to date, compared 4 months of neoadjuvant treatment with either letrozole or tamoxifen in 324 postmenopausal women with ER+ and/or progesterone-receptor-positive (PR+) breast cancer (18, 19). This study demonstrated that patients who were randomized to receive letrozole had a significant higher clinical response rate than tamoxifen (55% vs. 36%; $p < 0.001$). The response rates based on both ultrasound and mammographic assessment were also superior for letrozole (Table 3). Also, more patients in the letrozole-treated group compared with tamoxifen-treated patients, were able to undergo breast-conserving surgery (45% vs. 35%; $p = 0.022$). The only other factor apart from treatment that significantly influenced the chance of a patient undergoing breast-conserving surgery was the initial tumor size, with T2 tumors being much more likely to be suitable for breast-conservation surgery than other T stages ($p = 0.001$). In this study, letrozole was at least as well tolerated as tamoxifen. The higher efficacy of letrozole over tamoxifen in this large group of postmenopausal women with early breast cancer might well have implications for the adjuvant setting as well.

This study also demonstrated that letrozole was superior to tamoxifen across the whole range of ER expression (Fig. 1). A small number of patients had tumors

Table 3 Primary and Secondary Efficacy Endpoint Results of Trial P024 Comparing 4 Months of Neoadjuvant Letrozole vs. Tamoxifen, in All Study Patients

Efficacy endpoints	Letrozole (n = 154), %	Tamoxifen (n = 170), %	p value
Primary endpoint			
Clinical response (palpation)	55	36	<0.001
Complete	10	4	
Partial	45	32	
Secondary endpoints			
Ultrasound response	35	25	0.042
Complete	3	1	
Partial	32	24	
Mammographic response	34	16	<0.001
Complete	4	0	
Partial	30	16	
Breast-conserving surgery	45	35	0.022

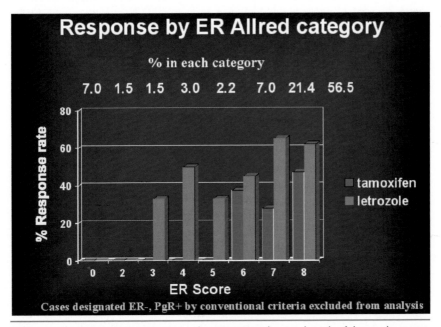

Figure 1 Response of patients in the P024 randomized trial of letrozole versus tamoxifen subdivided by ER Allred category score. Cases designated ER−, PR+ by conventional criteria were excluded from the analysis. (From Ref. 7)

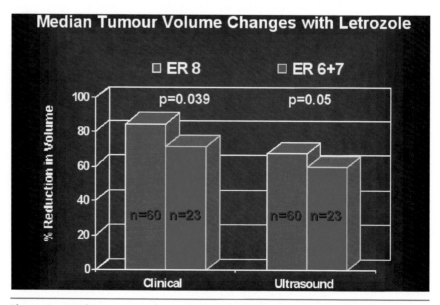

Figure 2 Median tumor volume changes by both clinical and ultrasound assessment in patients treated with 3 months of letrozole. Eighty-three patients were treated and the numbers with ER 8, 6, and 7 are shown. (From Ref. 20)

with low levels of ER expression, and in this group there were no patients responding to tamoxifen, but there was still a reasonable response rate to letrozole. Even at higher levels of ER expression, there was a better response rate to letrozole than tamoxifen. A subsequent study looking at treatment with neoadjuvant letrozole showed no significant difference in response rate in ER-rich tumors, which had Allred scores 6 and 7 vs. score 8, but this study did show that the median percentage reduction in tumor volume was greater for patients whose tumors had higher levels of ER (score 8) compared with those of scores 6 and 7 (Fig. 2) (20).

A second neoadjuvant study called IMPACT (IMmediate Preoperative Arimidex Compared with Tamoxifen) is comparing anastrozole 1 mg daily vs. tamoxifen 20 mg a day vs. anastrozole plus tamoxifen given for 3 months. This is a multicenter, randomized, double-blind trial that recruited 330 postmenopausal ER+ and/or PR+ breast cancer patients. The results of this study should be available later this year (21).

Data from the P024 study demonstrated that letrozole had a significantly higher response rate than tamoxifen in tumors that were ER+ and/or PR+ and also overexpressed EGFR or erbB2 (HER2/neu) (Table 4). Furthermore, there were significant reductions in proliferation in these tumors in patients treated by letrozole, but not in those treated by tamoxifen. Similar data have been presented with anastrozole, albeit in a very small collective. Of 23 patients treated with neoadju-

Table 4 Calculation of Odds Ratio of Clinical Response, Letrozole vs. Tamoxifen, in Subgroups of Patients with Tumors that were Either erbB1+ and/or erbB2+ (erbB1/2) and ER+ or erbB1– and erbB2– (erbB1/2–) and ER+

Category	Letrozole		Tamoxifen				
	No. of responders/ Total	%	No. of responders/ Total	%	Odds ratio (letrozole vs. tamoxifen)	95% CI	p
erbB-1/2+ ER+	15/17	88	4/19	21	28	4.5–177	0.0004
erbB-1/2– ER+	55/101	54	42/100	42	1.7	0.9–2.9	0.0780

This analysis ignored PgR status because none of the erbB-1/2+ cases was ER–, PR+.

vant anastrozole, six tumors were erbB2 3+ overexpressers. All six had a clinical response and all six showed significant reductions in proliferation over the three-month-study period (Fig. 3) (22).

These studies of neoadjuvant endocrine therapy have shown that, if patients are carefully selected and only those that are likely to respond (i.e., patients with ER-rich tumors) are treated, then response rates are high with few patients showing disease progression on treatment. Standard practice has been to

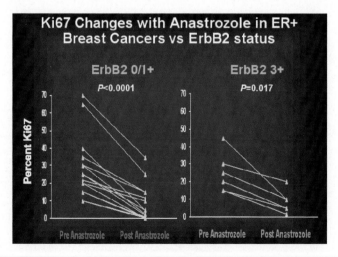

Figure 3 Changes in proliferation as measured by Ki67 in patients with ER-rich large operable locally advanced breast cancers treated with three months of anastrozole. Patients have been subdivided into whether the tumor was erbB2 0 or erbB2 3+. (From Ref. 22)

administer neoadjuvant chemotherapy between three and six cycles. The optimum duration of neoadjuvant endocrine therapy, however, has not been established. During initial studies, patients remained on tamoxifen until tumors became unresponsive and grew. Studies performed in Edinburgh, in a series of 100 patients who were more than 70 years old with ER-rich breast cancers treated with tamoxifen, showed that, after 3 months, 73 had responded based on ≥ 25% reduction in ultrasound volume, and 1 patient had progressive disease. The remaining 27 patients were continued on tamoxifen for an additional 3 months, and during this time, 18 remained static, 4 responded well, and 5 progressed (15). From these data it is evident that if a patient has not responded by 3 months, then the subsequent chances of response are small and the poor response-to-progression ratio does not warrant continuing treatment (15, 23). However, in patients who responded at 3 months, it is possible to continue treatment to shrink the tumor further so that surgery can either be completely avoided or any surgery performed can be less extensive.

V. LOCAL RECURRENCE AFTER NEOADJUVANT ENDOCRINE THERAPY

The data on local recurrence come from a series of patients treated in Edinburgh; 112 patients have been treated with neoadjuvant endocrine therapy followed by

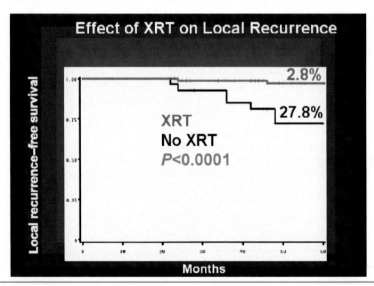

Figure 4 Local recurrence rates in 112 patients treated by neoadjuvant endocrine therapy (tamoxifen, $n = 47$; letrozole, $n = 34$; anastrozole, $n = 21$; exemestane, $n = 21$) followed by breast conserving surgery. Twenty-seven patients did not have radiotherapy following breast-conserving surgery; 85 did. Median follow-up is 62 months.

breast-conserving surgery. The median follow-up of this group is 62 months. At 5 years, the actuarial local recurrence rate of patients who had radiotherapy was 2.8% compared with 27.8% in patients who had no radiotherapy (Fig. 4) (15). There was no significant difference whether patients were treated with neoadjuvant tamoxifen or AIs.

VI. CONCLUSION

Neoadjuvant therapy appears safe. It can reduce the amount of surgery a patient requires. Converting a patient from needing a mastectomy to breast-conserving surgery does not increase local recurrence provided that breast-conserving surgery is followed by radiotherapy. Neoadjuvant endocrine therapy offers an alternative to neoadjuvant chemotherapy in older women with ER+ cancers. High RRs producing significant reductions in tumor volume are possible. The neoadjuvant setting provides the ideal opportunity to compare different agents and explore their effects on cancer cells. Studies have shown that letrozole is superior to tamoxifen in postmenopausal women with ER-rich breast cancers. Ongoing studies are evaluating how the AIs achieve such high RRs and how they influence gene transcription and protein expression in breast cancers.

REFERENCES

1. Richards MA, Smith IE. Role of systemic treatment for primary operable breast cancer. In: Dixon JM, ed. ABC of Breast Diseases. London: BMJ Publishing Group, 1995; pp. 38–41.
2. Bear H. Indications for neoadjuvant therapy for breast cancer. Semin Oncol 1998; 25(suppl 3):3–12.
3. Bonadonna G, Veronesi U, Brambilla C, Ferrari L, Luini A, Greco M, Bartoli C, Coopmans de Yoldi G, Zucali R, Rilke F. Primary chemotherapy to avoid mastectomy in tumours with diameters of three centimeters or more. J Natl Cancer Inst 1990; 82:1539–1545.
4. Veronesi U, Bonadonna G, Zurrida S, Galimberti V, Greco M, Brambilla C, Luini A, Andreola S, Rilke F, Raselli R. Conservation surgery after primary chemotherapy in large carcinomas of the breast. Ann Surg 1995; 222:612–618.
5. Mauriac L, Durand M, Avril A, Dilhuydy JM. Effects of primary chemotherapy in conservative treatment of breast cancer patients with operable tumours larger than 3 cm: results of a randomised trial in a single center. Ann Oncol 1991; 2:347–354.
6. Fisher B, Brown A, Mamouonas E, Wieand S, Robidoux A, Margolese RG, Cruz Jr. AB, Fisher ER, Wickerham D, Wolmark N, Decillis A, Hoehn JL, Lees AW, Dimitrov NV. Effect of preoperative chemotherapy on local-regional disease in women with operable breast cancer: findings from National Surgical Adjuvant Breast and Bowel Project B-18. J Clin Oncol 1997; 15:2483–2493.
7. Fisher B, Bryant J, Wolmark N, Mamounas E, Brown A, Fisher ER, Wickerham DL, Begovic M, DeCillis A, Robidoux A, Margolese RG, Cruz Jr. AB, Hoehn JL, Lees AW,

Dimitrov NV, Bear HD. Effect of preoperative chemotherapy on the outcome of women with operable breast cancer. J Clin Oncol 1998; 16:2672–2685.

8. Horobin JM, Preece PM, Dewar JA, Wood RAB, Cushieri A. Long-term follow up of elderly patients with locoregional breast cancer treated with tamoxifen only. Br J Surg 1991; 78:213–217.

9. Mustacchi G, Milani S, Pluchinotta A, De Matteis A, Rubagotti A, Perotta A. Tamoxifen or surgery plus tamoxifen as primary treatment for elderly patients with operable breast cancer: the GRETA trial. Anticancer Res 1994; 14:2197–2200.

10. Van Dalsen AD, De Cries J. Treatment of breast cancer in elderly patients. J Surg Oncol 1995; 60:80–82.

11. Bates T, Riley DL, Houghton J, Fallowfield L, Baum M. Breast cancer in elderly women: a Cancer Research Campaign trial comparing treatment with tamoxifen and optimal surgery with tamoxifen alone. Br J Surg 1991; 78:591–594.

12. Gazet JC, Ford HT, Coombes RC, Bland JM, Sutcliffe R, Quilliam J, Lowndes S. Prospective randomised trial of tamoxifen vs surgery in elderly patients with breast cancer. Eur J Surg Oncol 1994; 20:207–214.

13. Kenny FS, Robertson JFR, Ellis IO, et al. Primary tamoxifen versus mastectomy and adjuvant tamoxifen in fit elderly patients with operable breast cancer of high ER content. Breast 1999; 8:216.

14. Dixon JM, Anderson TJ, Miller WR. Neoadjuvant endocrine therapy of breast cancer: a surgical perspective. Eur J Cancer 2002; 38:2214–2221.

15. Dixon JM. Neoadjuvant therapy: surgical perspectives. In: Miller WR, Ingle JN, eds. Endocrine Therapy in Breast Cancer. New York: Marcel Dekker, 2002; pp. 197–212.

16. Cameron DA, Jack W, Forouhi P, Keen J, Dixon JM, Leonard RCF, Chetty U. Oestrogen receptor directed primary systemic therapy: a randomised trial compared with conventional therapy in operable breast cancer. Breast Cancer Res Treat 2002; 65, presented at the 25th Annual San Antonio Breast Cancer Symposium, San Antonio, Texas, December 2002.

17. Gazet JC, Ford HT, Gray R, McConkey C, Sutcliffe R, Quilliam J, Makinde V, Lowndes S, Coombes RC. Estrogen-receptor-directed neoadjuvant therapy for breast cancer: results of a randomised trial using formestane and methotrexate, mitozantrone and mitomycin C (MMM) chemotherapy. Ann Oncol 2001; 12:685–691.

18. Eiermann W, Paepke S, Appfelstaedt J, Llombart-Cussac A, Eremin J, Vinholes J, Mauriac L, Ellis M, Lassus M, Chaudri-Ross HA, Dugan M, Borgs M. Preoperative treatment of postmenopausal breast cancer patients with letrozole: a randomised double-blind multicentre study. Ann Oncol 2001; 12:1527–1532.

19. Ellis MJ, Coop A, Singh B, Mauriac L, Llombert-Cussac A, Janicke F, Miller WR, Evans DB, Dugan M, Brady C, Quebe-Fehling E, Borgs M. Letrozole is more effective neoadjuvant endocrine therapy than tamoxifen for erbB-1 and/or erbB-2 positive, estrogen-receptor-positive primary breast cancer: evidence from a phase III randomised trial. J Clin Oncol 2001; 19:3808–3816.

20. Dixon JM, Jackson J, Renshaw L, Cameron DA, Miller WR. Neoadjuvant letrozole: the Edinburgh experience. Breast Cancer Res Treat 2002; 65, presented at the 25th Annual San Antonio Breast Cancer Symposium, San Antonio, Texas, December 2002.

21. Smith I, Dowsett M on behalf of the IMPACT Trialists. Comparison of anastrozole vs tamoxifen alone and in combination as neoadjuvant treatment of estrogen-receptor-positive (ER+) operable breast cancer in postmenopausal women: the IMPACT trial. Breast Cancer Res Treat 2003; 82:56.
22. Dixon JM, Jackson J, Hills M, Renshaw L, Cameron DA, Anderson TJ, Miller WR, Dowsett M. Anastrozole demonstrates clinical and biological effectiveness in erbB2 ER positive breast cancers. Breast Cancer Res Treat 2002; 65, presented at the 25th Annual San Antonio Breast Cancer Symposium, San Antonio, Texas, December 2002.
23. Keen JC, Dixon JM, Miller EP, Cameron DA, Chetty U, Hanby A, Bellamy C, Miller WR. The expression of KiS1 and BCL-2 and the response to primary tamoxifen therapy in elderly patients with breast cancer. Breast Cancer Res Treat 1997; 44:123–133.

1

Therapy in Postmenopausal Women

Jacques M. Bonneterre and Henning T. Mouridsen, *Chairmen*

Monday, July 7, 2003

R. Santen: I wonder if I could start, with Mr. Chairman's permission, to ask a question of Bill Miller, to discuss an issue not previously covered. Bill, one of the issues that you raised is the dose-response curves with respect to the various aromatase inhibitors and the possibility that letrozole may be more potent than anastrozole in lowering estrogen levels. I want to ask you, because I think there is some controversy in the literature about measuring blood estrogen concentrations and how low you can actually suppress them with aromatase inhibitors. We know that with the isotopic kinetic techniques that you've showed us, there may be dose-response differences.

What we are really trying to do with an aromatase inhibitor is lower the level of estrogen in the breast to the lowest level possible. I was wondering whether you and Mike Dixon or Mitch [Dowsett] would have some data to let us know what percentage of estrogen reduction there is in the breast tumor itself when one looks at anastrozole, letrozole, and exemestane. This would give us dose-response curves that are a little more meaningful than measuring total aromatase or, potentially, aromatase in the blood?

W. Miller: I think that's a good point. I believe in the dose-response curves when one looks across individual inhibitors. The sort of data I showed you today, which came from Mitch Dowsett and Per Lonning, are fairly convincing. The effects on endogenous estrogens, aromatase, and the effects in vitro all go in parallel.

The concern that I have is that it relates to dose-response curves within individual aromatase inhibitors when it sometimes is very difficult to show those dose curves, once you go beyond a critical level. I guess your point is: Do we need more powerful aromatase inhibitors? What happens if we use them at increasing doses?

I worry about these things. I have deliberated in publications about the question: What is the actual percentage reduction in estrogens, particularly in the breast? The technology needed to address this is very difficult. If you use radioisotope methodology, and look for differences in counts in the tumor, you can, for example, measure maybe 20 dpm per gram of tissue before treatment and 1 [dpm per gram] with treatment, that represents 95% inhibition. But for a single count higher after treatment (i.e., 2), the inhibition then becomes only 90%.

I personally find it very difficult to do these studies. When you're looking at endogenous levels of estrogen in the breast, I think that was slightly different, and I hope Per [Lonning] might address this, [than] when you're looking at total body aromatase, and the clinical material you are dealing with is blood plasma rather than tumor.

P. Lonning: But when you look at estrone sulfate you may in theory detect only about 70–80% suppression, and for estrone and estradiol, in practice around 85–90% suppression, like we did in the study we published with Mitch [Dowsett] in Clinical Cancer Research in 2001.

M. Dowsett: Can I just make a couple of points about that? Firstly, when Bill [Miller] showed the data on the aromatase inhibition, he showed that letrozole had a value of 1.1% residual aromatase activity, which is the same way we generally present that. I think it's worthwhile remembering that we may be wrong to do this, but we always express undetectable data as equivalent to the detection limit. We give it a value of detection because we're trying to be conservative. That may not be the best way of doing things.

In fact in the publication, we put down the point estimates of each of those values. With letrozole in fact, if you take those values, I think it's 99.7% suppression. Thus, there is a 0.3% residual activity. It may be better if we express our estradiol levels like that as well because we express them as 2.1 if they're less than 2.1.

The extra point I wanted to bring from that in relation to using more potent aromatase inhibitors, is that if you look at the pharmacokinetics and the pharmacodynamics between letrozole and anastrozole, in fact 2.5 mg of letrozole per day is equivalent to 50 mg a day of anastrozole. It is 20-fold more potent in vitro, the pharmacokinetics are almost identical and if you look at the in vivo aromatization data, we derived from 0.5 mg of letrozole, that was equivalent to about 10 mg of anastrozole.

In essence, we have to say letrozole is a drug that has already given us 50-fold higher pharmacological effectiveness than anastrozole. I think there may be a marginal improvement with letrozole, but it's not a vast improvement. Do we need to get anything more potent than letrozole? I guess we probably don't. I hope that is understandable, it's really a rather convoluted argument.

R. Santen: Let's go into this issue a bit further. The fact that we now have neoadjuvant therapy means we have a tool to measure tissue estrogen levels in a more practical fashion. Previously, we had an indirect measure of what we were doing with aromatase inhibitors (and that's total body aromatization or estrogen levels in the blood). I think it's very important when we begin to ask these dose-response questions to get to the tissue that we need to measure, and that's the breast itself. I think we're beginning to get there.

That's really my only point to emphasize, that I think our measurements now need to be directly in the breast. We have a way of doing this. As Per [Lonning] said, we have assays that are probably sensitive enough to make those measurements.

P. Lonning: I think a very important issue in relation to what you have said is that I know that a couple of these patients, after developing acquired resistance on even the very potent aromatase inhibitors, are still sensitive to endocrine manipulation. That is based on your paper back in 1995. Based [on] your findings, that bell-shaped estrogen stimulation curve was actually the reason why we tried to treat a group of these patients with high dose estrogens after they failed on aromatase inhibitors. We found that 10 out of 32 patients achieved an objective response to therapy. There is no doubt clinically that a number of these tumors are still sensitive to hormonal manipulation. It may well be that to go further down with the estrogen levels in the tissue after they fail, letrozole or anastrozole could achieve a second response.

I. C. Henderson: My question is actually a corollary of this and [I am] directing this toward Bill, Dick, and Mitch. Do we really have evidence that the critical event here is the absolute level of estrogen as opposed to the perturbation of the hormone milieu? It always has seemed to me puzzling that we obtained these sequences of responses. In fact, they were in some ways more obvious in the 1970s when we had fewer choices, when we started by adding estrogen. We got a response by withdrawing estrogen. We further withdrew estrogen with an adrenalectomy. The only way it seemed to me that we could really explain that was that it wasn't the absolute level, it was the perturbation.

So in a way, this is a corollary of what Per [Lonning] was just saying. I'm pushing it a little bit further and saying: Do we really have evidence that the absolute level of estrogen suppression is a critical factor in vivo.

R. Santen: I could address that. I think it's very clear that breast cancer cells adapt. No matter what you do, if you treat them with Megace® or an aromatase inhibitor or tamoxifen, adrenalectomy, ovariectomy, those cells have a way of adapting so that they will respond to secondary, tertiary, or quaternary therapy. If one asks: What is the level of estrogen that induces an effect? you have to ask yourself: What is the level that does it acutely and what is the level that is necessary to have that same effect later on?

I think you really are focusing on a very important part. We really don't know that. But if, in fact, the tumor can respond to a minor reduction initially and a greater reduction of estrogen later on, then clearly the set point changes. One then needs to look at the time frame involved as well as the dose of estrogen. I don't think we have the answer to that question.

A. Howell: I'd like to ask Paul a question. Mitch [Dowsett] says in letrozole we may have the ultimate aromatase inhibitor but in exemestane we've got a drug that does other things, as you presented the flutamide data and the bone data. I'd like to ask you whether you feel that is correct and whether we may see something extra in terms of tumor efficacy by some other mechanism than aromatase inhibition with exemestane.

P. Goss: Tony, there will be more data in this regard soon. My belief is that the dual action of exemestane will be confirmed, and we will in time divide the aromatase inhibitors into "pure aromatase inhibitors" and "mixed action" drugs, like exemestane. The telling factor will be what actual steroidal effect exemestane will have at 25 mg a day.

It's easy in these animal models to show various effects where you're not exactly using the same milieu of dose and pharmacokinetics as in humans. I think that the clinical trial data actually suggests that there might be a slight advantage of exemestane over the other inhibitors in the metastatic setting. But I think it's also obscured by the fact that it's tested in the metastatic setting. The adjuvant trials will give us a clearer picture.

A. Bhatnagar: I think just to follow up on that, if I may, we mustn't forget that we have quite a wealth of data on a sister compound of exemestane, that's formestane. I think that all of the data from the formestane trials that Mitch [Dowsett] and the Marsden group generated will probably address this issue even better. But all the data from the Lentaron® trials didn't show that the added features of androgenicity, which Lentaron also has, of different effect or different lipophilicity, seem to make any difference in terms of its efficacy when you relate it to its potency as an aromatase inhibitor. So, I think if we are trying to speculate on what the exemestane results are going to show, the speculations have to be done [with] a backdrop of the information we already have. The Lentaron data are quite extensive.

H. Sasano: I have questions to Paul [Goss] and Bill [Miller]. Could you please clarify on bone-sparing effects of exemestane? Recently, limited data have indicated possible long-term benefits of this compound, which could act, at least in bone, like an androgen. However, adverse effects of androgens are well known and could be relevant if you apply this agent to chemoprevention or adjuvant therapy.

P. Goss: Are you asking about the mechanism by which it may have a bone-sparing effect?

H. Sasano: Right, and also its clinical relevance—namely low-dose androgenicity adding to an aromatase inhibitor activity. In other words, this seems to be a pure weak androgenic effect because the aromatase is completely blocked. So exemestane may exert some weak androgenic actions systemically. That could be an advantage or possibly a disadvantage. Could you please clarify on that point?

P. Goss: I think that's the point that I was making. Our hypothesis from the data is that there is a difference between giving exemestane as an aromatase inhibitor and a weak androgen simultaneously, [or] just giving a weak androgen to a postmenopausal woman. You increase bone resorption with the aromatase effect. What we've seen from the bone biomarkers is that both resorption and formation are decreased. So you have an effect similar to a bisphosphonate, at least in the first three-month study that we've conducted. With exemestane you reduce both resorption and formation, whereas with other inhibitors one sees an increase in formation [as a] consequence to the increase in resorption.

A. Bhatnagar: Could I just follow up on that, Paul, if I may. I would like Angela [Brodie] to address it as well. I mean the rat is a very unfortunate model to use here in this situation for the simple reason that we know very well that androgens are uterotropic in the female rat. Angela and I had that same discovery that we made in terms of Lentaron®, [i.e.,] that when you give Lentaron to mature female rats you get quite a large rise in uterine weight.

We also know that androgens have a disproportionate effect on bone in female rats as compared to the human situation. We're extrapolating from a model that was not built to extrapolate to the clinical situation because with Lentaron, again, we saw no effects on bone.

P. Goss: I don't understand why you don't. The model is a standard model for osteoporosis testing. This is the same model in which the bisphosphonates and raloxifene were tested. Raloxifene® is [a] hormone model.

A. Bhatnagar: The point I'm making is that the rat has a disproportionate androgenic effect on bone. It's the model that's used for estrogens, not androgens. When you use estrogens in the rat to show BMD changes, that is what is accepted. As concerns androgen effects, I'd like Angela [Brodie] to also respond to that because she actually did the same studies as we did and we had very similar results.

A. Brodie: It is a fact that androgens stimulate the myometrium of the rat uterus. However, we did not study the effects of formestane on BMD in the rat.

P. Lonning: I'd just like to add that with the different mechanism of action of the steroidal and nonsteroidal compounds, the evidence goes back to the formestane trials. It started with Robin Murray's study, published eight years ago, [which] showed that formestane worked after the patient failed on the aminoglutethimide. At that time people believed formestane was a more potent aromatase inhibitor compared to aminoglutethimide. All evidence collected afterwards has shown that this is not true.

Anyway, there were responders. I think the most striking evidence that there is a difference regarding the mechanism of action is a small study of Carlini et al., who showed that patients even failing on anastrozole and letrozole could respond to formestane afterwards. That shows that even though it is a less potent aromatase inhibitor, it may work as long as you give the steroidal after the nonsteroidal one. Obviously there must be something else going on.

J.-J. Body: I'm also not convinced that the rat model is the best one to study the bone effects. I would like to know if there have been any human studies so far. The second point I would like to ask the speakers is the following: Are there any data on the effects of pure antiestrogens on bone cells or on bone mass?

M. Dixon: We've got a study ongoing that should answer some of the questions. Patients are being randomized to either anastrozole, letrozole, or exemestane. We're looking at lipids and bone markers. We should get an idea whether what we see in the rat actually happens in the patient with breast cancer, and what sort of things, including chemotherapy, will interfere with their bone metabolism. One of the things to watch out for in all these studies is an enormous list of drugs these patients can't be on. It's actually quite difficult to get a clean study, but that's what we're doing at the moment.

S. Johnston: My understanding with the Faslodex® data is that there are preclinical data showing it's protective on bone in rats.

J.-J. Body: What were the precise effects on bone with a pure antiestrogen?

S. Johnston: I think with the ovariectomized model that the increasing doses were protective. Tony, you may want to expand on that.

A. Howell: That's true, but there are no data in humans. It's only the rat data from Alan Wakeling.

C. K. Osborne: To turn to a slightly different subject, maybe a practical one for those of us taking care of some of these patients. I guess if you add up the side effects of tamoxifen versus Arimidex® in the ATAC trial, sheer numbers are slightly favoring Arimidex. But when you take care of these patients day to day, I think I hear more complaints from the patients on the aromatase inhibitors than from those on tamoxifen.

I think that the musculoskeletal events are much more frequent than are reported. Maybe American patients complain about it more, but nearly every patient, if you ask them about it, has musculoskeletal, joint stiffness when they get out after riding in a car for a long time and so forth. There's not much you can do for that. Nonsteroidals don't help very much. They just have to learn to live with it.

What I am also concerned about is the ability of the breast tumor cell to adapt over time to very, very low concentrations of estrogen, 10^{-15} molar in some of Dick's [Santen] studies. Benita Katzenellenbogen's studies show stimulation of cells that have been estrogen deprived for a very long period of time.

What does that mean regarding dietary changes to our patients in terms of trying to get rid of any plant estrogens that might bind to the estrogen receptor. More importantly, although vaginitis is a big problem in these patients, can we believe that Vagifem® tablets or Estrace® are safe? It's said that absorption is very low, but you would not need much absorption to counteract the beneficial effect that you're seeing on the tumor cell. I wonder if we can have a little discussion on what people are doing about some of these side effects. Can we assume that the levels of estrogen absorbed with Estrace are not going to stimulate the tumor and what do you do?

H. Mouridsen: Could you just try and answer Kent's [Osborne] question rather briefly. I think we should devote approximately 15 minutes to the advanced disease and 15 to primary. We've got only half an hour left now. Please answer briefly to Kent's questions.

R. Santen: I can't answer his questions but I can address the issue of vaginal estrogen administration. We've done some fairly extensive studies regarding this. The Estring®, which is the silastic vaginal ring that delivers approximately 5 mcg of estrogen per day, gets absorbed by about 10%. Thus, about 500 nanograms of estrogen [are] absorbed. That's very, very little compared to the production rate in a postmenopausal patient. But it's still somewhat worrisome because there is some estrogen that is delivered. Clearly the other vaginal preparations, Estrace® cream, the 25 microgram Vagifem® tablet or the Premarin® cream deliver much more than that. If one wants to use vaginal estrogen and deliver the lowest dose which is still effective, use of the Estring is really the best way. However, I caution patients that we really don't know, particularly in patients taking aromatase inhibitors, whether this very small dose can exert some detrimental effects.

J. Ingle: Can I just make one comment about the musculoskeletal complaints. I think you're right, Kent, this could be disabling in some patients. Just one anecdote, I had a woman who was terribly disabled by musculoskeletal complaints. I switched her from anastrozole to exemestane. Her estimate was [that] in one month 70% of it went away. Now she still actually has some musculoskeletal complaints. I don't know if anybody else has experience with that.

M. Ellis: I can counter that with an anecdote where a switch didn't work.

M. Baum: Just before I address that particular issue, it's just to a question of mine which I gave up on, but it was resurrected, referring back to what Kent [Osborne] said. That is the corollary to Craig Henderson's corollary, which is the issue of the relevance of circulating estrogens versus the relevance of intratumoral or peritumoral estrogens. Some of the paradoxes that we've observed, as described by Craig Henderson, may be the fact that circulating estrogens per se are not important, but it's the gradient between the circulation and the tumor that's important.

I was going to address this question to Bill Miller. Is it conceivable that the benefits of aromatase inhibitors are not the effect on circulating estrogens but on endo tumoral and peritumoral estrogens and their gradient from the circulation to the tumor?

W. Miller: I guess the answer to your question is yes, it is conceivable. What I would have to caution, although the sensitivity of methodology is increasing all the time, we don't really have definitive methodology to measure very small amounts of estrogen in the breast. This may be a technical point but I think it is quite important. When you're doing some of these studies, us[ing] such a methodology as Per Lonning employs, then you can work on mililiters of blood or liters of urine. But when you're actually looking at events in the breast, you have a limited amount of material, and it's very difficult to be certain that your methodology is up to it.

What I can tell you anecdotally is that by and large the effects that you see in the circulation are mirrored in the breast. For example, you can show in premenopausal women that you reduce the circulation of estrogen following ovarian ablation. Levels fall in the tumor and you get responses. However, in postmenopausal women following treatment with aromatase inhibitors, when you actually look at individual patients, there are cases which show that while you can reduce the levels of estrogen in the circulation, you don't necessarily reduce them at the level of tumor.

That would go along with your perception that hormones may be exceptional at the local level of the breast. I think where things start to come unstuck a little bit is that you cannot always show the correlation by which, if you don't show reduction at the level of tumor, then you should not see a response. Sometimes you do. The definitive results to substantiate your hypothesis are not there.

I think I could add something to Craig Henderson's question. Craig Henderson is asking the question: Is it the estrogen or is it the estrogen signaling that matters? My suspicion is that it is neither one nor the other. In certain patients it will be the signaling; in certain patients, it will be the level.

I think the best way of teasing it out is to follow up [with] the patients who are going into these neoadjuvant studies in which you have sequential access to tumor material during short-term treatment and then, when patients come back with recurrence, you can look at the phenotype in the tumors. I think Mitch Dowsett presented some data fairly recently at ASCO to suggest that those people who come back with recurrent disease will have a change of phenotype in the tumor. This would suggest there are changes which have happened in the signaling. Others come back with the same phenotype at recurrence, which is perfectly compatible with the fact that the estrogen levels have not changed and are still low. There has to be some other mechanism to account for recurrent resistance.

H. Mouridsen: I think it is a very exciting discussion. After Mitch [Dowsett], I think we have to go and discuss some clinical aspects of advanced and primary breast cancer.

M. Dowsett: I wanted to really stay with this same issue that Craig [Henderson] brought up and Mike [Baum] returned to, as to whether or not it's just perturbation or is it degree of deprivation. There is a rationale that the more potent third-generation aromatase inhibitors are more effective than the second generation and first generation, since there is a greater degree of estrogen deprivation with the third-generation inhibitor in each of the studies that have been done. But it may just be the greater the perturbation, the greater response we get, rather than saying it's the degree of estrogen deprivation per se. If instead we were to give estrogen or more estrogen, we might get the same result there. It's interesting. Before coming here, I actually looked at one of Basil Stoll's books from 1971, where he addresses exactly the same question.

H. Mouridsen: We now again have too little time to discuss this because everybody has something to say. We have to go to the clinical situation. I'll start with advanced disease. Have you any questions about that?

J. Bergh: I'll return shortly to Mitch's [Dowsett] presentation at ASCO because I think that was an important one with reference to how stable are the expressions in the tumor. Although the study was limited, around 25% of the breast cancer patients, upon relapse, after receiving tamoxifen, had an altered expression of either HER2/neu or the receptor status. It could go in both directions. So when we are talking about advanced disease and the efficacy of new drugs, we should not forget to ask how we know for sure that the metastases are equivalent in their biological properties with reference to their primary tumors. I think we too often forget to biopsy [to] verify that they really contain the same properties as the primary tumor originally did. That reflects the difference among sophisticated mechanisms of action with reference to hormones. A basic thing, like the absence of receptors in the previous receptor positive tumor, could be the explanation of why the patient failed.

H. Mouridsen: Comments to that?

M. Ellis: As a follow-up to that, thinking about this mechanism of estrogen receptor downregulation in the instance of Mitch's [Dowsett] recent data with tamoxifen, I was quite struck from the neoadjuvant setting that some tumors do show very dramatic downregulation of estrogen-receptor when treated with tamoxifen. And certainly more frequently than when one treated with the aromatase inhibitor.

So if you see a patient relapsing on tamoxifen, and you biopsy that tumor and it's estrogen-receptor-negative, that might be purely a biochemical effect as the result of the presence of tamoxifen. Have you any data where you subsequently say you have done an estrogen withdrawal maneuver and a repeat biopsy which showed the estrogen receptor now reappeared, suggesting [that] tamoxifen really did cause a reversible biochemical down regulation? I'm a bit worried that if you biopsy a patient upon tamoxifen relapse and find it is estrogen-receptor-negative, it might be, in fact, estrogen-receptor-positive, but the presence of tamoxifen was obscuring that.

M. Dowsett: In that particular series, Matt, we emphasized and identified only patients that were actually still on tamoxifen. I would say that when we've done these three-month studies, and Bill [Miller] might want to comment on this as well, we do indeed see estrogen receptor downregulation with tamoxifen. We don't generally see in those three-month studies an absence of estrogen receptor. It's a run down in estrogen-receptor.

I think actually there are potentially two artifacts in that as well. One is that if you compare core cut biopsies and incision biopsy in those neoadjuvant studies, I think there are fixation artifacts which can actually lead to an apparent estrogen-receptor loss. When we look at core cuts, you do get a reduction, but it is not as great.

The other thing that perhaps Craig Allred might be able to respond to is whether the tamoxifen-estrogen receptor complex is immunologically and immunoreactively identical to an estrogen-estrogen receptor complex. Might we actually be seeing a parallel loss of estrogen receptor, which is in fact reflective of the fact that the shape of the estrogen receptor is different? I think I remember some of Pasqualini's stuff suggesting that was the case many years ago. Craig have you had any experience with that?

D. C. Allred: I don't know of anyone who has really studied that in a formal manner. There are older studies using ligand binding assays showing steric hindrance between tamoxifen and radio-labeled ligand (estrogen) when testing for estrogen receptor. With tamoxifen bound to estrogen receptor, the tumor would look like it was estrogen receptor negative when it was not, the steric hindrance of tamoxifen would result in a false-negative signal.

For immunochemistry, at least theoretically, I think the issue is different in that there are dozens of different antibodies with epitopes distributed along the length of the molecule. Those antibodies that are commercially available and popular have purposefully restricted their epitope targets away from the hormone binding domain. The thinking is that steric hindrance effect by tamoxifen wouldn't be an issue then by immunochemistry because the antibody is directed against a different part of the estrogen receptor molecule.

I. C. Henderson: I'd just like to make a point about metastatic disease and refer back to Carsten's [Rose] presentation. I guess Mitch [Dowsett] made the comment about aminoglutethimide versus third-generation aromatase inhibitors. I find the data very compelling and am quite willing to let it rest at that.

On the other hand, I think it would be inappropriate to take away too strong a message in the clinical trials that exist. As I recall from Carsten's presentation—and he may correct me in a second—there is really only one direct, randomized comparison of two aromatase inhibitors.

Secondly, in metastatic disease most of them are indirect comparison[s] of an aromatase inhibitor versus other drugs, such as Megace® and so on. You're shaking your head, so maybe I should turn this to Carsten. The point I was driving at is that, even when you're doing randomized trials, when you're doing trials that involve a relatively more toxic versus a less toxic therapy, you often end up with false positives on efficacy that are related to the toxicities. In other words, too early crossover, for example, and other effects that become important because you can't really do a double-blind trial and do a full evaluation.

[Although] on the one hand, the basic data seem to be overwhelming and the indirect comparisons are very compelling, I'm not so sure that the direct comparisons are sufficient for us to draw firm conclusions about at least the size of the differences among the different aromatase inhibitors.

C. Rose: You are not entirely right. There are more than two trials comparing directly aminoglutethimide and other aromatase inhibitors. I think we have to be aware that comparing aminoglutethimide with the newer generations implies that we're comparing 500 mg of aminoglutethimide. That is based on basically one reasonably large study from France, comparing 500 to 1,000 mg. If it is true that there is a dose-response relationship here, relating to letrozole and anastrozole, then this is not a fair comparison to aminoglutethimide. We will have fewer side effects, but in terms of efficacy you might overlook something. That is how it stands.

W. Eiermann: I was wondering about the figures in the P25 trial with a very low or relatively low response rate for tamoxifen of about 20%. Do we have to write the textbooks again because we usually expect 40–50% response rates in this situation? Is the reason for this a better evaluation of responses or is it a problem of the receptor determination in these patient groups? What is the explanation? 20% is first line, metastatic disease. It's very low— unexpectedly low.

H. Mouridsen: Carsten? You are expected to be the expert in advanced breast cancer, you start.

C. Rose: Being an expert, we always go back to the original investigator. Yes, I'm wondering too why we are seeing now this new generation of drugs and these low response rates. It's not only for this. Look back to the anastrozole comparison with Megace® and so forth. We have a very low response rate in populations of patients predominantly being estrogen-receptor-positive. That's the reason why I showed you the picture where we actually saw the higher response rate for those patients being positive to both estrogen and progesterone receptors. I have no good explanation for that. Maybe we should rewrite the textbook. This is a crucial question. We are all saying now that we have a revival of endocrine therapies. It is very safe to start out provided they have some degree of positivity for steroid receptors. I'm not so sure about that. Maybe Henning [Mouridsen] can explain why only 20% for tamoxifen.

H. Mouridsen: I don't have the explanation. On the other hand, if we look at the primary endpoint in Phase III trials and in clinical situations, the time to progression, it is very similar with the recent tamoxifen trials if we compare with trials from the past. Ingle did a trial once, 12 to 15 years ago, comparing tamoxifen with tamoxifen plus an androgen. Time to progression in the tamoxifen arm was exactly as time to progression in the P25 arm. The characteristics of the patients were quite similar.

It may be a problem of the definition of responses and reassessment of responses, etc., etc. Kent, you have a comment?

C. K. Osborne: I think it's probably what you say. That is, I think that over the years we finally agreed upon response criteria and applied them in a much more uniform way. It's not that patients are less responsive or [that] the drug has changed, it's simply that we're defining it better. I think on some of the earlier trials we mixed in a lot of stable disease patients and called them response. Stable disease didn't require six months duration. I think it's a definition thing. I think we're being more realistic now about what the real benefit is.

The more interesting question, though, is: Why are tamoxifen and Arimidex® so lousy in metastatic disease? It's curative in the adjuvant setting. That to me is the more interesting question.

I. Smith: Most of these newer trials were, at least to some extent, contaminated by adjuvant endocrine therapy, whereas the older studies weren't. Perhaps the better model is the neoadjuvant study. Matt Ellis' study would suggest higher response rates in neoadjuvant therapy; the IMPACT trial will have the results for that very soon. It may be that's giving you a purer picture, noncontaminated by previous adjuvant therapy. Otherwise you have to postulate that as the disease progresses it becomes less sensitive to hormone treatment.

A. Harris: One comment and one question. One comment might be the assessment of bone secondaries. Using modern criteria for the assessment, we may exclude patients to a large extent, and they could respond well. That's a comment on what might have changed.

The question really is to Per Lonning and to Bill Miller. Bill had a nice slide of mechanisms of resistance to aromatase inhibitors. We have the data that exemestane may work after nonsteroidals. What is the explanation for the lack of cross-resistance between those two molecules?

H. Mouridsen: Could I just suggest you have lunch together and you discuss it? Mike, you had a comment?

M. Baum: I want to offer a suggestion to Kent Osborne to explain the possible reason for this discrepancy of the potentially curative value in adjuvant setting versus the rather disappointing effect in the advanced setting. It's a hobbyhorse of mine. For a decade I think I've been concerned with the assumption that the advanced disease is a good model for the adjuvant disease. I really think we might have gone badly wrong in the past; that our whole strategy for developing adjuvant therapy has been predetermined by the effect on the advanced disease.

I believe just as there are long latency periods for the development in the primary, there are many of the so-called micrometastases that are not miniprimary diseases but could be a long period of latency for the metastatic disease. It's just possible the endocrine therapy has much greater effect on the latent disease than on the established primary disease. Where there is already an established microvasculature. My hypothetical model of a micrometastasis, a bunch of cancer cells and stromal cells without an established microvasculature.

T. Powles: I think another factor is that I know that in our earlier trials, when we didn't have a lot of treatment options, the median time to objective response was something like 14 months. That meant half the patients would not achieve objective response by 14 months. I think now with the other treatment options that are available in metastatic breast cancer, they're probably pulling out before those objective response rates are achieved. That's why your time to progression is the same, but your objective response rate is lower.

P. Lonning: I think Mike Baum is raising a very critical issue. What is actually happening with adjuvant therapy? Why do we give endocrine treatment or give the chemotherapy? I think perhaps one of the mistakes that we have done is that we have confused a clinical endpoint for a scientific endpoint. What influences relapse is not only tumor resistance, it's invasion of the metastasis, the growth rate. You have all these different characteristics of the tumor cells that could, more or less, potentially be influenced by treatment.

If you are really going to explore the use of microarrays and other biological techniques, the issue of, say, chemoresistance in patients, we need to define the type of clinical models where we can dissect these different characteristics from each other, such as using neoadjuvant therapy. You can directly assess the influence of treatment or the growth in tumor cells and so on. I think actually the adjuvant setting is a very, very poor model to study the biology of cancer.

H. Mouridsen: We haven't much time left, but could I just take the privilege here, as co-chairing this session, to ask Mike [Baum] a question? It is something related to selection of patients to be offered aromatase inhibitors in the adjuvant situation. I think that is a very critical question. To try and provoke you, I quote you the data now. We see approximately a 2% absolute difference, so a very, very small absolute difference between tamoxifen and aromatase inhibitors. As far as I've understood, the difference of benefit is observed only in local recurrence.

My next concern is that aromatase inhibitors are 30 times more expensive than tamoxifen. My last concern is that with tamoxifen, we saw a continued divergence between the control group and the tamoxifen group following discontinuation of therapy. With aminoglutethimide, we saw in

Trevor's [Powles] study, the benefit disappear immediately when the therapy was discontinued. I would be quite concerned that perhaps the benefit might disappear immediately upon discontinuation of the aromatase inhibitors. These are concerns for me to decide which patients should receive an aromatase inhibitor in the adjuvant situation. I'm very conservative just now.

M. Baum: You're absolutely right on one point there.

H. Mouridsen: Only one?

M. Baum: Yes. The relative costs of the drugs. The absolute differences in the estrogen-receptor-positive group are closer to 3% than 2%. You would find that these absolute differences are mirrored by almost any trial which is reporting dramatic relative risk reductions. It's just I'm one of the few people who describe the data in absolute terms in order to be conservative in their interpretation. In that way I am conservative.

As far as it only affecting local recurrence, again you're wrong in numerical terms. There is a numerical advantage for each of the breast cancer events except for contralateral DCIS. [For] each of the other breast cancers, there is a numerical advantage.

As far as predicting the future, it's very difficult to get a ten-year result. Unfortunately, you have to wait ten years. This is one of the major frustrations of my life! Sure, in the technology assessment report from ASCO they emphasize that, after stopping tamoxifen after five years, the curves continue to diverge. Yes, I share your conservatism. I would like to see what happens upon withdrawing anastrozole, whether there is a rebound effect. But you may come to a threshold where there is a significant difference in distant disease-free survival, and it might be quite difficult for one to wait long enough to look for these rebound effects because the dye is already cast, the outcome is already predetermined.

J. Ingle: Could I just ask, to reinforce your question to Trevor [Powles]? Could you interpret the duration question of aromatase inhibitors in light of your experience with your study?

T. Powles: It was obviously disappointing from our point of view. It was only a small trial, but the effect was lost. I thought that later on we would be seeing a bigger effect because of what had happened with tamoxifen. One of the few concerns I have with the adjuvant aromatase inhibitor trials, particularly Arimidex®, is that, if it is true that in the mechanism which occurs experimentally in humans, cancer cells adapt to growing in lower and lower levels of estrogen, and if we do give a long duration of an aromatase inhibitor like five years, then several things can happen. The consequences of having an agonist effect on hypersensitive cells from environmental factors and having an exaggerated, agonist response to tamoxifen, thus having a detrimental effect with tamoxifen, could produce a downside after we stop. It wouldn't be the same sort of thing that's occurring when there is an overexposure to tamoxifen.

I just think we really need to critically review what evidence we have at this stage, for example, of the effects of tamoxifen postaromatase inhibitors. I'm not familiar enough with those data. But is there evidence that tamoxifen is working as well post Arimidex or that we have activation of disease post aromatase inhibitors? Otherwise, I think we've really got to look very carefully at a possible rebound effect.

W. Jonat: Only one question. Contralateral breast cancer, the advantage, is it also true in the chemotherapy plus Arimidex® versus chemotherapy plus tamoxifen?

M. Baum: You ask me to tell you the results of the contralateral breast cancers that had . . .

W. Jonat: Chemotherapy plus Arimidex® versus chemotherapy plus tamoxifen.

M. Baum: That's a tiny subset. Only 20% of them.

A. Howell: We don't have those data. They're there but they wouldn't be interpretable because the number of events would be so few. The question is a good question.

I'd really like to ask Dick Santen what he thinks of what happens after you stop anastrozole. There is a separation of the curves with tamoxifen after you stop tamoxifen. That may be a withdrawal effect of tamoxifen. We don't know what it is. But when we stop aromatase inhibitors, we perturb the tumor to potentially be sensitive to very low levels of estrogen. When you stop the aromatase inhibitors, you increase the estrogen level to 20, 30, 40 pM, presumably. In your models would that be sufficient to inhibit the tumor and would you then think that there still may be separation of the curves with the aromatase inhibitors?

R. Santen: Tony [Howell] is asking a very good question. What we've observed, when you deprive MCF-7 cells of estrogen long term, they become hypersensitive to the stimulatory effects of estrogen. Paradoxically, when you increase the estrogen to physiologic concentrations, you actually turn on apoptosis and kill the cells, which is mediated through the Fas/Fas ligand death receptor pathway. Tony's [Howell] question is: If you treat a patient with an aromatase inhibitor for five years and then stop, would the rebound rise in estrogen that would occur after that be sufficient to trigger off a wave of apoptosis and actually be beneficial? I think that's the tenor of your question.

The level of estrogen that one achieves when you stop the aromatase inhibitor would be enough to trigger off apoptosis in the experimental MCF-7 cell model. Whether that would hold true in patients, of course, we don't know.

A. Brodie: Can I just interject a quick response to Tony's [Howell] comments? The aromatase tumor model—when we do get loss of inhibition with letrozole, we give the higher dose, and are able to induce responses again. This raises the possibility that you can increase the dose of letrozole. If tumor cells become sensitized to low levels of estrogen, we can still suppress them.

H. Mouridsen: Thank you.

C. K. Osborne: To get back to Trevor's [Powles] question about tamoxifen after aromatase inhibitors, there isn't very good data with the new aromatase inhibitors. We have anecdotal data. Ian, didn't you, in an early trial, do aminoglutethimide versus tamoxifen with a crossover? I'm not so sure that we have very good information about how well tamoxifen works after aromatase inhibitor.

J. Ingle: Henning, what is your data? You can answer that question.

H. Mouridsen: No, not directly. We don't have the exact data of response rate. I think it's so difficult to interpret these data because patients offered second line are not identical in the two arms. These are different patients because they are not randomized from the very beginning to the second-line therapy. They are highly selected. These patients are entering the second line according to response to the first-line therapy. It's very difficult to interpret that response data in this situation. But we know from the survival data and the time to progression data, that second-line patients who progressed on first-line tamoxifen and then received letrozole second line did significantly better than those receiving second-line tamoxifen following letrozole.

R. Santen: Can I comment on that? I don't remember precisely, but both of the North American and the European anastrozole-versus-tamoxifen trials had a secondary crossover on relapse. It's my understanding that both of those trials showed that the patients had a response to tamoxifen after they had failed initially on anastrozole.

J. Bonneterre: Unfortunately, there was no preplanned crossover. There was a retrospective analysis of patients treated with tamoxifen after anastrozole. It's even more difficult to interpret that data in highly selected patients.

A. Monnier: I want to come back to the ATAC trial and to make some comments. First, we know very well that the trial was initiated before the NIH consensus. When we look at the population, we can see that 34% of the population had node positive tumors. We can imagine that actually with the new consensus, 45% of the populations should receive chemotherapy and only 25 to 27, if I remember well, received chemotherapy in the trial.

The second point, you showed us on the first plot, was that there is no difference between tamoxifen and anastrozole for women receiving chemotherapy. But you have a difference in favor of anastrozole for women who did not receive chemotherapy. For my daily practice I am until now very skeptical concerning the benefit for anastrozole. I would be very happy if there was a retrospective analysis taking into account only women treated according to the new consensus in terms of chemotherapy.

M. Baum: If I understand the point that's being made—the results of the trial apply to the population in the trial. If you're treating that population, that's what you get. I'm sorry I'm not clear about the point that's being made here. The one thing that I tried to emphasize [is], that the effect of anastrozole and tamoxifen is equivalent after chemotherapy. In the current stage of analysis, they appear equivalent. But I think there is so much statistical noise in that— the confidence intervals are so wide—that I keep urging people to wait for another two years at least before [trusting] their sufficient events in the sub-population.

A. Monnier: Yes, but you have better results with anastrozole among women who did not receive chemotherapy.

M. Baum: Tests for heterogeneity are negative. There is no significant difference between those two groups, although one looks much better than the other. Again, I think it's because there are too few events in the chemotherapy. There is no significant difference between those two point estimates, even though they look impressive on the chart.

A. Monnier: You don't plan to make a retrospective analysis with women treated according to the actual consensus criteria, among your population?

M. Baum: No, this is nonsense as far as I'm concerned.

H. Mouridsen: This will be the last comment.

M. Kaufmann: The final question to Mike. Did you see fewer side effects or adverse effects for the combination?

M. Baum: As far as tolerability, side effects, the combination looks almost identical to tamoxifen alone, pretty much identical.

H. Mouridsen: I think we should close now.

7

Endocrine Therapy for Advanced Breast Cancer in Premenopausal Women

Walter Jonat
Universitatsklinikum Frauenklinik
Kiel, Germany

I. OVERVIEW

Relatively few data have been published on the use of endocrine therapy in premenopausal patients in the setting of advanced breast cancer. Although a common clinical assumption is that premenopausal patients can be rendered postmenopausal by either medical or surgical means, the validity of this assumption in terms of treatment outcomes has not been adequately explored. At present, the biology and behavior of breast cancer in premenopausal patients who have been rendered postmenopausal by ovarian suppression with luteinizing hormone-releasing hormone (LHRH) agonists are unknown. Similarly, questions about the use of combined vs. sequential therapy, or the selection of an optimal drug and sequence remain largely unanswered. This paper will review the published literature concerning these and other related issues.

II. INTRODUCTION

Over the last two decades, relatively few data have been published on endocrine therapy for advanced breast cancer in premenopausal women. To address this issue systematically, one might pose several key questions: 1) Is advanced breast cancer the same disease in pre- vs. postmenopausal women? 2) Is it the same disease in ovariectomized or LHRH-treated patients who are pre- vs. postmenopausal, or are there differences? 3) What is known about the efficacy of combined or sequential endocrine therapy? 4) What is the optimal drug and sequence? 5) Do novel endocrine therapies have a role? This chapter attempts to answer each of these questions based on the published literature.

III. PRE- VS. POSTMENOPAUSAL PATIENTS

Figure 1 shows the distribution of sex-hormone receptor status (concordant pairs) in breast carcinoma biopsies as a function of the potential for endocrine responsiveness (1). Although receptor status changes as a function of age, from 30 to 39 years up to those over age 80, there is no clear-cut difference in pre- vs. postmenopausal women. Those in the younger age groups, however, appear to be more receptor negative or hormone unresponsive compared to older patients. One might expect the hormone levels between the age cohorts to be comparable, although the receptor levels are totally different.

In order to investigate the possibility of breast cancer variants based on hormone-receptor expression, Anderson et al. reviewed breast cancer records from the National Cancer Institute's Surveillance, Epidemiology, and End-Results (SEER) database (2). The study included 19,541 non-Hispanic white women with node-negative breast cancer, in whom standard tumor cell characteristics and breast-cancer-specific survival were analyzed by independent estrogen receptor (ER), independent progesterone receptor (PR), and joint ER/PR phenotype. Age frequency density plots by joint ERPR phenotype are shown in Figure 2. The concordant ER/PR pair was characterized by a mix of early-onset (pre-

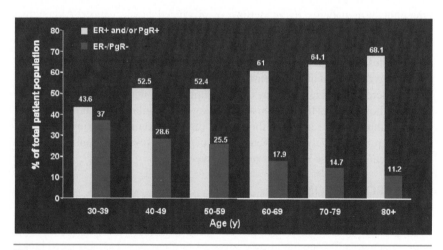

Figure 1   Sex hormone receptor status as a function of age. (From Ref. 1)

106

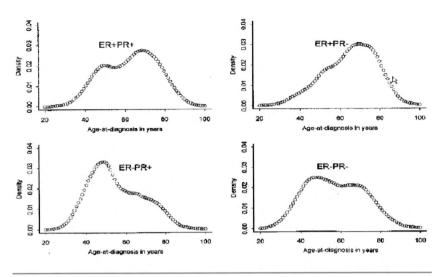

Figure 2 Age frequency density plot by joint ERPR phenotype. (From Ref. 2)

menopausal) and late-onset (postmenopausal) populations. Postmenopausal breast cancer dominated the ER+/PR+ phenotype, whereas the premenopausal peak was dominant in ER−/PR− expression. The discordant pair were shifted toward postmenopausal ages for ER+ PR− but toward premenopausal ages for ER− PR+. There was also a biologic gradient by joint ER/PR phenotypes for cancer-specific survival, with worsening chances of survival from ER+/PR+ to ER+/PR− to ER−/PR+ to ER−/PR− (Fig. 3). Rather than a single disease along a continuum, data from this study suggest two breast cancer variants with overlapping early- or late-onset etiologies based on hormone-receptor expression (2).

Experimental data suggest interaction between HER-2 and the ER pathways, with the possibility that HER-2 overexpression may serve as a marker of breast cancer resistance to endocrine therapy. A meta-analysis of seven studies involving patients with metastatic breast cancer ($n = 1,110$) was performed to evaluate the correlation between the response rate to endocrine therapy and HER-2 expression. For each study, the odds of disease progression was regarded as an indicator of tumor resistance to therapy, and the odds ratio for HER-2+ over HER-2− patients was calculated as an estimate of the predictive effect of HER-2. The overall odds ratio was 2.46 [95% Confidence Indicator (CI) = 1.81–3.34], indicating that metastatic breast cancers overexpressing HER-2 are resistant to endocrine therapy (3). Osborne has suggested that preclinical overexpression of HER-2 causes tamoxifen resistance; in turn, blocking HER-2 with tyrosine kinase inhibitors restores tamoxifen sensitivity. He concludes somewhat cautiously that tamoxifen may be less effective but it should not be withheld because it is not

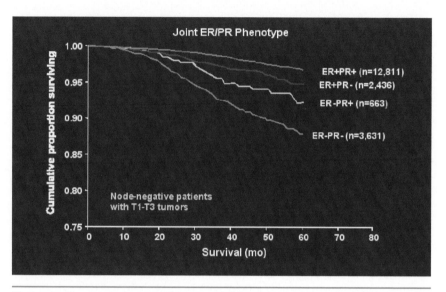

Figure 3 Breast cancer-specific survival by joint hormone receptor expression using data from the SEER database. (From Ref. 2)

ineffective. This applies to pre- as well as postmenopausal patients, although most of the data in this study and in the meta-analysis are based on post-menopausal patients (4).

Love et al. recently reported on a group of premenopausal patients ($n = 282$) participating in a randomized controlled trial of adjuvant oophorectomy and tamoxifen or observation, who had ER+ tumors that were evaluated for HER-2/neu overexpression. Women whose tumors were ER+ benefited from adjuvant as opposed to delayed ovarian ablation and tamoxifen. Among those who received adjuvant therapy, their data indicate little or no statistical difference in disease-free or overall survival for both the HER-2/neu/+ and HER-2/neu/− groups. However, the survival curves were much worse for the observation patients who were HER-2/neu/+ than for those who were HER-2/neu/−. The 3-year disease-free survival curves showed that HER-2/neu/+ patients received greater absolute benefit from adjuvant treatment (52% survival rate in observation patients vs. 82% treated) compared to HER-2/neu/− patients (observation, 73%; treated, 85%) (Table 1). The response in relation to HER-2/neu in premenopausal women to ovarian ablation and tamoxifen is contrary to results with tamoxifen alone in other settings (5).

Overall, evidence suggests that differences exist between premenopausal and postmenopausal advanced breast cancer, with potential implications for treat-

Table 1 Overall Survival in ER+ Patients According to HER-2/neu Status and Treatment with Adjuvant Surgical Oophorectomy and Tamoxifen or Observation

	DFS		OS	
Variable	RR	p	RR	p
Adjuvant oophorectomy/tam	0.59	0.11	0.76	0.50
HER-2/neu+ status	1.45	0.27	2.20	0.05
Interaction of HER-2/neu status and adjuvant treatment	0.38	0.18	0.21	0.07

Source: Ref. 5.

ment. Whether it is the same disease in both kinds of patients is not clear, but there are differences, for example, in biomarkers.

IV. OOPHORECTOMY/LHRH IN PREMENOPAUSAL PATIENTS

Another question to consider is the status of breast cancer in premenopausal patients who have been ovariectomized or treated with LHRH compared to post-menopausal breast cancer patients. Once again, is it the same disease in both groups?

Some of the earliest data relating to this question were published by Kaufmann et al., who studied the response of pre- and perimenopausal patients ($n = 134$) with breast cancer who were treated with goserelin. Mean serum estradiol levels fell into the range of castrated or postmenopausal women (< 30 pcg/ml) within 2 to 3 weeks, and suppression was maintained for the duration of therapy (up to 24 months). In addition, response rates (RR) and duration of remission produced by goserelin were comparable to those seen following oophorectomy (6). Nevertheless, the biology and behavior of breast cancer in a premenopausal patient who has been rendered postmenopausal by ovarian suppression with LHRH-agonists are currently unknown. There are relatively little data with which to address this question.

V. COMBINED/SEQUENTIAL ENDOCRINE THERAPY

A. Combined Therapy (Goserelin Plus Tamoxifen)

Data on the issue of combined endocrine therapy with goserelin and tamoxifen or goserelin alone in premenopausal patients are fairly well known. A meta-analysis of 29 Phase II clinical trials ($n = 228$ patients) concluded that goserelin provided effective, well-tolerated treatment for advanced breast cancer (7).

Nicholson et al. compared the endocrinologic effects and clinical efficacy of goserelin alone and goserelin plus tamoxifen in two separate groups of patients. Combination therapy resulted in more effective suppression of circulating concentrations of follicle stimulating hormone (FSH) and luteinizing hormone (LH), and a small but significant decrease in serum estradiol levels. The combination also prevented the uplift of FSH seen with goserelin alone. Although the incidence of static disease was increased in patients receiving goserelin and tamoxifen, perhaps at the expense of partial remissions, the time to progression (TTP) was extended in women receiving combination therapy. Remissions were primarily restricted to patients whose tumors were ER+, with only occasional responses seen in ER–disease (8).

In the largest such randomized trial to date, Jonat et al. compared the effect of goserelin with or without tamoxifen in 318 pre- and perimenopausal women. With a median follow-up of 93 weeks, 31% of goserelin-treated patients had ORs (complete objective regression, COR; partial objective regression, POR) compared with 38% of those receiving goserelin plus tamoxifen ($p = 0.24$). There was a modest benefit in favor of combination therapy in TTP of disease ($p = 0.03$), but not in survival ($p = 0.25$). Median times for disease progression and survival were 23 and 127 weeks in the goserelin alone group, and 28 and 140 weeks in the combination group, respectively. In a series of 115 patients, only those in a subset with musculoskeletal metastases receiving combination therapy showed significant differences in RR, TTP, and survival (9).

A meta-analysis by Klijn et al. combined evidence from four randomized clinical trials ($n = 508$) to compare combination therapy with LHRH and tamoxifen to LHRH alone in premenopausal women with advanced breast cancer. With a median follow-up of 6.8 years, there was a significant survival benefit (hazard ratio $= 0.78$; $p = 0.02$) and progression-free survival benefit (hazard ratio $= 0.70$; $p = 0.0003$) in favor of combination therapy (Table 2). The overall objective response (OR) rate was significantly higher for patients receiving combined treatment (OR $= 0.67$; $p = 0.03$). Although perhaps overly impacted by the single large trial by Jonat et al., the meta-analysis concludes that the combination of LHRH and tamoxifen is superior to LHRH alone in premenopausal women with breast cancer (10).

B. Goserelin vs. Oophorectomy

Goserelin, alone and in combination with tamoxifen, has been compared with oophorectomy. In an early study involving 81 perimenopausal women with advanced breast cancer, Boccardo et al. compared surgical castration (or ovarian irradiation), goserelin, surgical castration (or ovarian irradiation) plus tamoxifen, and goserelin plus tamoxifen in a 2×2 factorial randomized design.

Table 2 LHRH Agonist Plus Tamoxifen in Pre-/Perimenopausal Women with Advanced Breast Cancer: An EORTC Meta-analysis

Parameter	LHRH agonist ($n = 256$)	LHRH agonist + tamoxifen* ($n = 250$)	Odds/hazard ratio	p value
OR (CR+PR)	30%	39%	0.67	0.03
PFS (median)	5.4 mo	8.7 mo	0.70	<0.001
OS (median)	2.5 yr	2.9 yr	0.78	0.02

*The combination of LHRH agonist plus tamoxifen is superior to LHRH agonist alone in the treatment of advanced breast cancer in hormone-sensitive pre-/perimenopausal women

OR, Objective response; PFS, Progression-free survival; OS, Overall survival; Median follow-up of 6.8 years
Source: Ref. 10.

Despite the small sample size, oophorectomy or ovarian irradiation and the combination of goserelin plus tamoxifen were the most active regimens, yielding comparable OR rates. Although patient survival rates were statistically comparable regardless of treatment, the factorial design suggested that tamoxifen enhanced the activity of goserelin therapy but did not improve the efficacy of gonadal ablation (11).

A study by Taylor et al. compared failure-free survival and overall survival for premenopausal patients ($n = 136$) with ER+ and/or PR+ metastatic breast cancer treated with goserelin or surgical ovariectomy. Although initially designed as an equivalence trial with 80% power to rule out a 50% improvement in survival in patients who underwent ovariectomy, early termination resulted in a final power of 60% for the alternative hypothesis of equal survival distributions. Failure-free survival and overall survival were similar for goserelin and ovariectomy. The goserelin/ovariectomy hazaard ratios for failure-free survival and overall survival were 0.73 (95% CI: 0.51–1.04) and 0.80 (95% CI: 0.53–1.20), respectively. The test of 50% improvement in overall survival in ovariectomized patients was rejected at $p = 0.006$; median overall survival was 33 and 37 months for the ovariectomy and goserelin groups, respectively. Results from the study allowed the authors to rule out at least a moderate advantage for oophorectomy (12).

C. Goserelin Plus Other Agents

Relatively little is known so far about the efficacy of goserelin in combination with other agents. A small, open-label study by Dowsett et al. reported on the effects of the aromatase inhibitor (AI) vorozole in premenopausal women ($n =$ 10) with advanced breast cancer who received goserelin therapy for 4 weeks, followed by combined goserelin and vorozole therapy for 12 weeks, followed by goserelin therapy for another 4 weeks. When combined with goserelin, vorozole markedly enhanced suppression of serum levels of estrone, estradiol, and estrone sulfate over that achieved with goserelin alone (by a mean of 74%, 83%, and 89%, respectively) (13).

Overall, studies indicate that: 1) goserelin provides an effective alternative to oophorectomy for premenopausal women with hormone-sensitive advanced breast cancer; and 2) the efficacy of LHRH agonists in advanced disease is enhanced by the addition of tamoxifen.

VI. OPTIMAL DRUG AND SEQUENCE

Most clinicians would probably agree on a treatment algorithm for advanced breast cancer that splits into two paths: 1) endocrine therapy for hormone receptor-positive (HR+) breast cancer, switching to chemotherapy when the patient is either not responsive or clinically no longer a candidate for endocrine therapy; and 2) chemotherapy for hormone-receptor-negative (HR−) or highly progressive disease. From the list of potential endocrine agents, including antiestrogens, AIs and LHRH inhibitors, there are relatively little data in premenopausal patients on which to base either drug selection or sequence. Only few data suggest goserelin as first line, perhaps in combination with tamoxifen and/or anastrozole. A small study from Tan et al. supports this idea (14).

As part of a crossover design in the large study by Jonat et al., a subgroup of patients ($n = 71$) initially received goserelin, with tamoxifen added after first disease progression. Thirteen patients (18%) had an objective response (COR or POR), and 29 patients (41%) had stable disease. Median time from the addition of tamoxifen to second-disease progression was 20 weeks (range, 2–148 weeks). This result suggests that there may be no additional benefit of combined goserelin plus tamoxifen over sequential therapy, provided the second agent is given at progression (9).

Overall, optimal sequencing of available endocrine agents remains to be defined. There is unquestionably a need for large, randomized trials examining the roles of various new agents, including the ER down-regulator fulvestrant, and nonsteroidal and steroidal AIs, subsequent to therapy with goserelin plus tamoxifen.

VII. NOVEL AGENTS

With few exceptions, virtually no data exist on novel endocrine therapies in premenopausal advanced breast cancer. There is minimal data on use of aromatase inhibitors in premenopausal patients without ovarian ablation (medical or surgical).

Although it is possible to reduce estradiol production by the ovaries with AIs, the clinical outcome of this intervention is thus far limited to case presentations, with no studies to date. However, the first generation agent aminoglutethimide was not effective, perhaps because of its limited efficacy in reducing estradiol levels.

Similarly, there are no data on either selective estrogen receptor modulators (SERMs) or selective estrogen downregulators (SERDs). In particular, there are no efficacy and only limited safety data for fulvestrant in premenopausal patients, leaving the potential role for this agent and other SERMs to be defined. Studies are needed to compare alternative regimens of fulvestrant combined with ovarian ablation or LHRH analogue in premenopausal patients.

VIII. SUMMARY

Keeping in mind the paucity of data on treatment of advanced breast cancer in premenopausal women, it is possible to supply only limited answers to the original list of questions posed at the beginning of this chapter. Advanced breast cancer is probably not the same disease in premenopausal and postmenopausal patients, nor is it likely the same disease in oophorectomized or LHRH-treated pre- vs. postmenopausal patients. It appears that combined endocrine therapy is likely to be the approach of choice, especially considering the relatively high percentage of patients who have rapid progression of their disease and the difficulty of conducting adequate crossover studies. The optimal drug and sequence remains unknown, as do the roles of various new, and in some cases promising, novel endocrine therapies.

REFERENCES

1. Witliff J, Pasic R, Bland KI. Steroid and peptide hormone receptors. In: Bland KI, Copeland EM, eds. The Breast. 2nd ed. Philadelphia: Saunders, 1998; pp. 471.
2. Anderson WF, Chu KC, Chatterjee N, Brawley O, Brinton LA. Tumor variants by hormone receptor expression in white patients with node-negative breast cancer from the Surveillance, Epidemiology, and End Results database. J Clin Oncol 2001; 19:18–27.
3. De Laurentiis M, Arpino G, Massarelli E, Carlomagno C, Ciardiello F, Tortora G, Bianco AR, Bianco AR, De Placido S. A metanalysis of the interaction between HER-2 and the response to endocrine therapy in metastatic breast cancer. Proc Am Soc Clin Oncol 2000; 19:78a (A300).
4. Osborne CK, Schiff R, Fuqua SA, Shou J. Estrogen receptor: current understanding of its activation and modulation. Clin Cancer Res 2001 Dec; 7(suppl 12):4338s–4342s; discussion 4411s–4412s.
5. Love RR, Duc NB, Havighurst TC, Mohsin SK, Zhang Q, DeMets DL, Allred DC. HER-2/neu overexpression and response to oophorectomy plus tamoxifen adjuvant therapy in estrogen receptor-positive premenopausal women with operable breast cancer. J Clin Oncol 2003; 21:453–457.

6. Kaufmann M, Jonat W, Kleeberg U, Eiermann W, Janicke F, Hilfrich J, Kreienberg R, Albrecht M, Weitzel HK, Schmid H, et al. for the German Zoladex Trial Group. Goserelin, a depot gonadotrophin-releasing hormone agonist in the treatment of pre-menopausal patients with metastatic breast cancer. J Clin Oncol 1989; 7:1113–1119.

7. Blamey RW, Jonat W, Kaufmann M, Bianco AR, Namer M. Goserelin depot in the treatment of premenopausal advanced breast cancer. Eur J Cancer 1992; 28A(4-5):810–814.

8. Nicholson RI, Walker KJ, McClelland RA, Dixon A, Robertson JF, Blamey RW. Zoladex plus tamoxifen versus Zoladex alone in pre- and perimenopausal metastatic breast cancer. J Steroid Biochem Mol Biol 1990; 37:989–995.

9. Jonat W, Kaufmann M, Blamey RW, Howell A, Collins JP, Coates A, Eiermann W, Janicke F, Njordenskold B, Forbes JF, et al. A randomised study to compare the effect of the luteinizing hormone releasing hormone (LHRH) analogue goserelin with or without tamoxifen in pre- and perimenopausal patients with advanced breast cancer. Eur J Cancer 1995; 31A:137–142.

10. Klijn JGM, Blamey RW, Boccardo F, Tominaga T, Duchateau L, Sylvester R, for the Combined Hormone Agents Trialists' Group and the European Organization for Research and Treatment of Cancer. Combined tamoxifen and luteinizing hormone-releasing hormone (LHRH) agonist versus LHRH agonist alone in premenopausal advanced breast cancer: a meta-analysis of four randomized trials. J Clin Oncol 2001; 19:343–353.

11. Boccardo F, Rubagotti A, Perrotta A, Amoroso D, Balestrero M, De Matteis A, Zola P, Sismondi P, Francini G, Petrioli R, et al. Ovarian ablation versus goserelin with or without tamoxifen in pre-perimenopausal patients with advanced breast cancer: results of a multicentric Italian study. Ann Oncol 1994; 5:337–342.

12. Taylor CW, Green S, Dalton WS, Martino S, Rector D, Ingle JN, Robert NJ, Budd GT, Paradelo JC, Natale RB, Bearden JD, Mailliard JA, Osborne CK. Multicenter randomized clinical trial of goserelin versus surgical ovariectomy in premenopausal patients with receptor-positive metastatic breast cancer: an intergroup study. J Clin Oncol 1998; 16:994–999.

13. Dowsett M, Doody D, Miall S, Howes A, English J, Coombes RC. Vorozole results in greater oestrogen suppression than formestane in postmenopausal women and when added to goserelin in premenopausal women with advanced breast cancer. Breast Cancer Res Treat 1999; 56:25–34.

14. Tan SM, Cheung PC, Willsher PC, Blamey RW, Chan SY, Robertson JFR. Locally advanced primary breast cancer: medium-term results of a randomized trial of multi-modal therapy versus initial hormone therapy. Eur J Cancer 2001; 37(18):2331–2338.

8

Adjuvant Endocrine Treatment in Premenopausal Patients

Raimund Jakesz

Vienna General Hospital
Vienna, Austria

I. OVERVIEW

The role of adjuvant therapy in premenopausal women with breast cancer has been assessed by numerous randomized trials. New developments in hormonal blockade are often compared with traditional chemotherapy regimens as providing a more tolerable and efficacious treatment. With induction of amenorrhea as a goal in the adjunctive setting, ovarian ablation, antiestrogen and, more recently, aromatase inhibitors (AIs) contribute to the choice of treatments available for premenopausal women with hormone-responsive (HR) breast tumors. Overall results from past and recent trials favor ovarian ablation, with luteinizing hormone-releasing hormone (LHRH) analogues such as goserelin alone or in combination with the anti-estrogen tamoxifen, rather than with chemotherapy, in the adjuvant treatment of premenopausal patients with HR breast tumors.

Steroid hormone-receptor levels increasingly guide current selection of adjuvant therapy. However, emerging data suggest the role of new tumor markers, such as human epidermal growth factor (HER)-2/neu, in predicting prognosis and in selecting treatment regimens. Additionally, preliminary results from the Austrian Breast and Colorectal Cancer Study Group (ABCSG) 12 trial suggest the need for the addition of a bisphosphonate to adjuvant treatment involving ovarian-function suppression to prevent the deleterious effects on bone-mineral density. Despite current clinical evidence on the value of endocrine therapy in adjuvant therapy, future clinical trials must address numerous questions including the role of AIs in this setting.

II. INTRODUCTION

Breast cancer is the leading cause of death for women aged 20–59 years, with 1 in 229 women below the age of 39 in the United States developing the condition (1). Treatment of these patients attempts, in some situations, to induce remission while causing only a temporary cessation in menses and hence preserving fertility. Systemic adjuvant therapy following breast surgery consists of chemotherapy and endocrine treatment, the latter having less long-term harmful effects on reproduction. However, unlike postmenopausal women, few clinical trial data exist for adjuvant endocrine treatment in premenopausal patients. This chapter discusses the treatment options and the current clinical evidence available.

III. OVARIAN ABLATION

Ovarian ablation is an effective adjuvant therapy in patients with hormone-sensitive breast cancer. This can be achieved by a number of methods including surgery, radiotherapy, cytotoxic chemotherapy, and pharmacotherapy.

A continuing meta-analysis conducted by the Early Breast Cancer Trialists' Collaborative Group (EBCTCG) on randomized trials examining the effects of ovarian ablation on recurrence and death in women under the age of 50 years, now has information collected from 15 years of follow-up (2). The defined category of women under the age of 50 years was used rather than "premenopausal," as the menopausal status was not clearly ascertained across the trials. The meta-analysis incorporated trials with ovarian ablation by surgery, radiotherapy, and pharmacotherapy. Estrogen-receptor (ER) status was only defined in patient trials of ablation plus chemotherapy versus chemotherapy alone. Results showed 15-year survival with ovarian ablation in the absence of chemotherapy to be highly significant, with an overall 25% reduction in recurrence-free survival ($2p = 0.0005$) and 24% reduction in death ($2p = 0.0006$) compared with no adjuvant treatment. In trials with ablation plus chemotherapy, no significant benefit in survival or recurrence-free survival was seen, even in ER+ patients.

The efficacy of chemotherapy compared with ovarian ablation was also found to be insignificant in two other trials with 1,064 patients, though suboptimal chemotherapy regimen was used (3, 4). Despite this, ovarian ablation by cytotoxic chemotherapy is used in the adjuvant treatment of 30–70% patients with breast cancer.

The efficacy of any such adjuvant chemotherapeutic agent likely relies to a great extent on its ability to cause amenorrhea, with the induction of amenorrhea being age-dependent, and the amenorrheic state being of large prognostic value.

Ovarian ablation induced by luteinizing hormone-releasing hormone (LHRH) analogues such as goserelin, effectively generates a reversible amenorrhea, with patients regaining their menses once the drug is stopped. No placebo-controlled trial exists for the use of goserelin as an adjuvant agent.

A large trial, however, does exist in comparing goserelin with chemotherapy. The Zoladex Early Breast Cancer Research Association (ZEBRA) study assessed the efficacy of goserelin versus cyclophosphamide, methotrexate, and fluorouracil (CMF) chemotherapy as adjuvant treatments in premenopausal patients with node-positive breast cancer (5). Postoperatively, patients ($\leq$ 50 years of age, were randomized to receive either goserelin 3.6 mg every 28 days for 2 years, or six cycles of 28-day regimen of CMF. ER status of the patients was defined, with approximately one-fifth of the 1,493 patients identified as ER–. The patients were then followed up with an analysis performed after 684 events had been achieved. The median follow-up was 6 years.

The ZEBRA trial showed a correlation between ER status and treatment regimens. The overall survival was lower in goserelin-treated patients who were ER– compared with ER+ (hazard ratio = 1.77, 95% confidence interval (CI) = 1.19–2.63; and hazard ratio = 0.92, 95% CI = 0.76–1.28, respectively). Overall survival and disease-free survival between the treatments in ER+ patients were identical. This infers that additional CMF therapy is not required when administering goserelin in ER+ premenopausal patients with node-positive breast cancer. On the contrary, in ER– patients, goserelin was significantly inferior to CMF for disease-free survival (hazard ratio = 1.76, 95% CI = 1.27–2.44) (Fig. 1). Thus for this trial, CMF-treated patients had a markedly better prognosis, which suggests that endocrine therapy should not be given to patients with hormone-unresponsive tumors.

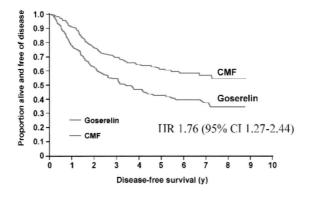

Figure 1 The ZEBRA study: Kaplan-Meier curve for disease-free survival in ER– patients demonstrates inferiority of goserelin compared with CMF chemotherapy. (From Ref. 5)

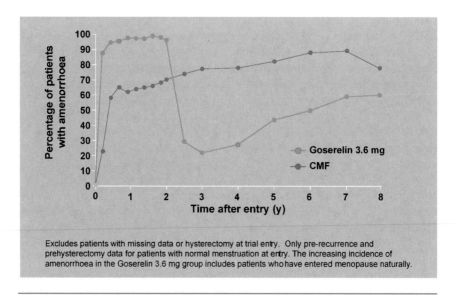

Excludes patients with missing data or hysterectomy at trial entry. Only pre-recurrence and prehysterectomy data for patients with normal menstruation at entry. The increasing incidence of amenorrhoea in the Goserelin 3.6 mg group includes patients who have entered menopause naturally.

Figure 2   The ZEBRA study: A greater percentage of patients treated with goserelin experienced amenorrhea compared with CMF chemotherapy. (From Ref. 5)

The ZEBRA study also demonstrated that a greater number of patients experienced amenorrhea induced by goserelin compared with CMF (approximately 95% and 65%, respectively after 6 months) (Fig. 2). Compared with CMF, not only did goserelin-treated patients achieve amenorrhea more successfully, but also a greater number of patients regained their menses more readily; only 22.6% of patients still remained amenorrheic after 3 years of follow-up versus 76.9% of CMF patients. This return of menses is an important benefit with regard to the impact on bone-mineral density, because the resumption of endogenous estrogen prevents osteoporosis.

Tolerability of goserelin was greater than for CMF, with more patients on CMF experiencing greater side effects, such as nausea/vomiting, infection, and alopecia. In conclusion, the ZEBRA study showed that in premenopausal patients with ER+ and node-positive breast cancer, goserelin is effective, well-tolerated, and, hence, an alternative to CMF. In ER− patients, chemotherapy is the recommended choice, with endocrine treatment reserved for patients with HR tumors. This trial demonstrates the importance of defining ER status and node status in any breast cancer trial design in order to determine the most beneficial therapeutic agents for each characteristic patient group.

The Zoladex in Premenopausal Patients (ZIPP) trial also examined the efficacy of goserelin as additional therapy to surgery and standard local therapy (6). Premenopausal patients were randomized following standard therapy, including chemotherapy if desired, to receive either goserelin or placebo, and a smaller proportion then further randomized to receive either tamoxifen or placebo. The ER status of patients was not a defined requirement. The results of the ZIPP trial demonstrated that the addition of goserelin to standard adjuvant therapy significantly improved overall and disease-free survival (hazard ratio = 0.82, 95% CI = 0.67–0.99; hazard ratio = 0.80, 95% CI = 0.69–0.92, respectively). More importantly, in patients receiving goserelin, there was a significantly reduced incidence of contralateral breast cancer (hazard ratio = 0.60; 95% CI = 0.35–1.00).

IV. ANTI-ESTROGEN

It was initially thought that ER antagonism offered no beneficial adjuvant therapy to premenopausal breast cancer patients. However, recent evidence from the EBCTCG shows that the anti-estrogen tamoxifen, given for 5 years, has a marked survival benefit in ER+ patients, even greater when indirectly compared with chemotherapy (7, 8). The analysis showed 45% reduction in recurrence and a 32% reduction in death. The current standard adjuvant therapy in the United States consists of a combination of chemotherapy and tamoxifen. However, insufficient trial data exist to support this regimen and further large, randomized trials are necessary.

V. ANTI-ESTROGEN PLUS OVARIAN ABLATION

As both the LHRH agonist, goserelin, and the anti-estrogen, tamoxifen, have been shown to be effective as adjuvant therapies (5, 7), one could predict that their combined use would be even more beneficial. Evidence in support of this theory has been shown in a meta-analysis by Klijn et al. (9) in the metastatic-disease setting. This analysis of four randomized clinical trials comparing the combined treatment of LHRH agonist and tamoxifen with LHRH agonist alone, in premenopausal women with advanced breast cancer, showed significant survival benefit with the combined treatments (Log rank $p = 0.02$). Progression-free survival was also greater with the combined treatment compared with LHRH agonist alone (Log rank $p = 0.0003$) (Fig. 3).

In the adjuvant setting, the Austrian Breast and Colorectal Cancer Study Group 5 (ABCSG V) took this one step further by comparing the combination of LHRH analogue and tamoxifen with chemotherapy in premenopausal patients with hormone-responsive breast cancer (10). The trial enrolled 1,034 patients, who where randomized to receive either 3 years of goserelin with 5 years of tamoxifen or six cycles of CMF. After 6 years, the overall total recurrence of breast cancer was 20% for all patients in the trial, with a 7.4% local recurrence and 10% death rate. The 6-year event-free survival was significantly in favor of the combined endocrine treatments ($p = 0.024$) (Fig. 4), as were the relapse-free and local recurrence-free survival compared with chemotherapy ($p = 0.037$ and

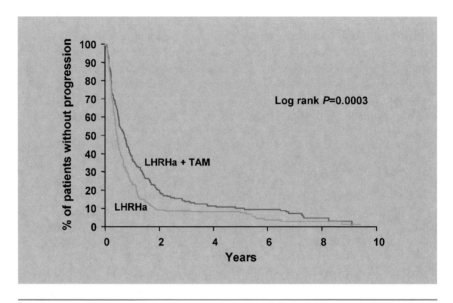

Figure 3   Progression-free survival was significantly better for combined treatment of LHRH agonist plus tamoxifen compared with LHRH agonist alone. (From Ref. 9)

$p = 0.015$, respectively). A similar beneficial, although insignificant trend for overall survival was also seen.

CMF does not represent the current standard of chemotherapy treatment for most premenopausal patients. A study conducted by Roche et al. looked at regimens

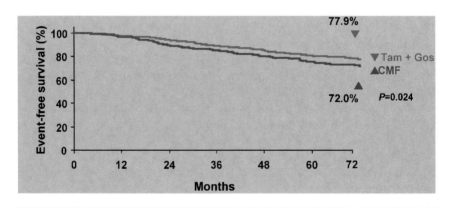

Figure 4   The Austrian Breast and Colorectal Cancer Study Group 5: Six-year event-free survival was significantly in favor of combined endocrine treatments ($p = 0.024$) compared with CMF chemotherapy. (From Ref. 10)

similar to the ABCSG V study (11). This study compared hormonal blockade with 3 years of LHRH agonist plus tamoxifen, versus six cycles of fluorouracil, epirubicin, and cyclophosphamide (FEC 50). The outcome effect was measured on disease-free survival and overall survival in premenopausal women with HR and node-positive breast cancer. Results of this study did not demonstrate any significant benefit of FEC 50 compared with hormonal blockade, but in both treatment arms, disease-free survival and overall survival rates were high.

VI. AIs AND OVARIAN ABLATION

The use of AIs in combination with ovarian ablation represents a new form of therapy for which clinical trial evidence has yet to emerge. The ABCSG 12 study is currently underway to determine the potential benefits of AIs in this setting. The trial aims to recruit 2,000 premenopausal women with HR breast cancer, randomized to receive 3 years of goserelin in combination with either tamoxifen or the AI, anastrozole. Patients will then be further randomized to receive either the bisphosphonate, zoledronic acid, or placebo, in an attempt to reduce the deleterious impact of complete endocrine blockade on bone-mineral density (BMD). Preliminary results from this trial indicate clearly that the combination of goserelin plus anastrazole has marked impairment on BMD, which can statistically be improved with the addition of zoledronic acid ($p < 0.02$ and $p < 0.0001$ for BMD in the trochanter and lumber spine, respectively) (12). BMD density is also impaired with the administration of tamoxifen, which once again improves with the addition of zoledronic acid. Little reduction in BMD was seen when anastrozole or tamoxifen plus goserelin were administered with zoledronic acid. These preliminary results show that the addition of zoledronic acid has a protective

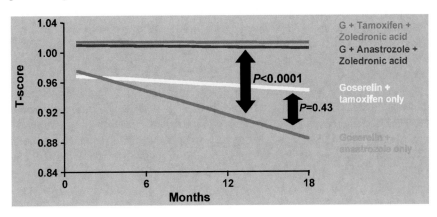

Figure 5 Addition of zoledronate has protective effect on bone-mineral density in the lumbar spine when endocrine blockade is given.

effect on BMD, especially in the lumbar spine, when endocrine-blockade is undertaken (Fig. 5).

VII. ST. GALLEN 2003 TREATMENT RECOMMENDATIONS

New information was presented at the St. Gallen meeting, emphasizing the administration of endocrine therapies in premenopausal patients with hormone-sensitive tumors (13). Consensus recommendations consisted of several treatment options for premenopausal patients with node-positive, hormone-responsive breast tumors > 2 cm. Ovarian ablation (with LHRH analogue) plus tamoxifen with or without chemotherapy or chemotherapy followed by tamoxifen was the consensus. Additionally, in node-negative patients with hormone-responsive breast tumors, tamoxifen or ovarian ablation alone is currently recommended.

VIII. CLARIFYING THE CONFUSIONS

What defines hormone-responsiveness and do data exist outlining hormone resistance? In the ABCSG V trial in which estrogen and progesterone status was defined and measured, multivariate analysis showed that the presence of progesterone receptors (PR) but not ER, had significant prognostic importance. This was true for overall survival and event-free survival (10).

Reiner et al. examined the prognostic importance of steroid hormone levels identified by immunocytochemical localization, in primary breast cancer (14). Immunocytochemical assay (ICA) results in this study showed that patients with ER− and PR− carcinomas had poorer prognosis than patients with only one negative receptor. As one could predict, patients with either ER ICA or PR ICA+ carcinomas demonstrated significantly better overall survival than patients with negative assays ($p < 0.00001$ and $p = 0.004$, respectively). This study demonstrated that hormone receptor status is a strong prognostic indicator, with clinical importance attributed to the proportion of receptor-positive tumor cells.

Data outlining hormone resistance were presented in a multivariate COX-analysis of the ABCSG V trial (10). In this analysis, HER-2/neu, a proto-oncogene cell surface receptor and an important marker in some epithelial carcinomas, was measured in 566 premenopausal patients with hormone-responsive tumors. The overall survival was significantly better for patients without HER-2/neu receptor markers compared with patients with HER-2/neu overexpression ($p = 0.007$) (Fig. 6) (10). Hence, HER-2/neu expression and overexpression are important prognostic factors.

Good clinical trial data have yet to emerge to define the efficacy of tamoxifen versus chemotherapy, and tamoxifen versus goserelin.

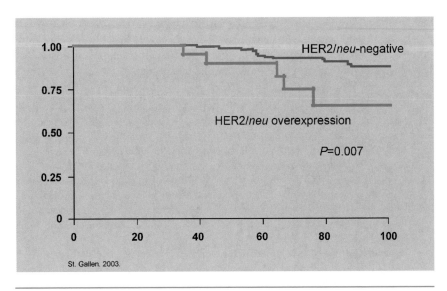

Figure 6 The overall survival was significantly better for HER-2/neu– patients compared with HER-2/neu overexpression ($p = 0.007$). (From Ref. 10)

The addition of endocrine blockade to premenopausal breast cancer patients receiving chemotherapy but not experiencing amenorrhea has yet to be confirmed. The Eastern Cooperative Oncology Group briefly highlighted this in their E5188, INT-0101 trial, a randomized trial in premenopausal, hormone-responsive, node-positive breast cancer (15). The 1,504 patients were randomized to receive one of the three treatment arms postoperatively; chemotherapy (cyclophosphamide, doxorubicin, 5-fluorouracil-CAF), CAF followed by 5 years of goserelin, and CAF followed by 5 years of goserelin plus tamoxifen. Results from this trial showed that in premenopausal women with node-positive, receptor-positive breast cancer, the addition of tamoxifen to CAF plus goserelin improves recurrence-free survival (hazard ratio = 0.73; $p < 0.01$). No significant effect on 9-year recurrence-free survival was demonstrated by the addition of goserelin to CAF. Amenorrhea was observed in 66% of women < 40 years and 95% of women ≥ 40 years at the end of CAF treatment. Hence, should goserelin or tamoxifen be administered to patients who are still not amenorrheic?

Finally, in an attempt to define the patients in which endocrine treatment is most suitable, the following characteristics may be proposed: Patients who are strongly receptor-positive, with no HER-2/neu overexpression, may be treated with endocrine treatment alone, without chemotherapy; patients who have HER-2/neu overexpression and are weakly receptor-positive, may benefit from the combination of chemo- and endocrine therapies. However, only future prospective, randomized, direct comparative trials, will be able to clarify the differences in beneficial outcomes provided by the current adjuvant treatments. Only then can more appropriate guidelines be designed.

REFERENCES

1. Jemal A, Thomas A, Murray T, Thun M. Cancer Statistics, 2002. CA Cancer J Clin 2002; 52:23–47.
2. Early Breast Cancer Trialists' Collaborative Group. Ovarian ablation in early breast cancer: overview of the randomised trials. Lancet 1996; 348:1189–1196.
3. Scottish Cancer Trials Breast Group and ICRF Breast Unit, Guy's Hospital, London. Adjuvant ovarian ablation versus CMF chemotherapy in premenopausal women with pathological stage II breast carcinoma: the Scottish trial. Scottish Cancer Trials Breast Group and ICRF Breast Unit, Guy's Hospital, London. Lancet 1993; 341:1293–1298.
4. Andersson M, Kamby C, Jensen MB, Mourisden H, Ejlertsen B, Dombernowsky P, Rose C, Cold S, Overgaard M, Andersen J, Kjaer M. Tamoxifen in high-risk premenopausal women with primary breast cancer receiving adjuvant chemotherapy. Report from the Danish Breast Cancer Co-operative Group DBCG 82B Trial. Eur J Cancer 1999; 35:1659–1666.
5. Jonat W, Kaufmann M, Sauerbrei W, Blamey R, Cuzick J, Namer M, Fogelman I, de Haes JC, de Matteis A, Stewart A, Eiermann W, Szakolczai I, Palmer M, Schumacher M, Geberth M, Lisboa B, Zoladex Early Breast Cancer Research Association Study. Goserelin versus cyclophosphamide, methotrexate and fluorouracil as adjuvant therpay in premenopausal patients with node-positive breast cancer: Zoladex Early Breast Cancer Research Association Study. J Clin Oncol 2002; 20:4628–4635.
6. Baum M, Houghton J, Sawyer W, Odling-Smee W, Rutqvist LE, Nordenskjold B, Mari E, Nicculuci A. Management of premenopausal women with early breast cancer: is there a role for goserelin? [abstr 103] Proc Am Soc Clin Oncol 2001; 20:27a.
7. Early Breast Cancer Trialists' Collaborative Group. Tamoxifen for early breast cancer: an overview of the randomised trials. Lancet 1998; 351:1451–1467.
8. Early Breast Cancer Trialists' Collaborative Group. Polychemotherapy for early breast cancer: an overview of the randomised trials. Lancet 1998; 352:930–942.
9. Klijn JG, Blamey RW, Boccardo F, Tominaga T, Duchateau L, Sylvester R, Combined Hormone Agents Trialists' Group and the European Organization for Research and Treatment of Cancer. Combined tamoxifen and luteinizing hormone-releasing hormone (LHRH) agonist versus LHRH agonist alone in premenopausal advanced breast cancer: a meta-analysis of four randomized trials. J Clin Oncol 2001; 19:343–353.
10. Jakesz R, Hausmaninger H, Kubista E, Gnant M, Menzel C, Bauernhofer T, Seifert M, Haider K, Mlineritsch B, Steindorfer P, Kwasny W, Fridrik M, Steger G, Wette V, Samonigg H, Austrian Breast and Colorectal Cancer Study Group 5. Randomized adjuvant trial of tamoxifen and goserelin versus cyclophosphamide, methotrexate and fluorouracil: evidence for the superiority of treatment with endocrine blockade in premenopausal patients with hormone-responsive breast cancer—Austrian Breast

and Colorectal Cancer Study Group 5. J Clin Oncol 2002; 20:4621–4627.

11. Roche H, Kerbrat P, Bonneterre J, Fargeot P, Fmoleau P, Monnier A, Chapelle-Marcillac I, Bardonnet M. Complete hormonal blockade versus chemotherapy in premenopausal early-stage breast cancer patients with positive hormone-receptor and 1–3 node-positive tumor: results of the FASG 06 trial [abstr 279]. Proc Am Soc Clin Oncol 2000; 19:72a.

12. Gnant M, Hausmaninger H, Samonigg H, Mlineritsch B, Taucher S, Luschin-Ebengreuth G, Jakesz R. Changes in bone mineral density caused by anastrozole or tamoxifen in combination with goserelin ($+/-$) zoledronate as adjuvant treatment for hormone receptor-positive premenopausal breast cancer: results of a randomized multicenter trial [abstr 12]. Breast Cancer Res Treat 2002; 76:S31.

13. Goldhirsh A, Wood WC, Gelber RD, Coates RD, Thurlimann B, Senn HJ. Meeting highlights: updated international expert consensus on the primary therapy of early breast cancer. J Clin Oncol 2003; 21:3357–3365.

14. Reiner A, Neumeister B, Spona J, Reiner G, Schemper M, Jakesz R. Immunocytochemical localization of estrogen and progesterone receptor and prognosis in human primary breast cancer. Cancer Res 1990; 50:7057–7061.

15. Davidson, NE, O'Neill A, Vukov A, et al. Effect of chemohormonal therapy in premenopausal, node-positive breast cancer. An Eastern Cooperative Group phase III intergroup trial (E5188, INT-0101) [abstr]. Breast 1999; 8:232–233.

9

Adjuvant Chemotherapy in Breast Cancer Patients with Hormone-Receptor-Positive (Responsive) Disease: Focus on Premenopausal Patients

Jonas C. S. Bergh
Karolinska Institute and Hospital
Stockholm, Sweden

I. OVERVIEW

Adjuvant polychemotherapy has for years been demonstrated to be the standard approach for the treatment of breast cancer patients with certain risk features, especially premenopausal patients. However, recent data from different types of hormonal therapy strategies partly challenge this view; indeed, some oncologists would consider certain premenopausal patients with receptor-positive disease as candidates for hormonal therapy only.

The outcome of adjuvant CMF (cyclophosphamide, methotrexate, 5-fluorouracil)-based polychemotherapy appears to be linked partly to the induction of amenorrhea in patients with receptor-positive disease; patients with amenorrhea have improved outcomes compared with those without. The efficiency of amenorrhea induction, however, differs with different chemotherapy regimens; classical CMF appears to be potentially more efficient at inducing amenorrhea compared with anthracycline-containing regimens. On the other hand, anthracycline- or taxane-containing regimens seem to offer a small but statistically significant survival gain, although outcomes have not been prospectively analyzed in relation to receptor status and induction of amenorrhea. Retrospective analyses indicate that taxane-containing regimens may have slightly more benefit in patients with receptor-negative disease.

Recent evidence supports the hypothesis that breast cancer is not a single disease, but rather comprises multiple diseases. This will imply more detailed subgrouping in addition to analyses of conventional prognostic factors and separation of patients into hormone-positive or -negative disease. Further developments will expand this, ultimately aiming at offering individual prognostic and predictive value.

II. INTRODUCTION

Different oncological therapeutic modalities have been used to significantly reduce the risk for breast cancer recurrence and to improve overall survival in younger breast cancer patients (1–4). The meta-analysis strategies by the Oxford team for the Early Breast Cancer Trialists' Collaborative Group (EBCTCG) have been instrumental for obtaining these data. Most patients have been included in studies using adjuvant chemotherapy. Chemotherapy versus nonsystemic therapy resulted in a relative reduction of recurrence of 34% (standard deviation ($\pm$ 4), with a corresponding relative mortality reduction of 27% ($\pm$5) (4). Ovarian ablation resulted in a 25% ($\pm$7) relative relapse reduction and a relative mortality reduction of 24% ($\pm$7). The earliest ovarian-ablation studies were hampered by the fact that receptor status was not determined; accordingly, hormone-receptor-negative (HR–) patients would very likely have been included, thus diluting the results. Tamoxifen alone for 5 years resulted in 45% ($\pm$8) and 32% ($\pm$10) relative reduction in recurrence and mortality, respectively (4). The addition of ovarian ablation to chemotherapy compared to chemotherapy alone resulted in an additional 10% ($\pm$9) and 8% ($\pm$10) reduction in recurrence and mortality, respectively.

Adjuvant chemotherapy alone in patients with (ER)-poor tumors resulted in a 35% ($\pm$9) relative mortality reduction. The potential of better efficacy of chemotherapy in patients with ER-poor disease is underlined by the fact that the corresponding relative mortality reduction for a patient with estrogen-receptor-positive (ER+) disease was 20% ($\pm$10). However, the confidence intervals are overlapping (3).

III. CHEMOTHERAPY COMPARED WITH OOPHORECTOMY

A. Amenorrhea-Related Effects

The effect of adjuvant chemotherapy on premenopausal patients with HR+ disease seems to be related to the induction of amenorrhea. This was demonstrated by data from Study VI of the International Breast Cancer Study Group, using classical cyclophosphamide, methotrexate and 5-fluorouracil (CMF) administered postoperatively for 3 or 6 courses, with or without re-induction at different time periods (5). A significantly improved disease-free survival ($p < 0.0001$) was recorded for patients with estrogen/progesterone-receptor-positive (ER+/PR+) disease obtaining amenorrhea, compared to those without. No difference was recorded in disease-free survival with respect to amenorrhea for the group with estrogen/progesterone-receptor-negative (ER–/PR–) disease.

Similar results were demonstrated in the Zoladex Early Breast Cancer Research Association (ZEBRA) study (6). In this study, premenopausal patients with axillary lymph node positive disease were randomized to receive goserelin subcutaneously every 28 days for 2 years compared with CMF given in 4 weekly schedules, with per oral cyclophosphamide and intravenous methotrexate and 5-fluorouracil on days 1 and 8, every cycle for 6 cycles. Patients with estrogen-positive, estrogen-negative and estrogen-unknown tumors were included in the ZEBRA study. Again, patients with amenorrhea at 36 weeks had a significantly better disease-free survival ($p = 0.005$) compared to those without (6) (Fig. 1). For patients with ER+ tumors, there was no difference between goserelin and CMF (6). Similar data have been reported from the Danish-Swedish study comparing

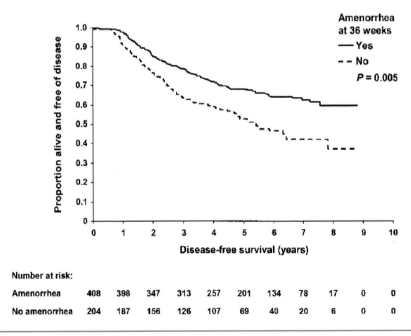

Figure 1 Effect of amenorrhea on disease-free survival over time in the CMF arm of the ZEBRA study. (From Ref. 6)

radiotherapy-induced oophorectomy (or surgical oophorectomy) to intravenous CMF given every third week for nine cycles for patients with estrogen- or progesterone-positive tumors (7).

The ZEBRA study, however, strongly underlined the need to include the correct patients in this type of study (6). ER– patients had a significantly worse survival rate in the goserelin group [hazard ratio = 1.77; 95% confidence interval (CI) = 1.19–2.63] (6). At 5 years there was a calculated 15% survival benefit for those randomized to CMF.

In conclusion, for premenopausal patients with receptor-positive breast cancer, the available data demonstrate an improved outcome for patients achieving amenorrhea. Amenorrhea can be induced by surgical oophorectomy, radiotherapy-induced oophorectomy or by the use of luteinizing hormone-releasing hormone (LHRH) analogues. CMF-based regimens result in equivalent outcomes in comparison with oophorectomy.

IV. ANTHRACYCLINE- AND TAXANE-CONTAINING REGIMENS

In an overview analysis by EBCTCG, anthracycline-containing polychemotherapy compared to CMF-like regimens resulted in a statistically significant relative survival improvement of 11% ($\pm$5) (3).

In the recently reported study 9344 from Cancer and Leukemia Group B (CALGB), 3,151 patients were randomized between doxorubicin at three different dose levels (60 mg/m^2, 75 mg/m^2, and 90 mg/m^2) and cyclophosphamide 600 mg/m^2 given for four cycles. These regimens were randomly compared with four additional cycles of paclitaxel (8). The eight-course regimens with paclitaxel, compared with the four-course regimens without paclitaxel, resulted in a significant survival advantage for those receiving paclitaxel ($p = 0.098$, unadjusted Wilcoxon) (8). Subgroup analyses revealed that paclitaxel conferred additional benefits regardless of nodal status, tumor size, and patient age, although the largest effect was seen in patients with receptor-negative disease and in those not receiving tamoxifen (8).

CALGB 9741, another recent study from CALGB with 2,005 randomized patients, compared concurrent and sequential doxorubicin, cyclophosphamide, and paclitaxel given every second or third week (9). The two-weekly schedules resulted in a significant survival advantage ($p = 0.013$, relative risk 0.69) at a short median follow-up of 36 months (9). Forty-eight to 50% of the patients were premenopausal in this study (9). The overall hazard reductions were 19% for patients with ER+ disease and 32% for patients with ER– disease (9).

Docetaxel has also been studied in the lymph-node-positive group of patients. In a study by the Breast Cancer International Research Group, a total of 1,491 patients were randomized to receive six courses of TAC (docetaxel 75 mg/m^2, doxorubicin 50 mg/m^2, cyclophosphamide 500 mg/m^2) versus six courses of FAC (5-FU 500 mg/m^2, doxorubicin 50 mg/m^2, cyclophosphamide 500 mg/m^2) (10). Sixty-nine percent of the patients had either ER+ or PR+ tumors and approximately 50% of the patients were defined as premenopausal. TAC therapy significantly improved disease-free survival ($p = 0.005$, relative risk 0.62) compared to FAC in patients with receptor negative disease (10). Patients with receptor-positive breast cancer also had a significant benefit ($p = 0.02$, RR 0.68) (10).

V. AMENORRHEA INDUCTION BY DIFFERENT REGIMENS

In many studies, detailed data on amenorrhea in relation to receptor status have not been reported. Classical CMF has been demonstrated to be very efficient in amenorrhea induction, with 61% of patients less than 40 years of age achieving amenorrhea by classical CMF (11) (Table 1). For patients 40 years and older, the corresponding figure was 95% (11). The previous U.S. standard regimen containing doxorubicin and cyclophosphamide has been demonstrated to induce amenorrhea in 34% of patients (12). The Canadian FEC regimen containing per oral cyclophosphamide, and epirubicin delivered on days 1 and 8, was described to induce amenorrhea in 51% of the treated patients (13). Nabholtz has compared the induction of amenorrhea by TAC versus FAC; the former induced amenorrhea in 51.4%, while the latter induced amenorrhea in 32.8% of patients (10) (Table 1).

Thus, classical CMF seem to be at least as good as conventional doxorubicin-containing regimens in amenorrhea induction (Table 1). In the overview comparison between CMF-like regimens and anthracycline-containing polychemotherapy, there was a slight benefit for the latter (3). However, these data are

Table 1 Efficacy of Amenorrhea Induction by Different Chemotherapy Regimens

Adjuvant chemotherapy	Incidence of amenorrhea (%)
Cyclophosphamide, methotrexate, fluorouracil (CMF)	61 (<40 years)
	95 (≥40 years)
Doxirubicin, cyclophosphamide (AC)	34
Fluorouracil, doxorubicin, cyclophosphamide (FAC)	32.8
Docetaxel, doxorubicin, cyclophosphamide (TAC)	51.4
Doxorubicin-based	59
Cyclophosphamide, epiribicin, fluorouracil (CEF)	51

Source: Ref. 20.

based on analyses on both receptor-negative and receptor-positive patients, so the conclusions, especially for patients with receptor-positive disease, must be treated with caution.

VI. SCANDINAVIAN BREAST GROUP STUDY 9401

The Scandinavian Breast Group Study 9401 (SBG 9401) was a randomized study in high-risk women under 60 years of age (14). The patients were estimated to have approximately 70% risk of relapse within 5 years, based on three Scandinavian registries (14). An individual-tailored and G-CSF-supported FEC-regimen was randomly compared to conventional FEC therapy followed by marrow-supported high-dose therapy with cyclophosphamide (6 g/m^2), thiotepa (0.5 g/m^2), and carboplatin (0.8 g/m^2) (14). Patients in the tailored arm received nine courses of FEC, while patients in the other arm received three (four) courses of FEC followed by the CTCb-regimen. Patients in the tailored regimens were given epirubicin doses varying from 38 mg/m^2 to 120 mg/m^2, and cyclophosphamide from 450 mg/m^2 to 1800 mg/m^2. 5-FU was administered from 300 mg/m^2 to 600 mg/m^2. Six different dose levels were used and patients received unchanged, escalated, or reduced doses based on the hematological toxicity recorded after 1, 1.5, and 2 weeks following each course (14). All patients were to be started at $F_{600}E_{75}C_{900}$ with G-CSF support from days 2 to 15 and prophylactic antibiotics from days 5 to 15 (14).

Patients in the G-CSF-supported and tailored FEC arm had statistically significantly fewer breast cancer relapses compared with standard FEC followed by marrow support (14). There was no difference in overall survival.

In a subanalysis of SBG 9401, the breast cancer relapse risk was calculated in relation to given doses; patients had similar breast cancer relapse risks, regardless of delivered dose levels. However, this does not mean that the dose level does not matter. The principle in this study was that each patient was treated according to the optimal dose that the patient required based on toxicity (14). The actual delivered dose level indicated that patients can receive markedly different dose levels if treated on the basis of equivalent toxicity.

The individually tailored therapy principle has recently been tested once more in the recently completed SBG 2000-1 study comparing seven courses of standard FEC versus tailored FEC without G-CSF support. By the end of the study in August 2003, 1,533 patients were randomized. The frequency of amenorrhea unfortunately was not recorded in the SBG 9401 study. However, it can be speculated that very few patients would not experience induction of amenorrhea unless they were very young, based on the very high cumulative doses of cyclophosphamide. The median dose of cyclophosphamide was 10,238 mg/m^2 and 8,400 mg/m^2 in the tailored FEC arm and standard FEC–CBCb high-dose arm, respectively (14). The corresponding epirubicin doses were 780 mg/m^2 and 181 mg/m^2, respectively (14).

VII. HORMONAL STATUS: THE BEST AND ONLY WAY FORWARD?

HR status in primary breast cancer is a powerful predictive instrument. Immunohistochemical determination of ER and PR status is today a widely accepted method to assign patients to different hormonal therapy modalities. It is recognized that the immunohistochemical expression in most tumors is markedly heterogeneous. The accepted cut-off level for receptor positivity in many studies is at least 10% positive cells, while a lower level of only 1% to 10% has also been indicated to be useful for the application of adjuvant endocrine therapy (15).

Hormonal status alone may not be enough to judge whether a patient should receive only hormonal therapy, a combination of hormonal therapy and chemotherapy, or chemotherapy alone. There is no question that the separation of breast cancer into hormone responsive (receptor positive) or unresponsive is valuable in clinical practice. However, it may not be the only way forward for therapy selections in the future because some patients with clearly hormone responsive disease will have no benefit from this type of therapy. In the future we must explore strategies for understanding the biology of small subgroups/individuals not behaving as expected according to present prognostic and predictive factors.

Current calculations of relapse risk and choice of therapy are based on group statistics from analyses of prospective and retrospective studies. However, judgment of this factor in the future may require more strategies for understanding the biology of smaller groups or even individual patients because present group statistics cannot predict who will relapse or respond to therapy.

Advances in research techniques and strategies may allow an increased understanding of breast cancer biology, thereby improving the potential for prognostic and predictive potential. For example, microarray-data using the HG U133 Affymetrix chips contain expression information from approximately 33,000 human genes (16). In a recent study on patients initially treated between 1994 and 1996, we found that around one-third of these genes were expressed in the breast cancer samples. ER– and PR– were found to have genes with discriminatory expression compared with ER or PR-containing tumors. These data further indicate that we may have to have additional information on patients with receptor-positive disease versus receptor-negative disease in our future therapy decisions. Breast cancer is a far more complex disease than the present separation of patients into hormone-responsive and hormone-unresponsive patients.

The more sophisticated separation of breast cancer into several subgroups has previously been illustrated in a study that classified breast carcinomas into five or six distinct diseases having a similar prognosis, based on variation of gene expression derived from microarray-expression data (17). It has also been demonstrated that the application of the array-technology will allow improved prognostic value for breast cancer patients (18). By the use of these 70 genes identified by the Dutch group, it was demonstrated that the gene-array-expression determination allowed a better risk separation of patients compared with the NIH or the commonly used St. Gallen criteria (19).

VIII. CONCLUSION

Polychemotherapy is very well documented for therapy of premenopausal patients with both axillary-lymph-node-negative and -positive disease. The mortality reduction by polychemotherapy is potentially higher in the receptor-negative group, compared to patients with receptor-positive disease. The reduction in relapse and improved survival by adjuvant chemotherapy in premenopausal patients with receptor-positive disease, especially with CMF-based regimens, appears to be related to the induction of amenorrhea.

Classical CMF is efficient in inducing amenorrhea in premenopausal patients. No upfront and randomized comparative studies exist between classical CMF and anthracycline-based regimens or taxanes in relation to the potential to induce amenorrhea and the relationship to outcome. Indirect comparisons indicate a potentially lower induction of amenorrhea by these regimens, but comparisons are difficult because different schedules and total doses have been used in different studies. However, regimens containing anthracyclines or taxanes or especially high-dose intensity of epirubicin offer an additional significant survival benefit compared with CMF-based therapy. However, outcomes in studies have not been prospectively analyzed for many of these anthracycline/taxane-containing regimens in relation to receptor status and induction of amenorrhea.

Recent microarray data strongly support the hypothesis that breast cancer no longer can be considered as a single disease entity, but rather as multiple-disease entities requiring separation into multiple subgroups in addition to the receptor-positive and receptor-negative groups. Further developments will allow further studies in this area, potentially with the addition of proteomic data, which may allow a deeper understanding of the different subgroup entities and potentially allowing the possibility of better and more tailored prognostic data and therapy prediction for each patient.

REFERENCES

1. Early Breast Cancer Trialists' Collaborative Group. Ovarian ablation in early breast cancer: overview of the randomised trials. Lancet 1996; 348:1189–1196.
2. Early Breast Cancer Trialists' Collaborative Group. Tamoxifen for early breast cancer: an overview of the randomised trials. Lancet 1998; 351:1451–1467.
3. Early Breast Cancer Trialists' Collaborative Group. Polychemotherapy for early breast cancer: an overview of the randomised trials. Lancet 1998; 352:930–942.
4. Emens LA, Davidson NE. Adjuvant hormonal therapy for premenopausal women with breast cancer. Clin Cancer Res 2003; 9:486S–494S.

5. Pagani O, O'Neill A, Castiglione M, Gelber RD, Goldhirsch A, Rudenstam CM, Lindtner J, Collins J, Crivellari D, Coates A, Cavalli F, Thurlimann B, Simoncini E, Fey M, Price K, Senn HJ. Prognostic impact of amenorrhoea after adjuvant chemotherapy in premenopausal breast cancer patients with axillary node involvement: results of the International Breast Cancer Study Group (IBCSG) Trial VI. Eur J Cancer 1998; 34:632–640.

6. Jonat W, Kaufmann M, Sauerbrei W, Blamey R, Cuzick J, Namer M, Fogelman I, de Haes JC, de Matteis A, Stewart A, Eiermann W, Szakolczai I, Palmer M, Schumacher M, Geberth M, Lisboa B. Goserelin versus cyclophosphamide, methotrexate, and fluorouracil as adjuvant therapy in premenopausal patients with node-positive breast cancer: The Zoladex Early Breast Cancer Research Association Study. J Clin Oncol 2002; 20:4628–4635.

7. Ejlertsen B, Dombernowsky P, Mouridsen H, Kjaer M, Rose C, Andersen K, Jensen M, Bengtsson N-O, Bergh J. Comparable effect of ovarian ablation and CMF chemotherapy in premenopausal high risk hormone receptor positive breast cancer (PHRP). Thirty-Fifth Annual Meeting of American Society of Clinical Oncology, Atlanta, GA, May 15–18, 1999.

8. Henderson IC, Berry DA, Demetri GD, Cirrincione CT, Goldstein LJ, Martino S, Ingle JN, Cooper MR, Hayes DF, Tkaczuk KH, Fleming G, Holland JF, Duggan DB, Carpenter JT, Frei E 3rd, Schilsky RL, Wood WC, Muss HB, Norton L. Improved outcomes from adding sequential Paclitaxel but not from escalating Doxorubicin dose in an adjuvant chemotherapy regimen for patients with node-positive primary breast cancer. J Clin Oncol 2003; 21:976–983.

9. Citron ML, Berry DA, Cirrincione C, Hudis C, Winer EP, Gradishar WJ, Davidson NE, Martino S, Livingston R, Ingle JN, Perez EA, Carpenter J, Hurd D, Holland JF, Smith BL, Sartor CI, Leung EH, Abrams J, Schilsky RL, Muss HB, Norton L. Randomized trial of dose-dense versus conventionally scheduled and sequential versus concurrent combination chemotherapy as postoperative adjuvant treatment of node-positive primary breast cancer: first report of Intergroup Trial C9741/Cancer and Leukemia Group B Trial 9741. J Clin Oncol 2003; 21:1431–1439.

10. Nabholtz J-M, Pienkowski T, Mackey J, Pawlicki M, Guastalla J-P, Vogel C, Weaver C, Walley B, Martin M, Chap L, Tomiak E, Juhos E, Guevin R, Howell A, Hainsworth J, Fornander T, Blitz S, Gazel S, Loret C, Riva A, Breast Cancer Intl Research LA, CA. Phase III trial comparing TAC (docetaxel, doxorubicin, cyclophosphamide) with FAC (5-fluorouracil, doxorubicin, cyclophosphamide) in the adjuvant treatment of node positive breast cancer (BC) patients: interim analysis of the BCIRG 001 study. Thirty-Eighth Annual Meeting of American Society of Clinical Oncology, Orlando, FL, May 18–21, 2002.

11. Goldhirsch A, Gelber RD, Castiglione M. The magnitude of endocrine effects of adjuvant chemotherapy for premenopausal breast cancer patients. The International Breast Cancer Study Group. Ann Oncol 1990; 1:183–188.

12. Bines J, Oleske DM, Cobleigh MA. Ovarian function in premenopausal women treated with adjuvant chemotherapy for breast cancer. J Clin Oncol 1996; 14:1718–1729.

13. Levine M, Bramwell V, Pritchard K, Norris B, Shepherd L, Abu-Zahra H, Findlay B, Warr D, Bowman D, Myles J, Arnold A, Vandenberg T, MacKenzie R, Robert J,

Ottaway J, Burnell M, Williams C, Tu D. Randomized trial of intensive cyclophosphamide, epirubicin, and fluorouracil chemotherapy compared with cyclophosphamide, methotrexate, and fluorouracil in premenopausal women with node-positive breast cancer. National Cancer Institute of Canada Clinical Trials Group. J Clin Oncol 1998; 16:2651–2658.

14. Bergh J, Wiklund T, Erikstein B, Lidbrink E, Lindman H, Malmstrom P, Kellokumpu-Lehtinen P, Bengtsson NO, Soderlund G, Anker G, Wist E, Ottosson S, Salminen E, Ljungman P, Holte H, Nilsson J, Blomqvist C, Wilking N. Tailored fluorouracil, epirubicin, and cyclophosphamide compared with marrow-supported high-dose chemotherapy as adjuvant treatment for high-risk breast cancer: a randomised trial. Scandinavian Breast Group 9401 study [in process citation]. Lancet 2000; 356:1384–1391.

15. Harvey JM, Clark GM, Osborne CK, Allred DC. Estrogen receptor status by immunohistochemistry is superior to the ligand-binding assay for predicting response to adjuvant endocrine therapy in breast cancer. J Clin Oncol 1999; 17:1474–1481.

16. Bjohle J, Pawitan Y, Skoog L, Shaw P, Amler L, Humphreys K, Huang F, Egyhazi S, Borg A-L, Hagerstrom T, Wedren S, Sandelin K, Hall P, Bergh J. Microarray studies on a population based breast cancer cohort: search for gene profiles with prognostic and predictive value. 25th Annual San Antonio Breast Cancer Symposium, San Antonio, TX, December 11–14, 2002; 76(suppl 1).

17. Sorlie T, Perou CM, Tibshirani R, Aas T, Geisler S, Johnsen H, Hastie T, Eisen MB, van de Rijn M, Jeffrey SS, Thorsen T, Quist H, Matese JC, Brown PO, Botstein D, Eystein Lonning P, Borresen-Dale AL. Gene expression patterns of breast carcinomas distinguish tumor subclasses with clinical implications. Proc Natl Acad Sci U S A 2001; 98:10869–10874.

18. van't Veer LJ, Dai H, van de Vijver MJ, He YD, Hart AA, Mao M, Petersen HL, van der Kooy K, Marton MJ, Witteveen AT, Schreiber GJ, Kerkhoven RM, Roberts C, Linsley PS, Bernards R, Friend SH. Gene expression profiling predicts clinical outcome of breast cancer. Nature 2002; 415:530–536.

19. van de Vijver MJ, He YD, van't Veer LJ, Dai H, Hart AA, Voskuil DW, Schreiber GJ, Peterse JL, Roberts C, Marton MJ, Parrish M, Atsma D, Witteveen A, Glas A, Delahaye L, van der Velde T, Bartelink H, Rodenhuis S, Rutgers ET, Friend SH, Bernards R. A gene-expression signature as a predictor of survival in breast cancer. N Engl J Med 2002; 347:1999–2009.

20. Minton SE, Munster PN. Chemotherapy-induced amenorrhea and fertility in women undergoing adjuvant treatment for breast cancer.Cancer Control 2002; 9:466–472.

2

Therapy in Premenopausal Women

Gini F. Fleming and Jan G. M. Klijn, *Chairmen*

Monday, July 7, 2003

J. Klijn: Thank you, Jonas [Bergh] for this last presentation. In line with your last remarks, I would like to show two slides to start the discussion. I have the first one. After the publication of the two trials, the ZEBRA trial and the Austrian study last year in the *Journal of Clinical Oncology* (December 15, 2002), Kathleen Pritchard wrote an editorial (J Clin Oncol 2002; 20:4611). You see these remarks: "While many questions remain to be answered, it seems clear that we must begin to think of endocrine therapy as a legitimate alternative to chemotherapy in the adjuvant treatment of women with receptor-positive breast cancer. This form of targeted therapy has probably been greatly under-used in North America and perhaps in other parts of the world as well. . . ."

What is really the key in hormone-receptor-positive patients will be endocrine treatment, certainly when we are able to improve the efficacy of endocrine treatment now and in the future.

C. K. Osborne: It seems like we've been focusing, particularly our European colleagues, on the issue that Dr. Pritchard raised there. That is, the underutilization of endocrine therapy perhaps by people in the United States, which I agree with. But that's not the important issue now. There is no question that endocrine therapy is important in premenopausal receptor-positive patients. Many of us use it all the time.

The real question is: For whom and when should we add on chemotherapy? That I still am confused about. Or when should we add endocrine therapy on to those who have gotten chemotherapy? Most people would treat those who have node-positive disease with chemotherapy. When do we add

137

on goserelin? Is it only in those that don't achieve amenorrhea? Would tamoxifen do just as well, chemotherapy plus tamoxifen, without any LHRH agonist or ovarian ablation?

Those are the questions that we still don't know the answers to. The Intergroup trial would have answered them if we'd been smart enough to have a fourth arm: chemotherapy plus tamoxifen. The issue now is who should get the combination of the two as opposed to either one alone? I think everyone would agree that if you're going to give chemotherapy or endocrine therapy in a low-risk patient, endocrine therapy would be the choice. It's at least as good and less toxic. But who should we give both to? That's the issue.

J. Klijn: May I have a question to Kent? How do you treat premenopausal estrogen-receptor-positive early breast cancer in daily clinical practice?

C. K. Osborne: Low-risk cancers I treat with tamoxifen alone; higher-risk ones I treat with both chemotherapy and tamoxifen. In some of those patients, particularly the younger ones and those at very high risk, I may give ovarian ablation of one sort or another along with tamoxifen, although I'm not certain that tamoxifen alone wouldn't be just as good.

W. Jonat: I would like to show two short slides from the ZEBRA trial focusing on the question which you just raised. One of the major points, of course, is still about chemotherapy and amenorrhea. We have analyzed this question a bit. What you can see here are patients who become amenorrheic. Patients who are amenorrheic due to CMF; patients who are amenorrheic due to hormone therapy alone; patients on CMF and nonamenorrheic, cytotoxic effect alone, hormone effect alone, combination of cytotoxic and hormone effect, showing superiority for the combination.

I think these data are previously unreported and although they are not randomized data, they more or less show what we are looking for. Of course, we need further data on age subgroups.

W. Eiermann: I would like to ask a question to Walter [Jonat] regarding the slide here. Is there any age dependency of the Zoladex® effect? Is the duration of amenorrhea with Zoladex age dependent?

W. Jonat: Of course this is just the whole group of all premenopausal patients and going into subgroups would make it too small.

A. Howell: This analysis is very problematic because basically what you're doing is comparing older patients with CMF versus younger patients with CMF. You haven't made the age adjustment, have you?

W. Jonat: We have. I didn't show these data.

A. Howell: In age-adjusted data do you get the same?

W. Jonat: We do. We can do age adjustment. It's just age groups looking at 35 to 40 and 40 to 45.

I. Smith: Can I ask you another question on that? We tend to be more confident giving chemotherapy in patients who are node positive. Can you split it down?

W. Jonat: These are all node-positive patients.

M. Ellis: The important next diagnostic step is to be able to differentiate ER+ endocrine-therapy-sensitive disease from estrogen-receptor-positive endocrine-therapy-insensitive. I believe a step has been made down that path by Filipits et al., from the Austrian Breast and Colorectal Cancer Study Group (ABCSG) Trial 5 presented at ASCO 2003. They examined P27^{Kip1} which looked quite promising as a predictor of sensitivity to goserelin/tamoxifen versus CMF in premenopausal women. Combination endocrine therapy was superior to CMF in patients with high P27^{Kip1} expression but not in those with low P27^{Kip1} expression.

P. Lonning: Did you also measure the cyclins? Was the P27 just a reflection of an increased level of cyclin D or cyclin E?

R. Jakesz: Yes, that's right. We have done that as well. P27 was the most differentiating one.

R. Santen: I'd like to ask a "Craig Henderson" question. Looking at existing data, one may ask whether chemotherapy works exclusively by chemical castration in ER+ premenopausal patients in the advanced setting. I've been trying to follow the data to see if we have an answer to that question now. In order to answer that question, we would have to take estrogen-receptor-positive, premenopausal patients with advanced disease, put them on a GNRH agonist and show that it clearly did lower the estrogen levels to postmenopausal levels with no FSH escape.

   After exposure to that manipulation for a period of time, one would add chemotherapy or placebo. It seems to me that's the only way to directly answer the question, which I've heard Craig Henderson ask multiple times over the past several years. Perhaps I have missed something? Do we have data now that incontrovertibly proves that chemotherapy adds something to ovarian ablation in that setting? I'm seeing a lot of no's. Do we have any positive data? Isn't it necessary that we obtain data to answer that question?

C. K. Osborne: That's indirect data right there.

R. Santen: But I think you have to block the ovaries first so that you have a patient who really is postmenopausal. At that time, when the tumor is quiescent, one then adds chemotherapy or placebo and observes the clinical outcome.

C. K. Osborne: In that case you may be counteracting the effectiveness of the chemotherapy with your hormone therapy. I think it's a more complicated issue to think about than you might think. You could argue the fact that chemo works very well in estrogen-receptor-negative patients which would suggest that there is a nonovarian ablation effect. That may be only in those tumors that are estrogen-receptor-negative. It may not be in those tumors that are estrogen-receptor-positive. That data that was just up there, the CMF ovarian ablation was a lot better than the Zoladex® ovarian ablation, which would implicate a chemotherapy effect. There are other indirect data. But it's not so simple to study because of the impact of ovarian ablation.

T. Powles: I want to ask a slightly different but related question. Do we have any evidence now from the trials that have been done with the use of Zoladex® that it will protect against permanent amenorrhea or protect against infertility? It's very relevant in our choice of treatment. I think the one single big factor is the loss of fertility when using chemotherapy in premenopausal women. Is there any evidence now?

I. Smith: There are two or three small uncontrolled studies, which tend to show very positive results at a very high rate of recurrence of ovarian function in patients who have had Zoladex® and then chemotherapy. We've been doing this ourselves and again in fairly small numbers, 30 or 35 women. We certainly don't see recurrence of ovarian function in anything like the 95% or so that's reported in the literature. It's not been looked at in a properly controlled group.

I. C. Henderson: Coming back to this question of the combination of therapies, I certainly did take the argument that Kent [Osborne] made for quite a few years. That is, if there is an effect, for example, in postmenopausal receptor-negative patients, and I think that's unequivocal, then it must have an effect against any receptor-negative tumor cells. However, there is something that strikes me just looking at the clinical data alone, and I think you could also make arguments based on preclinical data. Is the impact of endocrine therapy much greater than you would predict just looking at the estrogen-receptor positivity of the cells?

For example, I wrote in the early 1980s that we wouldn't have a big impact on survival (with hormone therapy) because I felt that you had to have close to 100% of the cells receptor positive. That definitely has not proven to be the case. That was sort of dogma in the early years of adjuvant therapy, that you had to somehow destroy something in excess of 99% of the cancer cells in order to have much of an impact on survival. That's not the case.

If we look at recent data coming from the Baylor group, tumors that have really a very, very small percentage of receptor-positive cells show regression that exceeds the amount that you would predict. I think that the question you raised, Dick [Santen], underscores the point that Kent [Osborne] made, that the complexity of this issue is quite a bit greater than we've thought. Sometimes our oversimplification leads us to conclusions that are inappropriate, such as that these therapies are always going to be additive. Maybe that comes back to what Matt [Ellis] was raising as an issue that the heterogeneity among what we call estrogen-receptor-negative and what we call estrogen-receptor-positive tumors, is in fact much more variable than we recognized thus far.

Going on from that, I'd like to ask a kind of practical question, picking up on one of the points that Kent [Osborne] made. That is, he said he would treat patients who are at low risk with tamoxifen alone. It seems to me that when we treat any group of patients we should at least offer them whatever is the optimal therapy, whatever gives them the greatest benefit. They may choose a therapy that has less toxicity and less benefit, but they certainly should be given the option of the therapy with the greatest benefit. Are you convinced that we have sufficient evidence right now that tamoxifen is as good as ovarian ablation in patients with endocrine sensitive tumors? Do we have sufficient evidence to conclude that?

C. K. Osborne: It is probably better but we don't have the evidence.

I. C. Henderson: It seems to me that was a mistake in the take-home point from the overviews. By putting all the patients together and comparing tamoxifen versus no tamoxifen, it has resulted in a lot of patients who have been made postmenopausal (by chemotherapy) in that group. It's such a heterogeneous group to begin with that I wonder if we're short-changing patients. Have we closed our minds to this issue prematurely in younger premenopausal women?

W. Eiermann: I don't want to make things still more complicated with amenorrhea. Amenorrhea does not mean that this patient is in a postmenopausal situation. Amenorrhea means that there is no more cyclic ovulation. The estrogen values can be higher than postmenopausal values. So the symptom of amenorrhea does not necessarily mean a patient is postmenopausal. We have to reexamine these patients, for example, to look at the real estradiol values they have. They still can be premenopausal. This makes the discussion more complicated.

R. Santen: I was going to make this comment before because it's come up several times in the discussion. I think it's very important to focus on some new physiology that we know about normal breast. Normal breast only has about 1–2% of cells that are estrogen-receptor positive.

Several Speakers: 20%

R. Santen: OK, so let's say 20%. I'm quoting Jose Russo's and Bob Clark's data. But basically the cells in the breast that are estrogen-receptor-positive are not the cells that are dividing. The cell that is estrogen-receptor-positive resides next to [the] cell that is Ki67+. In the normal breast situation, estrogen is really working via a paracrine mechanism. The best explanation is that estrogen binds to the estrogen receptor and stimulates growth factors. Those growth factors then travel to and bind to the cells that are surrounding the normal estrogen-receptor-positive cells and stimulate proliferation of cells lacking estrogen-receptor but containing growth-factor receptors.

   Marc Lippman and others presented data regarding MCF-7 cells many years ago, suggesting that estrogen could directly stimulate cell proliferation in breast cells. These data may be a bit misleading. These observations would suggest that a breast cell has to work in an autocrine or an endocrine fashion, where the estrogen is acting directly on the cell where the estrogen is made. If we take the concept that you have a few estrogen-receptor-positive cells, and it may be as few as 5% in a tumor, those few cells are really the drivers. Those are the cells that respond to estrogen and stimulate the remaining breast cancer cells through paracrine, growth-factor-mediated mechanisms.

   When we begin to analyze immunohistochemistry and say that 5% of the cells in that tumor are receptor positive and, therefore, hormone sensitive, 95% are receptor negative and, therefore, hormone insensitive, this is not really a concept that we can hold onto any further. Clearly, estrogen can bind to the cells that have estrogen receptor and drive the proliferation of others. I think that's a very important concept when we begin to look at these kinds of data.

C. K. Osborne: We'd better be cautious in interpreting immunohistochemical data. First of all, we've known for a long time, even from the days of biochemical data, that we always used a cut off of undetectable values to be positive or negative. Values between 3 and 10 fmol per milligram protein were considered to predict good response rates to hormonal therapy. I'm not sure why people raised the cutoff to 10, but it became routine. We weren't surprised when we saw very low percentages of hormone receptor cells still being able to predict benefit from tamoxifen adjuvant therapy. In fact, the biggest difference is between less than 1% of cells and between 1 and 10% of cells. That's a much bigger difference than the higher and higher levels of estrogen-receptors in terms of tamoxifen benefit in our study.

   We're looking at the percent of cells that have estrogen receptor at that moment. We know that estrogen receptor is cell cycle dependent. We're also looking at the limits of detection of the assay. It may be that when you detect a tumor that has some estrogen-receptor-positive cells, that means that the majority of those cells at some point in the cell cycle do express estrogen-receptor and would be sensitive to hormone therapy. Or that even in those cells where we can't measure it, the fact that we can see it in some cells means that they all have it below the limits of detection of the assay and they respond. While I think the things that you bring up are certainly more likely the possibility, I think we don't know for sure whether these other cells are, in fact, estrogen responsive because they have receptor at some other point in time that we're not seeing, or that they have very low levels of receptor that are still biologically relevant.

R. Santen: Just to respond quickly if I can. Gerald Cunha has done some beautiful work, mixing estrogen-receptor-negative cells and estrogen-receptor-positive cells obtained from transgenic animals. This model represents benign, not malignant, tissue. But I think his model really gets around the concept that you're raising that a cell might have a receptor at one time, and not at another. He clearly shows that estrogen-receptor-positive cells can stimulate surrounding estrogen-receptor-negative cells in a paracrine fashion. These experiments represent the benign situation, and it seems also to be true in prostate cancer and in other types of cancer that one can show this important paracrine mechanism. We need to think about this paradigm because we fairly routinely interpret the kinds of data that we've seen with a different explanation.

A. Howell: If I could just complete what you're saying, Dick. As you know, we were the first to show this separation between estrogen-receptor-positive and estrogen-receptor-negative cells in normal breast. In tumors, you find that estrogen-receptor-positive cells proliferate. Almost one of the first changes that one sees in ADH and DCIS is that separation is lost.

Our interpretation is that there is a paracrine effect in tumors because there are estrogen-receptor-positive and estrogen-receptor-negative cells within the tumor. But also estrogen is directly stimulating some of the estrogen-receptor-positive cells in the tumor as well as there being a potential paracrine effect in the cells.

C. K. Osborne: Regarding that, I forgot about a paper that we published back in the early '80s where we took estrogen-receptor-positive cells and mixed them with estrogen-receptor-negative cells and put them in a mouse. The hypothesis originally was that the estrogen-receptor-negative cells would release paracrine factors which would cause the estrogen-receptor-positive cells to grow in the absence of estrogen, and vice versa. If we didn't supplement the mice with estrogen, the only cells that grew out were estrogen-receptor-negative. If we did supplement the mouse with estrogen, the only cells that grew out were estrogen-receptor-positive. We weren't able to show the paracrine effect in either direction. It was a publication in one of the first issues of Breast Cancer Research and Treatment.

J. Klijn: Can you suggest any other factors, Kent, apart from the receptor, which may be important in tumors with only 5% positive estrogen-receptor cells?

C. K. Osborne: I think there are a couple of possibilities. Dick [Santen] mentioned one. When you shut off the estrogen-receptor in the estrogen-receptor-positive cells, you shut off the expression of the TGF alpha and EGF and IGF2 in some tumors that then would feed the estrogen-receptor-negative cells. That's certainly one possibility.

The other possibility is that the majority of the cells do have estrogen-receptors, if you were able to measure it over time. If you had a movie with live cells, which people are now starting to be able to do, you might find that this cell, 12 hours later in the cell cycle, does now express estrogen-receptor whereas it didn't at this time. Those are important issues that perhaps just now we have the technology to begin to look at.

M. Baum: In the same way, the other side of the coin may be the response to tamoxifen that could explain bystander effects, in that there is upregulation and induction of transforming growth factor beta and downregulation of insulin like factor 1 by using tamoxifen. Anthony Coletta in my lab some years ago suggested the induction of TGF beta from fibroblasts. So, just as it is complex to look at the estrogen effect, it's equally complex in interpreting the response to tamoxifen in cancers with a minority of receptor positive cells.

H. Sasano: I'd like to comment from the standpoint of a pathologist. I believe that one of the most important things is, as Dr. Osborne mentioned, that more than 1% receptor-positive cells may be the cutoff for prediction of benefit from hormone therapy in the patients with breast cancer. However, it is true that the great majority of pathology laboratories depends merely on the percentage of the positive cells. Recently, the intensity of each positive cell has also been shown to be important in predicting response to endocrine therapy or other biological treatments.

I believe that standardizations of both the scoring and the staining system of estrogen receptor immunohistochemistry are now becoming more important than before, considering recent development of endocrine therapy in the patients with breast cancer. In this regard, the scoring system as Professor Craig [Allred] had developed, which is a combination of intensity and also the absolute number of the cells, probably satisfies some of the questions that clinical colleagues raised in this discussion. I would like to emphasize again that the scoring system incorporating the number and intensity of positive carcinoma cells may also be a better evaluation method for estrogen-response protein such as EBAC 9 or efp, as well as cyclin-related protein. These four scoring methods probably select some patients' responses to the therapy. These scoring methods can select the patients who may respond to endocrine therapy with more precision. However, whatever markers will be introduced, the important thing is the standardization of procedure.

C. K. Osborne: I think you're absolutely right. In the United States in the early 1980s there was a major, federally funded program to standardize ligand binding assays. By the end of the 1980s everybody was doing it exactly the same way. If you got 50 femtomoles in this lab, you'd get 40 to 60 in that lab.

Now with immunohistochemistry, we're back to where we were in 1979 or 1980. According to the studies from the U.K., 30% of estrogen receptors are wrong by immunohistochemistry in the routine average laboratory. Craig will tell you the same thing is true in the United States I think there are a lot of patients who are not receiving potentially life-saving adjuvant endocrine therapy simply because their laboratory hasn't paid attention to how they do the receptor. They think it's an easy test. You just do it; get the cheapest antibody you can and run it.

R. Jakesz: We have made quality control. We run it continuously over all departments of pathology in Austria. It's a small country so it's easy to do. It's only twenty departments. But we are doing that continuously.

J. Ingle: For completeness sake, in the early-stage disease, some of the questions that Kent [Osborne] and other people have raised about the importance of amenorrhea in outcome, the role of aromatase inhibitors, what is the role of chemotherapy? Clearly things that people face every day. There is a triad of studies, I'm sure everybody is aware of, that will address these issues: SOFT, TEXT and PERCHE. These were developed with the IBCSG taking the lead and involvement of the Breast International Group and the North American Breast Intergroup. They are absolutely crucial studies that people have come to acknowledge to address important questions.

J. Klijn: Mitch, and then I would like to go for the last 10 minutes to clinical questions.

M. Dowsett: I really wanted to just go back to the postmenopausal setting and an analogous situation in the premenopausal setting. Perhaps the best clinical data we've got regarding the ability of breast tumors to acquire hypersensitivity to estrogens are with a GnRH agonist. Look at the patients who respond to a GnRH agonist and then relapse. When we add an aromatase inhibitor, these patients will respond in many cases. There was a very small study which Charles Coombes did back in about 1989 that showed that four out of six patients responded in those circumstances.

I'm just thinking about the adjuvant effects of oophorectomy. In those studies there are major separations of the lines in the overview analysis, and the lines do not come back together in this premenopausal situation when we're depriving the patient of estrogen. I just wonder whether that might be slightly reassuring to Kent [Osborne] in his consideration of the aromatase inhibitors in the postmenopausal situation. If the biology in the premenopausal woman is that we're sort of sensitizing these tumors to estrogen, yet those lines are not coming back together, can that reassure us in the postmenopausal setting? Can you respond to that, Kent?

C. K. Osborne: I don't know which way it's going to go in the postmenopausal setting. I think there are arguments that it could be beneficial by killing off cells or that it could also be detrimental. I think one of the reasons that I haven't switched over to aromatase inhibitors as a standard adjuvant therapy is that we don't know. We have many, many years of experience with tamoxifen. I'm intrigued that only two years of ovarian ablation in the German studies represent very good therapy. That's attractive for patients. I don't know which way it's going to go.

M. Dowsett: Can I just ask Dick [Santen] a very simple question. You said two words which provoked thought. In the goserelin-treated patients, you do get increases in FSH. This happens in male patients with prostate cancer as well. Can you just say a couple of words about the significance? How frequent that is? How frequently does it cause increases in estrogen levels? Is it sufficient for us to think that's really distinct from an oophorectomy?

R. Santen: I really can't answer that. The studies that I was referring to were mainly in men with prostate cancer. It was clear that the FSH levels went up over time, probably because of inhibin effects on negative feedback and effects on the testes. Clearly it occurs in premenopausal patients as well. I don't think that's been studied carefully enough to know what the effects on estrogen are in that situation or even whether systematic measurements of FSH levels have been adequately performed.

R. Jakesz: We're doing that routinely and we have never seen that.

M. Dowsett: You have never seen?

R. Jakesz: Never seen that LH or FSH goes up.

M. Dowsett: We published two papers on that several years ago. One was for Zoladex® and one was with Lupron®. LH levels stayed flat. They don't escape at all. FSH levels steadily increased. In the first study, we managed to do a little statistical investigation, sort of an exploratory analysis. We correlated the fact where their FSH increases were highest, the estrogen levels also increased. The estrogen levels didn't become premenopausal, but the levels were higher after six months than they were after four weeks.

R. Jakesz: But not with tamoxifen. We are measuring only with tamoxifen.

M. Dowsett: I think actually that's interesting data. If you give tamoxifen, the FSH no longer rises. The estrogen levels, therefore, stay low.

R. Santen: We need to concentrate a bit on the physiology here. In postmenopausal women, tamoxifen is an estrogen agonist on the pituitary. Clearly postmenopausal women on tamoxifen will have suppression of both LH and FSH. Here we are talking about premenopausal patients. This represents an open loop feedback situation. When you lower the level of estrogen with the GNRH superagonist analogue, by lowering LH and FSH, you'll lower ovarian inhibin levels. Inhibin is an alternate negative feedback regulator for FSH but not for LH. The physiology of FSH going up in the individuals with GNRH superagonist analogues is pretty well understood.

I don't know the data regarding what effect that rise of FSH has on the endogenous level of estrogen being made in those patients.

J. Klijn: In line with this discussion, it is very important to discuss what the optimal duration of treatment is with an LHRH agonist. It is now unknown. So a question to Walter Jonat. You showed that a certain number of women get recurrence during Zoladex® treatment. My question is, since recurrence was seen at 36 months of follow-up, does that mean that one year after stopping Zoladex® the patients [would be] having a recurrence in the Zoladex-only arm?

W. Jonat: Once again, it's just a question of age groups that you're looking into. We have looked into the question of being on Zoladex® in women over 35 years of age, as you would say, after 2.5 years. Half a year off Zoladex treatment, there was still an amenorrheic group and one group that did get the menstrual bleeding back. If we are comparing those two groups and the outcome, then there was no difference in the outcome.

So the amenorrheic group and the nonamenorrheic group are totally the same. Have in mind the sample size, only 327 patients. Of course it is of importance to look into the age subgroups. Once again, if we are looking at women 40 to 45 years, the curves are still exactly the same.

I. C. Henderson: How many patients in each of those two groups?

W. Jonat: This is exactly one of the points. The distribution is not exactly right. Of course there are more on Zoladex® who get menstrual bleeding. The proportion is one-third to two-thirds.

I. C. Henderson: One-third is permanent or not?

W. Jonat: Not permanent.

A. Howell: This is the remarkable result. Two years of amenorrhea is as good as permanent amenorrhea. The question is whether you are giving two or three endocrine therapies at the same time. You get amenorrhea for two years and then the estrogen goes up à la Dick Santen. Is that another endocrine therapy in which those patients may subsequently go through menopause and get a third endocrine therapy? That may be why the two years is as good as permanent amenorrhea.

R. Santen: Can I make a comment? I think there are a couple of very interesting things. One, we know that there is a carry-over effect of tamoxifen. Five years of tamoxifen use results in continuing benefit at 15 years. I don't think that we've focused sufficiently on the fact that these endocrine therapies may actually be cytotoxic. They trigger off apoptosis. We know that reduction of estrogen will kill cells through this mechanism. Is it possible as an explanation that if you give two years of depo Zoladex® and you have residual micrometastases or local hormone sensitive cells, you're basically killing the cells that are there via apoptosis?

Then when you stop, you don't have any cells left that can be hypersensitive and you don't have cancer cells left. What you've really done is destruction of a subset of cells. This concept obviously isn't proven, but it's very important when we start thinking about prevention of breast cancer. A lot of patients that we're treating with tamoxifen for breast cancer prevention probably have pre-existing small tumors. Some of those, we may be in essence curing through this pro apoptotic mechanism. Although we have to speculate about what may be going on, it is important not to implicate just one potential explanation for the effects seen with two years of depo Zoladex.

J. Klijn: For the last few minutes, let's focus on the role of aromatase inhibitors. Dick, do you think that when you have very low estrogen levels by the combination of LHRH agonists plus aromatase inhibitor that in that case more tumor cells will die than during the LHRH agonist treatment alone? Or do you expect no difference?

R. Santen: I can only speculate. I think we need data to find that out. Clearly when one lowers estrogen levels in MCF-7 cells, there is a dose-response curve to enhance apoptosis. In that setting it would suggest that further reduction of estrogen under some circumstances might kill more cells than a lesser reduction. That's really a major leap, extrapolating that in vitro data to predict the effects of the combination in women. My guess is yes, blockade of estrogen action and of ovarian synthesis of estrogen may be more effective. Or the aromatase inhibitors, where you're lowering the levels even further, may be even more effective.

I think that's only speculation at this point. We need to think about that. We need to test it to find out what our therapies are doing.

J. Klijn: There is one small Spanish study, presented in Paris, and data in the abstract book of the San Antonio Breast Cancer Conference last year which show that a combination of an LHRH agonist plus an aromatase inhibitor is more effective in metastatic disease than the combination of LHRH agonist with tamoxifen. My question to you as experts is: What do you expect of the application of aromatase inhibitors in premenopausal breast cancer? What is the role for aromatase inhibitors? Will it replace tamoxifen or not?

A. Howell: I'm waiting for the Austrian result.

J. Klijn: Indeed, these are very important.

R. Santen: I was very impressed with Steve Johnston's presentation this morning. I've seen these data previously. If you take the nude mouse xenograft model of breast cancer, the results from a comparison oophorectomy with a SERM, such as tamoxifen, are quite interesting. Lowering of estrogen as a result of oophorectomy is always more effective than any of the SERMs. I don't think that's been emphasized enough before. These results indicate to me that when one gives a SERM, it still has some estrogen-agonistic effects, even though it has a major estrogen-antagonist effect. These preclinical data comparing castration with tamoxifen suggest that there is some residual estrogen agonistic effect of the SERM under these circumstances.

You could apply these concepts to patients who have their ovaries medically downregulated by GNRH superagonist analogues. Under these circumstances, you could ask whether tamoxifen or an aromatase inhibitor might be better. I would be very concerned that under those circumstances, you still would have some estrogen agonistic effect of tamoxifen, which you don't have with an aromatase inhibitor. I think the data Steve [Johnston] showed is really very important in this regard.

C. K. Osborne: I think we should stop thinking of tamoxifen as an anti-estrogen. It's not. It is a weak estrogen. When you load the receptor with a weak estrogen, you have a little tiny bit of agonist activity but you're able to counteract the more potent 17-beta estradiol that was on the receptor. That amount of agonist activity, which in most breast cancers is a very small amount, can be made bigger by certain things that happen in the cell, to the point where tamoxifen could be bad or deleterious by stimulating the tumor.

149

It's a lot easier to explain the ATAC data, if you think of tamoxifen as being in most patients a weak estrogen, not an antiestrogen. It almost always has a little bit of agonist activity even in breast cancer cells. Cross-talk with growth factor pathway and then stress pathways is one of the mechanisms that can boost up its relative amount of agonist activity.

R. Santen: Steve [Johnston] showed another slide this morning that he didn't comment on. Tamoxifen, in the face of no estrogen, exerts primarily estrogen-agonistic properties. Tamoxifen in the presence of a lot of estrogen acts as an antagonist. He showed a beautiful slide where, with castration, tamoxifen stimulated uterine weight up to a given level. The intact animal, given tamoxifen, inhibited uterine weight down to the same level that tamoxifen stimulated it.

The condition of very low estrogen levels is exactly the setting in which tamoxifen will become an agonist, particularly as seen in the ATAC trial in which one is markedly lowering the estrogen levels with the aromatase inhibitor. I think when Mitch Dowsett and I objected to the combination, this was really the reasoning. The worst situation in which to add tamoxifen to an aromatase inhibitor is the one where there is very little estrogen present.

C. K. Osborne: Estrogen for the tamoxifen to antagonize.

S. Johnston: Therefore, do you think it would be a worthwhile approach if the SERMs were to have any resurgence, to take something that had very little agonist activity and put it on a background of low estrogen levels with aromatase inhibitors? I don't see anybody necessarily jumping up and down wanting to do that. There might be benefit in early disease, adjuvant setting, or prevention setting in having that combination. It's quite a high-risk strategy to go down a major development route going that way.

M. Dowsett: Perhaps someone else can answer this. I heard of a study which is a raloxifene plus one of the aromatase inhibitors in advanced disease. Does anybody else know of that and can anyone give an update on that?

J. Ingle: It's at Memorial Sloan Kettering. I think Maura Dickler is doing exemestane plus raloxifene. It's a neoadjuvant study.

Unidentified Speaker: Plus raloxifene; why raloxifene?

J. Ingle: Yes, it's a combination.

M. Dowsett: One does sort of wonder whether there could be a rationale there.

J. Klijn: Before closing this session, one last question.

I. Smith: It just relates to the discussion that Dick [Santen] and Kent [Osborne] have been having. In premenopausal advanced disease, overview trials of LHRH agonists alone versus the addition of tamoxifen show that the addition of tamoxifen is beneficial there. I just can't quite see how that works in view of these other discussions we've been having and in view of the ATAC data.

C. K. Osborne: The estrogen levels vary much with ovarian ablation. You still have aromatase there that is making a lot of estrogen in the tumor.

R. Santen: Remember that 30 years ago we knew that surgical adrenalectomy was effective when used in sequence after medical oophorectomy. The concept has now been raised. The tumors become more sensitive to estradiol after exposure to low levels following oophorectomy. Some people call this phenomenon the estrostat. That is, as the estrogen levels go down, the tumors become more sensitive to this. When you use the GNRH superagonist analogue and put the patient into menopause, the levels of estradiol are about 10 picograms per ml. That's just the situation where tamoxifen works in postmenopausal patients when you antagonize that amount of estrogen. So it seems that you are antagonizing a good deal of estrogen that is still present in that setting. Remember that the level of estrogen in the breast in a postmenopausal woman is about the same as the estrogen level in the breast in a premenopausal patient. There is really plenty of estrogen there to antagonize further. I think that's probably the most likely explanation.

J. Klijn: I'm sorry. I have to close this session. Maybe we can continue this discussion tomorrow. I wish you good afternoon.

10

Biology of Premalignant Lesions and Pathogenesis

D. Craig Allred

Baylor College of Medicine
Houston, Texas, U.S.A.

I. OVERVIEW

All invasive breast cancers evolve from premalignant lesions. The biological alterations behind this evolution represent potential prognostic factors for progression to invasive disease and, perhaps more importantly, targets for prevention. This paper reviews which lesions are the most important in terms of premalignant potential, their biological characteristics in terms of standard biomarkers, and the implications of pathological findings for chemoprevention. Little is known about the biological evolution of premalignant lesions into invasive disease, and progress in prevention depends on a better understanding of this biology, which should be a fundamental research priority.

II. INTRODUCTION

Because all invasive breast cancers arise from premalignant lesions, the biological alterations behind this evolution are potential prognostic factors for progression to invasive disease. Perhaps more importantly, such lesions may be potential targets for breast cancer prevention strategies. This chapter focuses on a few key issues of clinical relevance: 1) which lesions, from the many that exist, appear to be the most important in terms of premalignant potential and the evidence for their status; 2) the biological characteristics of these lesions, particularly as they relate to standard detectable biomarkers; and 3) the clinical implications of histological findings in terms of risk and prevention strategies.

III. MAJOR PREMALIGNANT LESIONS

Among the hundreds of permutations and combinations of proliferative breast lesions in humans, only a relatively small number are thought to be premalignant (Fig. 1). They include normal terminal duct lobular units (TDLU) simply because this is thought to be the stem cell compartment for all the other proliferative lesions (Fig. 1a). One of the earliest histological abnormalities with significant premalignant potential is the hyperplastic unfolded lobule (HUL), sometimes identified as

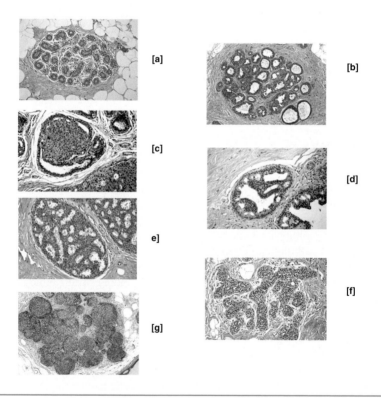

Figure 1 Major types of human premalignant breast lesions: (a) Terminal duct lobular units (TDLU). (b) Hyperplastic unfolded lobule (HUL). (c) Usual ductal hyperplasia (UDH). (d) Atypical ductal hyperplasia (ADH). (e) Ductal carcinoma in situ (DCIS). (f) Atypical lobular hyperplasia (ALH). (g) Lobular carcinoma in situ (LCIS).

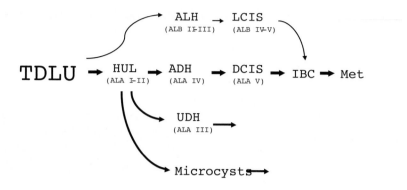

Figure 2 Evolutionary model for development of invasive breast cancer from premalignant lesions. (See legend to Fig. 1 for abbreviations.) (From Ref. 1)

clonal alteration of lobules or blunt duct adenosis (Fig. 1b). Other early lesions include usual ductal hyperplasia (UDH), also known as hyperplasia of the usual type (HUT) (Fig. 1c), atypical ductal hyperplasia (ADH, Fig. 1d), ductal carcinoma in situ (DCIS, Fig. 1e), and their lobular counterparts, atypical lobular hyperplasia (ALH, Fig.1f), and lobular carcinoma in situ (LCIS, Fig. 1g), each with its own unique histological features.

Although published nearly 30 years ago, the evolutionary model proposed by Jensen and Wellings based on the idea of histological continuity remains the most consistent with accumulated laboratory data (1). In their evolutionary scheme, TDLU play the central role as the stem cell repository for everything else that ensues (Fig. 2). There are two main lineages in the evolution toward invasive breast cancer: 1) the central lineage—evolving to so-called ductal carcinomas and accounting for 85% of invasive breast cancer—where TDLU gives rise to HUL, which gives rise to ADH and beyond; and 2) a second histologically independent, smaller evolutionary pathway, involving the so-called lobular neoplasias, where ALH evolves to LCIS and eventually invasive breast cancer. Some of the competing contemporary models for breast cancer evolution have placed UDH on the direct lineage to invasive breast cancer, but most recent thinking is that it represents a side branch on the evolutionary tree, with some importance at least as a risk factor because of shared ancestry through other lesions in the evolutionary scheme.

IV. EVIDENCE FOR AN EVOLUTIONARY MODEL OF PREMALIGNANCY

Virtually all of the evidence that exists regarding an evolutionary schema for premalignant lesions is correlative and indirect in nature. There is very little direct

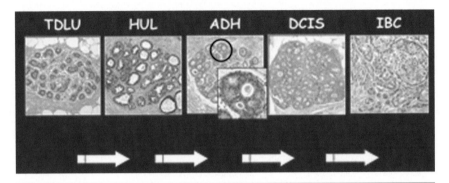

Figure 3 Histological continuum for the development of invasive breast cancer (IBC) from TDLU. (See legend to Figure 1 for abbreviations.) (From Ref. 1)

evidence, simply because the development of breast cancer in humans cannot be observed and animal models do not seem to be especially representative of the process in humans.

A. Histological Continuum

One of the most compelling arguments for the evolution of invasive breast cancer from a relatively small group of premalignant lesions remains the idea of histological continuity, perhaps best illustrated by focusing on the development of ductal carcinomas. As shown in Figure 3, the process starts with TDLU, which is a small terminal duct emanating from a subsegmental duct in the breast, and ending in a grapelike cluster of blind secretory acini. Each acinous is lined by a single layer of cuboidal secretory cells, scattered among which reside the stem cells.

A substantial subpopulation of TDLU cells undergo hyperplasia, i.e., relatively uncontrolled proliferation, until they evolve to a lesion called HUL, whose general overall shape is very similar to TDLU. Volumetrically, however, HUL are 100- to 1,000-fold larger, involving tens of thousands more cells. HUL are extraordinarily common, to the point where they are sometimes considered part of the spectrum of normal breast epithelium. In a subset of HULs, the epithelium continues to proliferate, accumulating within the acini and often expanding them in a cribriform growth pattern known as ADH. As that process continues in extent, it becomes DCIS. Eventually, a substantial subset of DCIS invades to become invasive breast cancer.

B. Frequency of Premalignant Lesions

Data from autopsy and mastectomy studies have shown that specific lesions are much more common in cancerous than noncancerous breasts. A review by the author of 24 mastectomy/autopsy studies performed since 1930 and involving about 5,300 patients indicates anywhere from a two-fold increase in the incidence of HUT to an approximately 20-fold increase in DCIS. In breasts without invasive cancer, the incidence of HUT, ADH, and DCIS were 25%, 5%, and 5%, respectively, compared to 50%, 50%, and 90%, respectively for those with invasive breast cancer (2, 3).

C. Risk Factors

Other pathological and epidemiological studies have demonstrated conclusively that premalignant lesions are risk factors for developing invasive breast cancer. Nearly all these studies are retrospective in nature and have calculated the relative risk, compared to age-matched controls, of eventually developing invasive breast cancer in patients who have had an excisional biopsy containing specific lesions. Again, a review by the author of 30 studies since 1960 involving over 120,000 patients indicates an approximately two-fold increase for HUL, a five-fold increase for ADH and a ten-fold increase in the incidence of DCIS in patients who develop invasive breast cancer compared to those who do not (2, 3). These findings are consistent with a large study by Dupont and Page (4).

D.   Genetic Evidence

The most recent types of evidence come from laboratory studies showing that these putative premalignant lesions share identical genetic abnormalities with synchronous invasive breast cancer in the same breast. To illustrate the idea of clonal evolution for important carcinogenic events, the author has reviewed more than 30 studies assessing allelic imbalance (loss of heterozygosity or LOH), and comparative genomic hybridization (CGH) at more than 100 loci on 17 chromosomes. From 40% to 90% of lesions involved in this evolutionary progression contain allelic imbalances, sometimes a dozen or more in a single lesion, such as high-grade DCIS at the far end of the spectrum. Among that subset of premalignant lesions that contain LOH and CGH, when they occur in the breast with invasive breast cancer, they share those identical genetic abnormalities in 50% to 90% of cases. Although LOH and CGH are relatively low resolution assays, the rate of sharing is virtually the same with defects examined using higher resolution assays.

V.   BIOMARKERS

Although evidence points to specific premalignant lesions as being involved in the development of invasive breast cancer, the important issue clinically is how to interfere with that process. One important strategy is to target specific biological alterations; unfortunately, very little is known about these evolutionary alterations

Table 1 Biological Characteristics of Premalignant Lesions

Characteristic	TDLU (%)	HUL (%)	UDH (%)	ADH (%)*	DCIS (%)**
Proliferation rate	2	5	5	5	20
ER (any + cells)	98	100	98	98	80
ER (% + cells)	30	90	60	90	50
HER-2 amplification	0	0	0	0	30
P53 mutation	0	0	0	0	30

*ALH = ADH.
**LCIS = DCIS (low-grade).
DCIS is a biological continuum.

at the biological level. Instead, most of what is known in a comprehensive fashion involves standard biomarkers with predictive significance in invasive breast cancer that have retrospectively been evaluated in premalignant disease, usually by immunochemistry.

Table 1 summarizes information about the standard biomarkers. Although a dynamic process, the proliferation rate is quite low in TDLU (2%), and significantly higher but still relatively low for ADH (5%). Not until the far end of the spectrum with DCIS (20%) does the rate of proliferation increase substantially.

The estrogen receptor (ER) has been studied extensively and been shown to have important alterations. If one defines estrogen-receptor positivity (ER+) as the presence of any positive cells, then nearly all premalignant lesions are ER+, with the exception of a relatively small subset of DCIS. Where premalignant lesions differ is in the proportion of ER+ cells. In general, the proportion of ER+ cells is much higher in the premalignant lesions compared to their adjacent, normal counterparts (i.e., TDLUs).

HER-2 alteration—amplification of the gene or overexpression of the protein—has been studied very thoroughly, as has P-53 mutation, using immunohistochemistry as a surrogate for mutation in most studies. Very little evidence exists for alteration of these genes in early premalignant disease; it is not until the very late stages in a subset of DCIS that they play any kind of significant role. In trying to document the biological characteristics of most premalignant lesions, proliferation is relatively low, ER+ is high, and HER-2 and P-53 appear normal (2, 3).

VI. BREAST CANCER EVOLUTION AND PREVENTION

The following comments address a handful of issues that are often overlooked or misunderstood but are still very important in terms of breast cancer evolution, risk, and prevention.

A. In Situ Risk

A strong argument can be made that the true in situ risk of developing invasive breast cancer associated with these premalignant lesions is probably much higher than generally believed. Most substantial studies that have established this risk were retrospective in nature, based on excised lesions in patients—many of whom were probably cured by the surgery. From a clinical perspective, the challenge is really one of detection and subsequent treatment to interfere with the process of cancer development.

B. Hyperplasias/In Situ Carcinomas

Despite the distinctions inherent in the classification scheme, atypical hyperplasias and in situ carcinomas are essentially the same disease. They vary on a continuum only in terms of extent, with the distinction between ADH vs. DCIS, and ALH vs. LCIS based on somewhat arbitrary rules that remain a subject of discussion among pathologists. In a biological sense, the difference has very little meaning, although the clinical implications in terms of therapy are very profound.

C. Lobular Neoplasia

Lobular neoplasia, which is the term applied to the spectrum of evolution from ALH to LCIS, is a serious disease; it is a precursor rather than simply a risk factor, which is how many clinicians think of it today. For example, 20–30% of patients with lobular neoplasia on excisional biopsy eventually develop invasive breast cancer. Almost always it is an infiltrating lobular-type carcinoma or one with very striking lobular features, located in the ipsilateral breast by a ratio of three- or four-to-one (5). Similarly, 10–15% of patients with lobular neoplasia in a core needle biopsy have more advanced disease (DCIS/invasive breast cancer) on surgical excision, suggesting that this subgroup be treated as candidates for follow-up excision (6).

D. ER+ in Premalignant Disease

ER+ is very high in nearly all types of premalignant lesions—a point that is important enough to warrant further discussion. Figure 4 summarizes data from a study by Allred et al. involving several hundred patients that was designed to measure ERs in premalignant lesions (7). The histograms show the proportion of ER+ in terms of frequency of cases. Despite obvious variability in content, the overwhelming majority of all premalignant lesions, with the exception of a small subset of generally high-grade DCIS, have high ER content (8). Globally, over 90% of lesions are highly ER+; it approaches a biological abnormality, suggesting that prevention strategies with hormonal therapies are a good idea. If, as might be hypothesized,

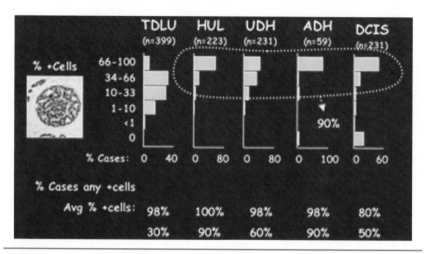

Figure 4   Histograms showing the proportion of ER+ in terms of frequency of cases. (See legend to Fig. 1 for abbreviations.) (From Ref. 5)

most of the small ER− subsets of premalignant lesions evolve through various mechanisms from ER+ DCIS, then eventually a reduction in ER− breast cancer should follow from hormone prevention strategies.

E.   DCIS vs. Invasive Breast Cancer

Unlike the other premalignant lesions, DCIS is a histological and biological continuum very similar to invasive breast cancer. Pathologists specializing in breast disease have recognized for a long time that DCIS varies on a continuum from very well-differentiated lesions definable as ADH, to very high-grade lesions that are associated with aggressive biological features. The convention of dichotomizing DCIS into low-grade noncomedo and high-grade comedo type is incorrect.

Various grading methods have been designed to convey this histological diversity on more of a continuum. At Baylor College of Medicine, we grade DCISs using the Scarff–Bloom–Richardson method that has been used for decades to grade invasive breast cancer—slightly modified to take into account the extent of necrosis that has played such an important role historically in classifying DCISs. Using this method, we conducted a study of 400 consecutive DCISs correlating histological grade with standard biomarkers for invasive breast cancer (Fig. 5) (8). The dotted line indicates a fairly even distribution of cases along the histological continuum, underscoring the impossibility of dividing them into low-grade vs. high-grade lesions. Hormone receptor (HR) expression is relatively high at the very well-differentiated or low end of the grading scale, gradually decreasing to very low levels at the high end of the spectrum. Proliferation gradually increases

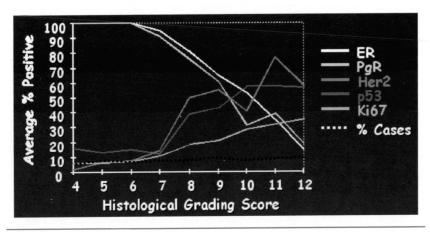

Figure 5 Biomarkers for DCIS based on grade showing that DCIS is a histological and biological continuum. (From Ref. 6.)

from low levels in well-differentiated lesions to relatively high levels in poorly differentiated lesions. P-53 and HER-2 abnormalities are rare in well-differentiated lesions, but gradually increase to fairly high levels in the higher grade lesions. Overall, these data emphasize a highly correlated histological and correlated biological continuum (8).

This study was extended to provide data on the prognostic value of these biomarkers by comparing their frequencies in pure DCIS to the DCIS component associated with invasive breast cancer. There were no significant differences in any of these phenotypes, with the exception of a trend toward accumulating lower histological grade in association with invasive breast cancer. This not only runs counter to the notion that high grade lesions are the most likely to progress but also suggests that these features are not very useful in predicting the clinical course of disease (8). Data from a prospective study by Solin et al. also confirm that low-grade DCIS is a potentially serious disease. They examined the rate of local recurrence in patients with high- vs. low-grade DCIS treated by lumpectomy and radiation. At relatively short follow-up (5 years), there is indeed a statistically significant difference in the rate of local recurrence, but with long-term follow-up (10 years), the difference is not significant (9).

By definition, all DCIS is harmless, if it is truly non-invasive and can be excised within adequate margins. Unlike invasive breast cancer, relatively little is known about prognostically significant biomarkers in noninvasive disease. Perhaps most important, however, is that little is currently known about the biological evolution of premalignant lesions into invasive disease. Progress in prevention depends on a better understanding of this biology, which should be a fundamental research priority.

REFERENCES

1. Wellings SR, Jensen HM, Marcum RG. An atlas of subgross pathology of the human breast with special reference to possible precancerous lesions. J Natl Cancer Inst 1975; 55:231.
2. Allred DC, Mohsin SK. Biological features of premalignant disease in the human breast. J Mammary Gland Biol Neoplasia 2000; 5(4):351–364.
3. Allred DC, Mohsin SK, Fuqua SAW. Histological and biological evolution of human premalignant breast disease. Endocr Relat Cancer 2001; 8:47–61.
4. Dupont WD, Page DL. Risk factors for breast cancer in women with proliferative breast disease. N Engl J Med 1985; 312:146–151.
5. Pope DL, Schuyler PA, Dupont WD, Jensen RA, Plummer WD, Simpson JF. Atypical lobular hyperplasia as a unilateral predictor of breast cancer risk: a retrospective cohort study. Lancet 2003; 361:125–129.
6. Arpino G, Allred C, Mohsin S, Weiss H, Conrow D, Elledge R. Atypical lobular hyperplasia (ALH) and lobular carcinoma in situ (LCIS) on core needle biopsy clinical significance [abstr 361]. Proc Am Soc Clin Oncol 2003; 22:90.
7. Mohsin SK, Hilsenbeck SG, Allred DC. Estrogen receptors and growth control in premalignant breast disease. Mod Pathol 2000; 13:145.
8. Berardo M, Hilsenbeck SG, Allred DC. Histological grading of non-invasive breast cancer and its relationship to biological features. Lab Invest 1996; 74:68.
9. Solin LJ, Kurtz J, Fourquet A, Amalric R, Recht A, Bornstein BA, Kuske R, Taylor M, Barrett W, Fowble B, Haffty B, Schultz DJ, Yeh IT, McCormick B, McNeese M. Fifteen-year results of breast-conserving surgery and definitive breast irradiation for the treatment of ductal carcinoma in situ of the breast. J Clin Oncol 1996; 14:754–763.

11

Estradiol-Induced Carcinogenesis via Formation of Genotoxic Metabolites

Richard J. Santen,[1] Wei Yue,[1]
Wayne Bocchinfuso,[2] Kenneth Korach,[3] Ji-Ping Wang,[1]
Eleanor G. Rogan,[4] Yubai Li,[1] Ercole Cavalieri,[4] Jose Russo,[5]
Prabu Devanesan,[6] and Michael Verderame[7]

[1]University of Virginia Health System, Charlottesville, Virginia
[2]Eli Lilly & Co., Research Triangle Park, North Carolina
[3]National Institute of Environmental Health Services,
Research Triangle Park, North Carolina
[4]Eppley Institute, Nebraska Medical Center, Omaha, Nebraska
[5]Fox Chase Cancer Center, Philadelphia, Pennsylvania
[6]PPD Discovery, Morrisville, North Carolina
[7]Penn State University, Hershey, Pennsylvania

I. OVERVIEW

Long-term exposure to estradiol is associated with an increased risk of breast cancer but the mechanisms responsible are not firmly established. The prevailing theory postulates that estrogens increase the rate of cell proliferation by stimulating estrogen receptor (ER) mediated transcription and thereby the number of errors occurring during DNA replication. An alternative theory suggests that estradiol is metabolized to quinone derivatives, which directly remove base pairs from

163

DNA through a process called depurination. Error prone DNA repair then results in point mutations. We postulate that these two processes—increased cell proliferation and genotoxic metabolite formation—act in an additive or synergistic fashion to induce cancer. If correct, aromatase inhibitors (AIs) such as letrozole, anastrozole, or exemestane would block both processes whereas anti-estrogens would only inhibit receptor-mediated effects. Accordingly, AIs would be more effective in preventing breast cancer than use of anti-estrogens.

Our initial studies demonstrated that catechol-estrogen metabolites are formed in MCF-7 human mammary cancer cells in culture. We then utilized an animal model that allows dissociation of ER-mediated function from that of the effects of estradiol metabolites. Knock-out of ER-alpha in Wnt-1 (ERKO/Wnt-1) transgenic mice allows examination of the effect of estrogen deprivation in the absence of ER in animals with a high incidence of mammary tumors. In the mammary tissue of these ERKO/Wnt-1 transgenic mice, we demonstrated formation of genotoxic estradiol metabolites. The ERKO/Wnt-1 mammary extracts contained picomole amounts of the 4-catechol estrogens (CE), but not their methoxy-conjugates nor the 2-CE and their methoxy-conjugates. The 3,4 estradiol quinones, conjugated with glutathione and its derivatives, were also detected in picomole amounts in both tumors and hyperplastic mammary tissue. We also examined the incidence of tumors formed in ERKO mice bearing the Wnt-1 transgene. To assess the effect of estrogens in the absence of ER, animals were castrated at day 15; half the animals were given back estradiol and the other half were given a vehicle by silastic implant. The absence of estradiol markedly reduced the incidence of tumors and delayed their onset.

In aggregate, our results support the concept that metabolites of estradiol may act in concert with ER-mediated mechanisms to induce mammary cancer. This finding supports the possibility that AIs might be more effective in preventing breast cancer than use of antiestrogens.

II. INTRODUCTION

A variety of experimental and epidemiological data suggest that estrogens contribute to the development of mammary cancer, but the mechanisms responsible have not been conclusively established (Fig. 1 and 2) (1–9). The most commonly held hypothesis is that estrogens bind to ER-alpha or -beta and stimulate the transcription of genes involved in cell proliferation (8–9) (Fig. 3A). With each cycle of new DNA synthesis during the cell proliferative process, the chances for errors in DNA replication increase, and permanent point mutations result if DNA repair is insufficient. As the process continues, several mutations accumulate (10–11). When these mutations involve critical regions needed for cellular proliferation, DNA repair, angiogenesis, or apoptosis, neoplastic transformation results (12). A more controversial hypothesis is that estradiol can be metabolized to genotoxic

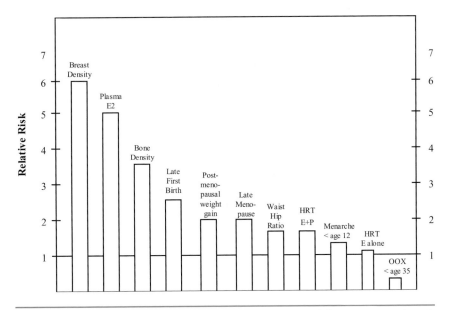

Figure 1 Hormonal indicators and risk of breast cancer. Each bar represents the relative risk of breast cancer with respect to factors reflecting exposure to estradiol. (From Ref. 30)

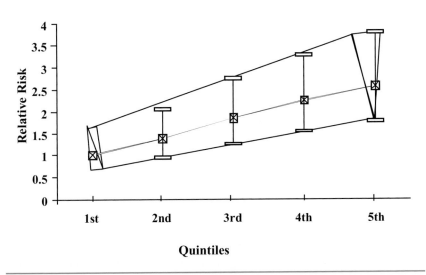

Figure 2 Free estradiol levels and risk of breast cancer. (Adapted from the pooled analysis of nine studies relating the risk of breast cancer to level of free estradiol levels in postmenopausal women.) (Reprinted from Ref. 31)

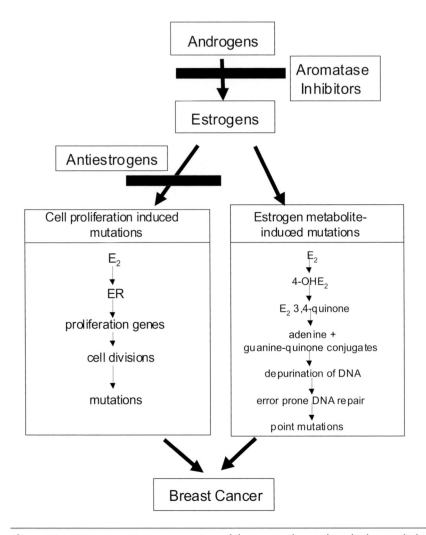

Figure 3A Diagrammatic representation of the two pathways by which estradiol is postulated to cause breast cancer. The anti-estrogens block only the ER-mediated pathway, whereas the AIs block the formation of genotoxic metabolites as well as the ER-mediated pathway.

metabolites and directly damage DNA (Fig. 3A) (10–11, 13–14). Cytochrome p450 1B1 catalyzes the hydroxylation of estradiol, to 4-OH-estradiol, which is then further converted to the 3,4 estradiol quinone. This compound can bind covalently to guanine or adenine and results in destabilization of the glycosidyl bond, which links these nucleotides to the DNA backbone. (Fig. 3B).

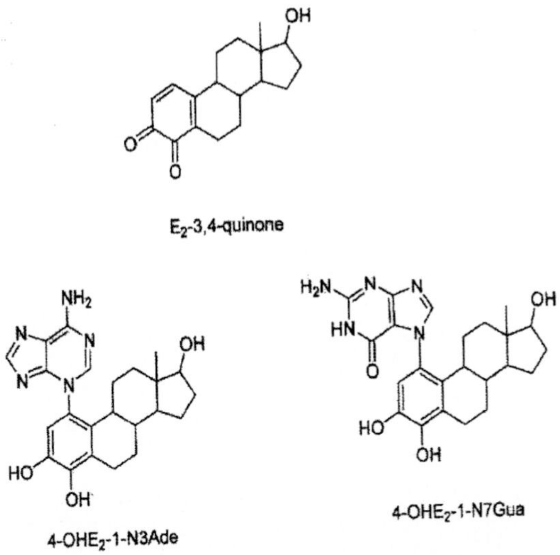

Figure 3B   Structure of the key molecules involved in the genotoxic effects of estradiol.

Adenine and guanine, which are bound to estradiol, exit the DNA backbone and form 4-OH-estrone (estradiol)-1-N7-guanine (Fig. 3B) or 4-OH-estrone (estradiol)-1-N-3-adenine, two depurinated products that leave behind a naked site on DNA. Through the process of error-prone DNA repair, these sites now form point mutations that serve as potential initiators of neoplastic transformation (14). Our working hypothesis is that estradiol acts on both pathways shown in Figure 3 in an additive or synergistic fashion to induce breast cancer.

Experimental evidence regarding estradiol genotoxicity derives from in vitro studies. Liehr and colleagues, using the V-79 cell carcinogenicity assay, found that low doses of estradiol in the tenth to the eleventh and twelfth molar ranges, causes a 3.8- to 4.2-fold increase in rate of genetic mutations (15). In other experiments, Russo et al. administered estradiol to benign MCF-10F breast cells in vitro in doses ranging from 0.007 nM to 1 mM (16, 17). They found that even very low estradiol concentrations induced loss of heterozygosity (LOH) at chromosomal sites (11 q23.3, 11q23.1–25, 3p21, 3p21–21.2, 3p21.1–14.2, 3p14.2–14.1) at which human breast cancers commonly exhibit LOH. They also documented the neoplastic transformation of these cells by demonstrating an increase in anchorage-independent colony formation and loss of duct differentiation (Fig. 4). Taken together, these recent data provide support for the genotoxic hypothesis.

In the studies described herein, we sought further evidence of the validity of the estrogen genotoxic hypothesis. Initially, we wished to demonstrate that human

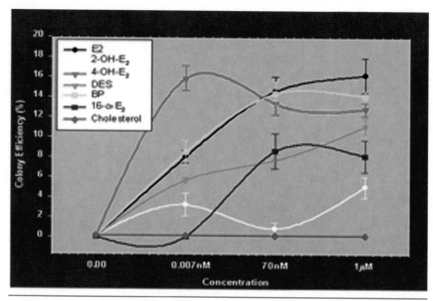

Figure 4   Effects of estrogens and benzepyrine (BP) on the colony plating efficiency of benign MCF-10 F cells in agar methocel. (From Ref. 17)

mammary cancer cells contain the enzymes necessary for conversion of estradiol to estradiol quinones and that depurination can occur. For these studies we utilized MCF-7 cells containing a stably transfected aromatase gene and measured genotoxic products after incubation with estrogen substrates (13, 18–19). In addition, we used an ERKO animal model (20–23). These animals express no ER-beta in mammary tissue as demonstrated by RNase protection assay. In this model system, estradiol cannot act via receptor-mediated effects on breast and any neoplastic changes induced by estrogens must work through ER independent pathways. Taken together, these studies demonstrated that mammary cancer cells can convert estradiol to genotoxic metabolites and that nonreceptor mediated mechanisms involving estradiol can modulate the process of mammary cancer development.

III.   SUMMARY OF OUR RECENT RESULTS

A.   Aromatase Transfected MCF-7 Cells

We initially determined whether enzymes responsible for formation of depurinating metabolites were present in human MCF-7 human breast cancer cells (Fig. 5A and B). 10 μM of 4-OH estradiol were incubated for 24 hours before collecting media for later measurement of the various metabolites. As shown in Fig. 6A,

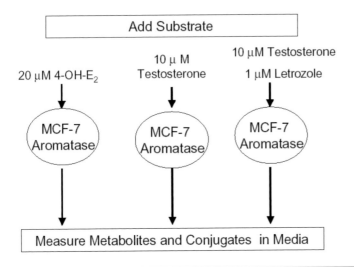

Figure 5A   Diagrammatic representation of the experimental design of the studies demonstrating formation of metabolites in aromatase-transfected MCF-7 cells.

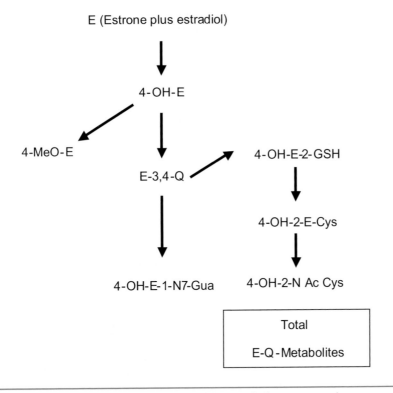

Figure 5B   Diagrammatic representation of the metabolites measured.

we detected large amounts of 4 methoxy-estradiol as well as substantial amounts of the quinone conjugates and the depurinated species, 4-OH-estrone (estradiol)-1-N7-guanine. We then determined in these aromatase-transfected MCF-7 cells whether they could aromatize a sufficient amount of testosterone to estradiol to result in formation of the depurinating species. As shown in Figure 6B, we detected 131 pg/ml of estrogen indicating the production of estrogens from aromatization. The 4-OH-estrone (estradiol)-1-N7-guanine species was also present at a total concentration (E1 plus E2) of 0.17 pg/ml as were the glutathione, cystein, and n-acetyl-cystine conjugates of 3,4 estradiol quinone. Finally, the AI, letrozole, inhibited estrogen formation from a total of 131 pg/ml of E1 and E2 (Fig. 6C) to 2.8 pg/ml and their downstream metabolites to undetectable levels in most cases.

B. Measurements in Human Breast Tissue

As previously reported and shown in Fig. 7A and B, the levels of estradiol plus estrone in breast cancer tissue approximated 5 pMol/gm of tissue and, in the surrounding normal breast, 2 pMol/gm. Expressed as pg/ml these values would represent 1,650 and 660 pg/ml (24). The levels of the 4-OH, 2-OH, and 16 alpha-OH catechol-estrogen metabolites are similar in magnitude. As evidence that the human breast can synthesize the quinone derivatives of estradiol, the total E1 and E2 conjugates of the estrogen quinones are in the range of 2 pM in the surrounding normal tissue and 8 pM in the cancer itself.

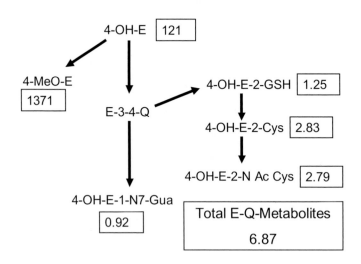

Figure 6A   Formation of metabolites when 20 μM of 4-OH estradiol are added. The boxes represent the amount of metabolite measured and represented as pg/ml.

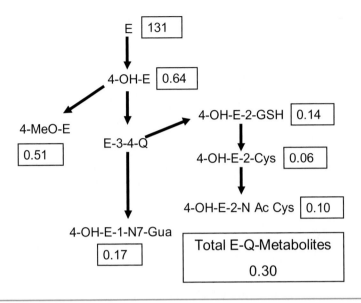

Figure 6B Formation of metabolites when 10 μM of testosterone are added.

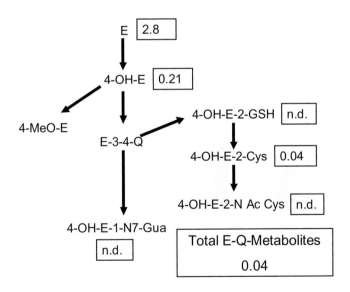

Figure 6C Formation of metabolites when 1 μM of letrozole is added to 10 μM of testosterone.

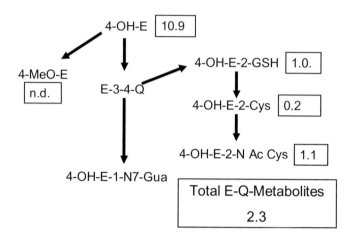

Figure 6D Measurement of metabolites in the hyperplastic mammary tissue of ERKO/Wnt-1 double transgenic mice.

C. Measurements in ERKO/Wnt-1 Mammary Tissue

ERKO/Wnt-1 mammary tissue exhibits an altered metabolic balance (25). Formation of 4-OH-estrogen metabolites are favored over those of the 2-OH species and the catechol-O-methyl-transferase pathway appears to be relatively inactive (Fig. 6D). As summarized in Figure 7, we detected 10.9 pM/gm of

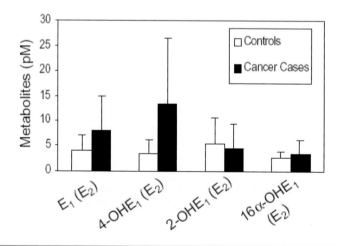

Figure 7A Levels of estrone and estradiol, 2- and 4-OH estrone and estradiol, and 16 alpha-OH-estrone and estradiol in 77 breast cancer tissues (Cancer Cases) from women and the benign tissue distant from the tumors from the same breasts (Controls).

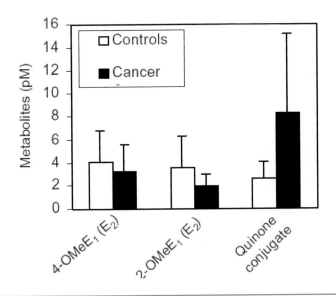

Figure 7B Levels of 2- and 4-methoxy-estrone and estradiol and the quinone conjugates in these same samples. (From Ref. 24)

4-OH E2 and E1 in mammary tissue as well as a total of 2.3 pM/gm of total conjugated quinone. No 4-methoxy-estrogen metabolites were present.

D. Tumor Incidence in ERKO/Wnt-1 Animals

Bocchinfuso et al. had previously shown that ERKO/Wnt-1 animals exhibit a delayed onset of tumor development compared to animals expressing the ER-alpha. Nonetheless, they observed a nearly 100% incidence of mammary tumors even in the absence of ER-alpha and -beta (20–21). To directly determine the effect of estradiol in the absence of ER, we castrated animals at age 15 and treated half with silastic implants containing estradiol and the other half with implants of cholesterol. After 100 weeks of observation, the estradiol-treated animals developed more tumors (12/15 vs 4/10), which appeared earlier than in animals receiving cholesterol implants (50% of tumors at 50 weeks versus 25% of tumors at 100 weeks) ($p < 0.004$) (unpublished results). These data provide evidence that estradiol exerts effects both through an ER-alpha-dependent pathway as well as an ER-independent pathway to produce breast tumors.

IV. DISCUSSION

Studies in vitro in animals and in women provide compelling evidence that estrogens contribute to the development of breast cancer (1–11). The commonly held mechanism of carcinogenesis is that estrogens stimulate cell proliferation, increase the number of genetic mutations in proportion to the number of mitotic divisions, and promote the propagation of these mutations by stimulating growth (9, 26). An alternate hypothesis suggests that estrogens may be metabolized to directly genotoxic compounds (10–11, 13, 27). Our working construct is that these two pathways act in concert in an additive or synergistic fashion to cause breast cancer (Fig. 3A). We sought to provide evidence in support of the genotoxic hypothesis by demonstrating the formation of genotoxic metabolites in cell culture and in human breast tissue. In addition, we utilized a double transgenic mouse model to provide proof of the principle that estrogens can influence breast tumor development in the absence of functioning ERs.

We demonstrated that MCF-7 cells can convert 4-OH-estradiol and testosterone both to the 4-OH-estrone (estradiol)-1-N7-guanine depurinated product and to estrogen quinones. We also demonstrated that the incidence of breast tumor development in ERKO/Wnt-1 transgenic animals could be enhanced by administration of estradiol to oophorectomized animals. These new data provide direct evidence of the biological importance of the genotoxic pathway.

Our first aim was to demonstrate that human breast cancer cells convert testosterone or 4-OH estradiol to genotoxic products. We clearly demonstrated this in an MCF-7 cell model system by using a highly sensitive and specific assay for steroid measurements. A commonly expressed criticism of the genotoxic hypothesis is that supraphysiological amounts of estrogen are needed to form genotoxic metabolites of estradiol (11). Our in vitro experiments can be criticized on the same basis. However, we believe that biological endpoints of this process provide a higher level of sensitivity than do biochemical measurements. This reasoning is supported by studies that examined the biological effects of estrogen under similar in vitro conditions. Russo et al. have shown that 0.007 nM estradiol can induce neoplastic transformation as evidenced by increased colony formation in benign MCF-10 cells that lack a functional ER (17). This treatment also reduced the formation of ducts, another parameter indicative of neoplastic transformation. Similar concentrations induce loss of heteozygosity in benign, non-ER breast cells at hot spots for LOH in breast cancer tissue. Such low concentrations can also induce mutations in V-79 cells (15). As further evidence of the ability of physiological amounts of estrogen to serve as substrate for these genotoxic metabolites, human breast cancer tissue and surrounding benign breast tissue contain large amounts of these metabolites. Taken together, the tissue measurement data and the findings from incubated cells in vitro clearly demonstrate that human breast tissue can form substantial amounts of the genotoxic metabolites of estradiol.

The ERKO/Wnt-1 animals provide a powerful model for studying the effect of estrogen in the absence of a functioning ER. These animals have circulating estradiol levels in the range of 325 pg/ml.* This is approximately 30- to 50-fold higher than normal as a consequence of the absence of estradiol negative feedback on the pituitary and the resultant rise in LH levels. In addition, the breast tissue from these animals appears to convert little 4-OH estradiol to 4-methoxy-estadiol, a metabolite that is thought to be inactive and to obviate further conversion to genotoxic metabolites. In a prior report, we called this metabolic pathway unbalanced because of the propensity for estrogens to be converted to the depurinating, 4-OH-genotoxic-quinones (25).

We consider it highly relevant with respect to prevention of breast cancer to determine whether the genotoxic pathway is biologically important. Anti-estrogens act only to block ER-mediated function, whereas the AIs reduce estradiol levels and consequently block both ER mediated as well as genotoxic pathways. Theoretically, AIs would then be much more efficacious for prevention of breast cancer than the anti-estrogens (8). Data from the recently reported ATAC trial can be interpreted in light of the genotoxic hypothesis (28–29). In this trial, the AI, anastrozole, resulted in a 50% greater reduction of invasive contralateral breast cancer ($p < 0.05$) at 4 years than did the anti-estrogen, tamoxifen. Although there are other explanations for this difference, the magnitude of greater effect of the AI is substantial. This observation, when taken together with the biological data presented in this chapter, highlight the compelling need to determine conclusively whether the genotoxic hypothesis of estradiol-induced carcinogenesis is operative.

REFERENCES

1. Zumoff B. Does postmenopausal estrogen administration increase the risk of breast cancer? Contributions of animal, biochemical, and clinical investigative studies to a resolution of the controversy. Proc Soc Exp Biol Med 1998; 217:30–37.
2. Gunson DE, Steele RE, Chau RY. Prevention of spontaneous tumours in female rats by fadrozole hydrochloride, an aromatase inhibitor. Br J Cancer 1995; 72:72–75.
3. Trichopoulos D, MacMahon B, Cole P. Menopause and breast cancer risk. J Natl Cancer Inst 1972; 48: 605–613.
4. Feinleib M. Breast cancer and artificial menopause: a cohort study. J Natl Cancer Inst 1968; 41:315–329.
5. The Endogenous Hormones and Breast Cancer Collaborative Group. Endogenous sex hormones and breast cancer in postmenopausal women: reanalysis of nine prospective studies. J Natl Cancer Inst 2002; 94: 606–616.
6. Fisher B, Costantino JP, Wickerham DL, Redmond CK, Kavanah M, Cronin WM, Vogel V, Robidoux A, Dimitrov N, Atkins J, Daly M, Wieand S, Tan-Chiu E, Ford L, Wolmark N. Tamoxifen for prevention of breast cancer: report of the National Surgical Adjuvant Breast and Bowel Project P-1 Study [see comments]. J Natl Cancer Inst 1998; 90:1371–1388.

*Korach K. Personal communication, 2002.

7. Cummings SR, Eckert S, Krueger KA, Grady D, Powles TJ, Cauley JA, Norton L, Nickelsen T, Bjarnason NH, Morrow M, Lippman ME, Black D, Glusman JE, Costa A, Jordan VC. The effect of raloxifene on risk of breast cancer in postmenopausal women: results from the MORE randomized trial. Multiple Outcomes of Raloxifene Evaluation. JAMA 1999; 281:2189–2197.
8. Santen RJ. To block estrogen's synthesis or action: that is the question. J Clin Endocrinol Metab 2002; 87:3007–3012.
9. Preston-Martin S, Pike MC, Ross RK, Jones PA, Henderson BE. Increased cell division as a cause of human cancer. Cancer Res 1990; 50:7415–7421.
10. Liehr JG. Dual role of oestrogens as hormones and pro-carcinogens: tumour initiation by metabolic activation of oestrogens. Eur J Cancer Prev 1997; 6:3–10.
11. Liehr JG. Is estradiol a genotoxic mutagenic carcinogen? Endocr Rev 2000; 21:40–54.
12. Hahn WC, Weinberg RA. Rules for making tumor cells. N Engl J Med 2002; 347:1593–1603.
13. Cavalieri E, Frenkel K, Liehr JG, Rogan E, Roy D. Estrogens as endogenous genotoxic agents—DNA adducts and mutations. J Natl Cancer Inst Monographs 2000; 75–93.
14. Chakravarti D. Evidence that error-prone DNA repair converts dibenzo(a,l)pyrene-induced depourinating lesions into mutations. Mutation Res 2000; 456:17–32.
15. Kong LY, Szaniszlo P, Albrecht T, Liehr JG. Frequency and molecular analysis of hprt mutations induced by estradiol in Chinese hamster V79 cells. Int J Oncol 2000; 17:1141–1149.
16. Russo J, Tahin Q, Lareef MH, Hu FF, Russo IH. Neoplastic transformation of human breast epithelial cells by estrogens and chemical carcinogens. Environ Mol Mutagen 2002; 39:254–263.
17. Russo J, Hu YF, Tahin Q, Slater C, Lareef MH, Russo IH. Carcinogenicity of estrogens in human breast epithelial cells. APMIS 2001; 103:S95–108; discussion S109–111.
18. Yue W. In situ aromatization enhances breast tumor estradiol levels and cellular proliferation. Cancer Res 1998; 58:927–932.
19. Yue W, Santen RJ, Wang JP, Hamilton CJ, Demers LM. Aromatase within the breast. Endocr Relat Cancer 1999; 6:157–164.
20. Bocchinfuso WP. A mouse mammary tumor virus-Wnt-1 transgenic induces mammary gland hyperplasia and tumorigenesis in mice lacking estrogen receptor-alpha. Cancer Res 1999; 59:1869–1876.
21. Bocchinfuso WP. Mammary gland development and tumorigenesis in estrogen receptor knockout mice. J Mammary Gland Biol Neoplasia 2002; 2:323–334.
22. Lubahn DB. Alteration of reproductive function but not prenatal sexual development after insertional disruption of the mouse estrogen receptor gene. Proc Natl Acad Sci USA 1993; 90:11162–11166.
23. Couse JF, Korach KS. Contrasting phenotypes in reproductive tissue of female estrogen receptor null mice. Ann NY Acad Sci 2001; 948:1–8.
24. Rogan EG, Badawi AF, Devanesan PD, Meza JL, Edney JA, West WW, Higginbothan SM, Cavalieri EL. Relative imbalances in estrogen metabolism and conjugation in breast tissue of women with carcinoma: potential biomarkers of susceptibility to cancer. Carcinogenesis 2003; 24:697–702.

25. Devanesan P, Santen RJ, Bocchinfuso WP, Korach KS, Rogan EG, Cavalieri E. Catechol estrogenmetabolites and conjugates in mammary tumors and hyperplastic tissue from estrogen receptor alpha knock out (ERKO)/Wnt-1 mice; implications for initiation of mammary tumors. Carcinogenesis 2001; 22:1573–1576.
26. Henderson BE, Feigelson HS. Hormonal carcinogenesis. Carcinogenesis 2000; 21:427–433.
27. Jefcoate CR, Liehr JG, Santen RJ, Sutter TR, Yager JD, Yue W, Santner SJ, Tekmal R, Demers L, Pauley R, Naftolin F, Mor G, Berstein L. Tissue-specific synthesis and oxidative metabolism of estrogens. J Natl Cancer Inst Monographs 2000; 95–112.
28. The ATAC Trialists' Group. Anastrozole alone or in combination with tamoxifen versus tamoxifen alone for adjuvant treatment of postmenopausal women with early breast cancer: first results of the ATAC randomised trial. Lancet 2002; 359:2131–2139.
29. Baum M. Four year update of the ATAC trial. Endocrine Therapy in Breast Cancer. In press.
30. Santen RJ. Breast and prostate cancer. In: Larsen PR, Kronenberg HM, Melmed S, Polonsky KS, eds. Williams' Textbook of Endocrinology. 10th ed. Philadelphia:WB Saunders, 2003; pp. 1797–1833.
31. Santen RJ. Endocrinology of breast and endometrial cancer. In: Barbieri RL, ed. Reproductive Endocrinology. 5th ed. Philadelphia:WB Saunders, 2003. In press.

12

Beyond Tamoxifen: Results of Clinical Trials

Norman Wolmark
Allegheny General Hospital
Pittsburgh, Pennsylvania, U.S.A.

I. OVERVIEW

Results from the National Surgical Adjuvant Breast and Bowel Project (NSABP) Breast Cancer Prevention Trial Protocol (BCPT; P-1) indicated a 50% decrease in the frequency of breast cancer in women who received tamoxifen. Two other smaller European studies failed to show any benefit, perhaps because of differences in study population. More recently, the International Breast Cancer Intervention Study (IBIS-I) confirmed NSABP P-1 findings, with results showing that prophylactic tamoxifen reduced the incidence of breast cancer by about one-third. The benefit of tamoxifen therapy, however, is tempered by significant increases in the risk of endometrial cancer and thromboembolic events.

In this chapter, information from the major tamoxifen breast cancer prevention trials and from more recent, ongoing clinical trials is examined. The goal is to help develop a strategy for finding safer, more effective alternatives, such as selective estrogen receptor modulators (SERMs) or aromatase inhibitors (AIs), for breast cancer prevention.

II. INTRODUCTION

In this chapter, a number of major prevention trials are reviewed, with an eye toward the future of breast cancer prevention, e.g., use of SERMs or AIs, especially in postmenopausal women. Data from the National Surgical Adjuvant Breast and Bowel Project NSABP (P-1 showed clearly that tamoxifen reduced the incidence of invasive breast cancer in the prevention setting. On the basis of these data, tamoxifen was approved by the United States Food and Drug Administration (FDA) for use in high-risk women as defined by the Gail model. However, the benefits of tamoxifen therapy are accompanied by risks, suggesting the need to go beyond therapy with tamoxifen and perhaps even outside the class of SERMs as a whole. At the same time, recent publication of data from the Women's Health Initiative (WHI) study, showing that the risks of hormone replacement therapy (HRT) outweighed the benefits, has changed the backdrop against which future breast cancer prevention studies will be conducted in the United States because patients on HRT were not eligible to participate in NSABP trials. The resulting treatment void in that setting can potentially help to evolve new strategies in breast cancer prevention.

III. THE NSABP P-1 BREAST CANCER PREVENTION TRIAL

The NSABP P-1 trial tested the hypothesis that tamoxifen might play a role in breast cancer prevention. Women ($n = 13,388$) who had increased risk for breast cancer based on the Gail algorithm (age 60 years or older, age 35–59 years with a predicted risk of at least 1.66%, or history of lobular carcinoma in situ) were randomly assigned to receive either tamoxifen (20 mg/day) or placebo. Subjects who entered the study were required to stop the use of HRT. The primary endpoint in P-1 was the incidence of invasive breast cancer. Thirty percent of patients were age 60 or older, 30% were age 50–59, and 40% were under age 50; thus young, premenopausal women were well represented in the study. There was a mean follow-up of 4.7 years.

As shown in Figure 1, there was a highly significant reduction (49%) in the incidence of invasive breast cancer in the tamoxifen group that was independent of age, year of follow-up, or level of risk at the time of randomization into the study. In particular, tamoxifen reduced the incidence of estrogen-receptor-positive (ER+) tumors by 69% (130 events for placebo vs. 40 for tamoxifen). There was no significant difference in the incidence of estrogen-receptor-negative (ER–) tumors. Among women who were at increased risk because of either lobular carcinoma in situ or atypical hyperplasia, the risk of invasive breast cancer was reduced by 56% and 86%, respectively. The incidence of noninvasive breast cancer also was reduced by 50%, and there was a 19% reduction in the incidence of osteoporotic fractures among women who received tamoxifen (1).

In terms of risks, there was a 2.53% increase in the rate of endometrial carcinoma, and the rates of stroke, pulmonary embolism (PE), and deep vein thrombosis (DVT) were elevated in the tamoxifen group. Although the benefits of tamoxifen therapy applied to all age groups, the risks were age dependent. For those over

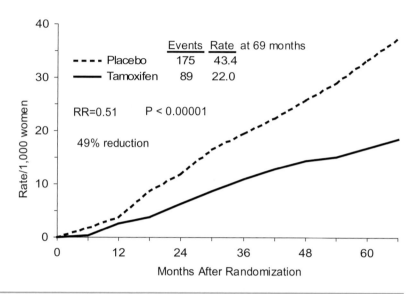

Figure 1 Cumulative rate of invasive breast cancer in patients receiving tamoxifen or placebo. (From Ref. 1)

age 50, for example, the risk of endometrial cancer was increased nearly four-fold, while the rates of stroke, PE, and DVT were increased by 1.75%, 3.19%, and 1.71%, respectively, in those who received tamoxifen (Fig. 2). There was no excess of ischemic heart disease, including myocardeal infarction (MI), in the

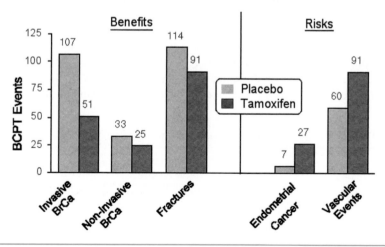

Figure 2 Risk of various outcomes in patients 50 years or older receiving tamoxifen or placebo. (From Ref. 1)

tamoxifen group. Overall, then, tamoxifen reduced the incidence of invasive and noninvasive breast cancer by half in women of all age groups (35 years or older) and at all levels of breast cancer risk. Thus, the risks and benefits must be weighed before a woman is prescribed tamoxifen. However, this drug appears to be of clear benefit in specific subsets of patients, including women who have had a hysterectomy, women with atypical ductal hyperplasia or lobular carcinoma in situ, and women under 50 (1).

IV. THE EUROPEAN PREVENTION TRIALS

Results from two smaller prevention trials in Europe have demonstrated less favorable results for tamoxifen, as indicated by the event summary for prevention trials shown in Table 1. Recruitment for the Italian National trial, which randomized 5,408 hysterectomized women to either tamoxifen (20 mg/day) or placebo, was stopped early as a result of the large number of study dropouts. Primary endpoints were the incidence of breast cancer and resulting mortality. After a mean follow-up of 46 months, this study found no difference in the frequency of breast cancer between the placebo (22 cases) and tamoxifen (19) arms, and there were no deaths attributed to breast cancer. At the same time, there was a significantly increased risk of vascular events in women who took tamoxifen compared to those who took placebo. Overall, tamoxifen was shown to have no protective effects in the cohort of women studied. It is important to note that these women were at low-to-moderate risk, as suggested by the relatively low frequency of primary events, compared to women in the P-1 trial who were at higher risk (2).

In the Royal Marsden Hospital trial of 2,471 healthy women 30–70 years of age and with a family history of breast cancer, subjects were randomized to receive tamoxifen (20 mg/day) or placebo. The primary endpoint of this study was the occurrence of breast cancer. There was a mean follow-up of 70 months, although few women in the study took the entire 5-year course of tamoxifen. As in the Italian trial, the overall frequency of breast cancer was similar for women on tamoxifen or placebo, with a low event rate (Table 1) again indicating a study

Table 1 Summary: Major Tamoxifen Prevention Trials

		Invasive breast cancer (no events)		
Study	*n*	Placebo	Tamoxifen	HRT allowed
NSABP P-1	13,388	175	89	−
IBIS-I	7,152	85	64	+
Italian National	5,408	22	19	+
Royal Marsden	2,471	36	34	+

population at relatively low risk compared to the NSABP P-1 cohort (3). Another possible confounding factor was the use of HRT by subjects in the Royal Marsden Hospital study (4).

V. RECENT TRIALS

A. IBIS-I

The International Breast Cancer Intervention Study (IBIS-I) randomized 7,152 women aged 35–70 years who were at increased risk for breast cancer to tamoxifen (20 mg/day) or placebo. The primary outcome measure in this trial was the frequency of breast cancer (including ductal carcinoma in situ), after a median follow-up of 50 months. As shown in Table 1, there were 149 cases of invasive breast cancer (85 in the placebo group vs. 64 in the tamoxifen group) for a reduction of 25%. When ductal carcinoma in situ is included, there was a 32% decrease (170 total; 101 for placebo vs. 69 for tamoxifen). Age, degree of risk, and the use of HRT did not affect the rate of reduction. In terms of risks, there was a nonstatistically significant increase in endometrial cancer, while thromboembolic events were significantly increased by 2.5%, particularly after surgery. There was also a significant increase in the total number of deaths from all causes in the tamoxifen group (11 for placebo vs. 25 for tamoxifen) (5).

Although IBIS-I had a different design and entry criteria—for example, women taking HRT were allowed to participate—data from this study appear to complement findings from the NSABP P-1 trial and to be in the same range. The finding of an unexpected increase in all-cause mortality in IBIS-I is troubling. Most of the risk and all of the deaths in the tamoxifen group occurred after surgery. Hence, the excess risk of thromboembolic events seen in the major clinical trials, and the increased number of thromboembolic deaths both in IBIS-I and in the NSABP P-1 trial indicate that thromboembolism is the most important risk associated with tamoxifen use (5). Combined data from IBIS-I and NSABP P-1, nevertheless, argue convincingly for the efficacy of tamoxifen in reducing the incidence of invasive breast cancer. Additional trials are not likely to add anything further based on numbers of events.

This rationale is consistent with the decision to drop the tamoxifen arm from IBIS-II, which will compare the (AI) anastrozole (1 mg/day), with placebo alone in women who are at increased risk of breast cancer or who are diagnosed with ductal carcinoma in situ. The target accrual for IBIS-II is 6,000 postmenopausal women, aged 40–70 years. Follow-up will extend to 5 years (6).

B. The NSABP STAR Trial

In contrast to IBIS-II, the design of the NSABP Study of Tamoxifen and Raloxifene (STAR) trial reflects the efficacy data generated by the NASBP P-1 trial and the possibility of finding a safer and more effective alternative to tamoxifen. STAR will compare the ability of tamoxifen (20 mg/day) or raloxifene (60 mg/day) to reduce the incidence of breast cancer. Women will take either of these two drugs for a period of 5 years, and there will be at least a 2-year follow-up period. Entry criteria are the same as those of the NSABP P-1 (age 35 years or older, lobular carcinoma in situ or 5-year risk of invasive breast cancer of at least 1.67%), except that STAR is limited to postmenopausal women. After 4 years of recruitment, 16,770 women have been randomized of the required 19,000. The median age of randomized women is 58 years, with a median 5-year risk of breast cancer of 3.3%. Hysterectomy was reported by 52.5% of subjects, and lobular carcinoma in situ by 8.4% (7).

C. The MORE Trial

A key issue related to STAR concerns the use of raloxifene, which was selected on the basis of results from the Multiple Outcomes of Raloxifene Evaluation (MORE) trial. MORE compared raloxifene, a SERM approved for prevention and treatment of postmenopausal osteoporosis, at 60- and 120-mg/day doses, and placebo (2:1) in 7,705 women. The mean age of women in this study was 66.5 years at entry, they were an average of 19 years post menopause, and had

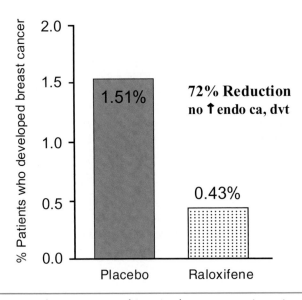

Figure 3 MORE trial: 4-year rates of invasive breast cancer in patients receiving raloxifene or placebo. (From Ref. 8)

been diagnosed with osteoporosis. After 4 years, there was a 72% reduction in the incidence of invasive breast cancer in women who took raloxifene compared to those who took placebo (Fig. 3), primarily a result of the highly significant reduction (84%) in invasive ER+ cancers. There was no increase in endometrial cancer, although thromboembolic disease (including DVT and PE) occurred significantly more often with raloxifene than placebo (1.44, 3.32, and 3.63 events per 1,000 woman years for placebo, and raloxifene 60 mg/day or 120 mg/day, respectively) (8).

VI. HRT AND BREAST CANCER TRIALS

The WHI was a randomized, controlled trial that included 16,608 postmenopausal women aged 50–79 years with an intact uterus at baseline who were allocated either to a combination of conjugated equine estrogens (0.625 mg/day) and medroxyprogesterone acetate (2.5 mg/day), or placebo. The primary outcome measured in this study was coronary heart disease (CHD) (nonfatal MI and CHD death), with invasive breast cancer as the primary adverse outcome. A global index summarizing the balance of risks and benefits included the two primary outcomes in addition to stroke, PE, endometrial cancer, colorectal cancer, hip fracture, and death from other causes. The trial was stopped early, after a mean of 5.2 years of follow-up, when the test statistic for invasive breast cancer exceeded the stopping boundary for this adverse outcome and the global index statistic supported risks exceeding benefits (9–12).

Figure 4 summarizes principal results from the WHI trial according to relative risks and benefits. Women who took HRT had a 1.29% increased risk of CHD, a 1.41% increased risk of stroke, and a 1.26% increased risk of breast cancer, which tended to be diagnosed at a more advanced stage. There was also a 2.11% increased risk of vascular events and a 1.90% increased risk of dementia. In terms of benefits, there was a 0.63% decrease in the proportion of patients who developed colorectal cancer and a 0.66% reduction in hip fractures, which, other than the increased risk of breast cancer, was perhaps the only expected finding from the study. No differences were found in the incidence of endometrial cancer or overall mortality (9, 10).

It has generally been accepted, at least in the United States, that conjugated estrogens negate the benefits of tamoxifen. However, postmenopausal women taking estrogen for menopausal symptoms have been reluctant to stop HRT in order to enter a clinical breast cancer trial. This has posed a barrier to breast cancer prevention trials in the United Sates that, with publication of the WHI results, has been lowered. From a public health perspective, the void that now exists for treatment of menopausal symptoms might be utilized in evolving new prevention strategies for the approximately 10 million women who, under the Gail algorithm, are eligible to participate in breast cancer prevention trials.

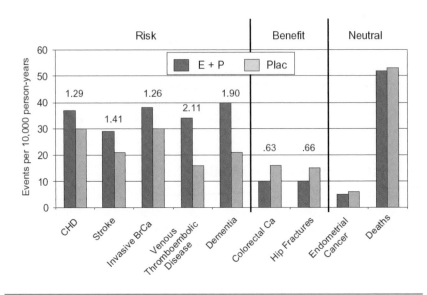

Figure 4   Summary of risks and benefits of HRT therapy from the WHI trial. (From Ref. 9)

VII.   SUMMARY

Accrual to STAR will be completed in 2004, and results will be available 2 to 3 years later. Meanwhile, in thinking about the direction of clinical trials to date, one might ask the extent to which we are prepared to move beyond tamoxifen and perhaps even the entire family of SERMs. Perhaps the next logical step might be to compare raloxifene with an AI in women who are at increased risk of invasive breast cancer. There are now enormous opportunities to make significant gains in prevention, provided that we correctly apply the information already learned.

REFERENCES

1.   Fisher B, Costantino JP, Wickerham DL, Redmond CK, Kavanah M, Cronin WM, Vogel V, Robidoux A, Dimitrov N, Atkins J, Daley M, Wieand S, Tan-Chiu E, Ford L, Wolmark N. Tamoxifen for prevention of breast cancer: Report of the National Surgical Adjuvant Breast and Bowel Project P-1 Study. J Natl Cancer Inst 1998; 90:1371–1388.
2.   Veronesi U, Maisonneuve P, Costa A, Sacchini V, Maltoni C, Robertson C, Rotmensz N, Boyle P, on behalf of the Italian Tamoxifen Prevention Study. Prevention of breast cancer with tamoxifen: preliminary findings from the Italian randomized trial among hysterectomised women. Lancet 1998; 352:93–97.

3. Powles T, Eeles R, Ashley S, Easton D, Chang J, Dowsett M, Tidy A, Viggers J, Davey J. Interim analysis of the incidence of breast cancer in the Royal Marsden Hospital tamoxifen randomized chemoprevention trial. Lancet 1998; 352:98–101.

4. Costantino JP, Vogel VG. Results and implications of the Royal Marsden and other tamoxifen chemoprevention trials: an alternative view. Clin Breast Cancer 2001; 2:41–46.

5. Cuzick J, Forbes J, Edwards R, Baum M, Cawthorn S, Coates A, Hamed H, Howell A, Powles T; IBIS Investigators. First results from the International Breast Cancer Intervention Study (IBIS-I): a randomised prevention trial. Lancet 2002; 360:817–824.

6. Cuzick J. Aromatase inhibitors in prevention-data from the ATAC (Arimidex, Tamoxifen Alone or in Combination) trial and the design of IBIS-II (the Second International Breast Cancer Intervention Study): recent results. Cancer Res 2003; 163:96–103.

7. Vogel VG, Costantino JP, Wickerham DL, Cronin WM. National Surgical Adjuvant Breast and Bowel Project update: prevention trials and endocrine therapy of ductal carcinoma in situ. Clin Cancer Res 2003 (suppl); 9:495S-501S.

8. Cauley JA, Norton L, Lippman ME, Eckert S, Krueger KA, Purdie DW, Farrerons J, Karasik A, Mellstrom D, Ng KW, Stepan JJ, Powles TJ, Morrow M, Costa A, Silfen SL, Walls EL, Schmitt H, Muchmore DB, Jordan VC. Continued breast cancer risk reduction in postmenopausal women treated with raloxifene: 4-year results from the MORE trial. Breast Cancer Res Treat 2001; 65:125–134.

9. Rossouw JE, Anderson GL, Prentice RL, LaCroix AZ, Kooperberg C, Stefanick ML, Jackson RD, Beresford SA, Howard BV, Johnson KC, Kotchen JM, Ockene J; Writing Group for the Women's Health Care Initiative. Risks and benefits of estrogen plus progestin in healthy postmenopausal women. Principal results from the Women's Health Initiative randomized controlled trial. JAMA 2002; 288:321–333.

10. Chlebowski RT, Hendrix SL, Langer RD, Stefanick ML, Gass M, Lane D, Rodabough RJ, Gilligan MA, Cyr MG, Thomson CA, Khandekar J, Petrovich H, McTiernan A; for the WHI investigators. Influence of estrogen plus progestin on breast cancer and mammography in healthy postmenopausal women. The Women's Health Initiative randomized trial. JAMA 2003; 289:3243–3253.

11. Rapp SR, Espeland MA, Shumaker SA, Henderson VW, Brunner RL, Manson JE, Gass MLS, Stefanick ML, Lane DS, Hays J, Johnson KC, Coker LH, Dailey M, Bowen D;for the WHIMS investigators. Effect of estrogen plus progestin on global cognitive function in postmenopausal women. The Women's Health Initiative Memory Study: A randomized controlled trial. JAMA 2003; 289:2663–2672.

12. Hays J, Ockene JK, Brunner RL, Kotchen JM, Manson JE, Patterson RE, Aragaki AK, Shumaker SA, Brzyski RG, LaCroix AZ, Granek IA, Valanis BG; for the WHI investigators. Effects of estrogen plus progestin on health-related quality of life. N Engl J Med 2003; 348:1839–1854.

13

Clinical Trials with Aromatase Inhibitors for the Prevention of Breast Cancer

Mitch Dowsett

The Royal Marsden Hospital
London, England

I. OVERVIEW

With the acceptance of the feasibility of risk-reduction (generally called preventive) therapy for breast cancer, it has now become increasingly important to identify optimal treatment paradigms to improve prognosis. As few as one-third of the high-risk women selected in preventive trials of tamoxifen benefited from therapy. New generations of trials with aromatase inhibitors (AIs)—which have a low incidence of side effects and an early promise in preventing contralateral tumors—are investigating the effects of these drugs on surrogate markers of breast cancer, including bone and lipid metabolism and breast density. Other trials of AIs are seeking new ways of treating patients through the partial elimination of estrogen production. What remains clear, however, is that without better patient selection, the identification of women who will benefit most from preventive therapy will remain low and, as such, new therapies will not reach their full potential.

II. TAMOXIFEN—WHERE ARE WE NOW?

A review of the outcomes from the four main breast-cancer prevention trials with tamoxifen reported that while breast-cancer incidence could be reduced, these reductions came at a cost (1). The review covered randomized trials with tamoxifen:

189

International Breast Cancer Intervention Study I (IBIS I) (2); National Surgical Adjuvant Breast and Bowel Project (NSABP) P-1 study (3); Royal Marsden Study (4); and the Italian Tamoxifen Prevention Study (5, 6); as well as the trial of raloxifene in postmenopausal women with osteoporosis; from the Multiple Outcomes Raloxifene Evaluation (MORE) study (7).

Overall, tamoxifen reduced the incidence of breast cancer by 38% ($p < 0.0001$). This reduction in incidence occurred regardless of age. No reduction was seen in estrogen-receptor-negative (ER−) breast cancers, while a 48% reduction was seen in estrogen receptor-positive (ER+) tumors ($p < 0.0001$). The MORE trial, comparing raloxifene with placebo, reported a 64% reduction in overall breast-cancer incidence ($p < 0.0001$).

Allied with these reductions were increases in adverse events. In the tamoxifen studies, the relative risk (RR) of thromboembolic events was 1.9 ($p < 0.0001$), with a similar increase observed in the raloxifene group ($p = 0.003$). Endometrial cancer rates were increased in both prevention trials and in the adjuvant trials with tamoxifen. Consensus RR for endometrial cancer in the prevention trials was 2.4 ($p = 0.0005$), while in adjuvant trials, the hazard ratio was 3.4 ($p = 0.0002$). It is important to note that these increased risks of thromoboembolism and endometrial cancer were age-related with greater absolute increases in tamoxifen-induced incidence in the older-than-50 group. This provides a better therapeutic index for tamoxifen in the preventive setting in younger high-risk women.

Although overall mortality in the tamoxifen groups was no different than placebo, there was a significant increase in all-cause mortality in the IBIS I tamoxifen arm. The number of deaths reported in this study of 7,152 patients were 25 (0.70%) and 11 (0.30%), respectively ($p = 0.028$) (2). However, it seems likely that this is an aberrant result because exhaustive analysis has revealed multiple causes for the excess deaths mostly unassociated with tamoxifen's known effects.

The data from the meta-analysis provide strong support for tamoxifen's reduction of the incidence of ER+ breast cancer. Using the pooled data, Cuzick et al. (1) predicted an 18% reduction in the 10-year risk of death from breast cancer in high-risk women similar to those entered into the trials. This predicted gain needs to be weighed against the high risks of a venous thromboembolism and the increased risk of endometrial cancer. In light of the adverse events which accompany tamoxifen, the authors concluded that tamoxifen cannot yet be recommended as a preventive treatment.

The American Society of Clinical Oncology (ASCO) has published a technology assessment of breast cancer risk reduction (8) that suggested that women with a 5-year projected cancer risk of ≥1.66% could be offered tamoxifen as preventive therapy. The authors went on to state that the greatest benefits would be seen in patients who were younger (as noted earlier), had no uterus, and had a higher risk of breast cancer. The available data were summarized as not yet suggesting that tamoxifen provides an overall health benefit in this context.

Overall, the data indicate that, while tamoxifen may offer some benefits to selected groups of high-risk women, these benefits are associated with a significantly increased risk of adverse events. It is, therefore, important that new therapeutic options and algorithms be developed for breast cancer risk reduction. One therapeutic option of major current interest is the use of AIs.

III. AIs

The effect of hormonal agents on the incidence of contralateral breast cancer during adjuvant therapy is an important marker of their likely effects in the prevention of breast cancer. An overview analysis of adjuvant trials by the Early Breast Cancer Trialists Cooperative Group (EBCTCG) suggested that 5 years of tamoxifen adjuvant therapy was associated with a 47% RR reduction of contralateral breast cancer ($p < 0.00001$) (9). More recently, the Arimidex (anastrozole), Tamoxifen, Alone or in Combination (ATAC) trial found that the AI anastrozole produced a greater reduction in the incidence of contralateral breast cancer than tamoxifen (odds ratio $= 0.42$; $p = 0.007$) (10) after 33 months median follow-up. The difference after 47 months median follow-up was marginally less but still significant (Fig. 1). Furthermore, data from the ATAC trial indicated that anastrozole was significantly better tolerated than tamoxifen as measured by the prespecified reporting of adverse events (Table 1). Importantly, thromboembolic events, cere-

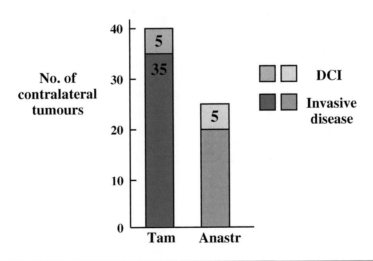

Figure 1 Occurrence of contralateral breast cancer after 47 months follow-up in the ATAC trial.

Table 1 Occurrence of Prespecified Adverse Events in the ATAC Trial That Differed Significantly Between the Anastrazole-Alone and Tamoxifen-Alone Arms

	Anastrazole (A) (n = 3092)	Tamoxifen (T) (n = 3094)	A + T (n = 3097)
Hot flashes	1060 (34.3%)*	1229 (39.7%)	1243 (40.1%)
Musculoskeletal disorders	860 (27.8%)*	660 (21.3%)	685 (22.1%)
Vaginal bleeding	138 (4.5%)*	253 (8.2%)	238 (7.7%)
Vaginal discharge	86 (2.8%)*	354 (11.4%)	357 (11.5%)
Endometrial cancer	3 (0.1%)‡	13 (0.5%)	6 (0.3%)
Fractures	183 (5.9%)*	115 (3.7%)	142 (4.6%)
Ischemic cerebrovascular events	31 (1.0%)†	65 (2.1%)	51 (1.6%)
Any venous thrombo-embolic event	64 (2.1%)†	109 (3.5%)	124 (4.0%)
Deep-venous thrombo-embolic event	32 (1.0%)‡	54 (1.7%)	63 (2.0%)

*$p < 0.0001$ vs. tamoxifen; †$p = 0.0006$ vs. tamoxifen; ‡$p = 0.02$ vs. tamoxifen.

brovascular events, and endometrial cancer incidence were significantly lower with anastrozole although there were significantly more fractures and musculoskeletal disorders.

Thus, it is possible that AIs might offer greater risk reduction of breast cancer than tamoxifen as well as better tolerability. However, it must be recognized that AIs will not be without some detrimental effects, increased bone loss having already been established (11). It is therefore appropriate that clinical trials with these agents should be conducted in order to establish their potential in the preventive setting, but it is prudent that these trials should include careful monitoring of potential side effects. The early development of strategies to avoid or manage such side effects will be important in allowing the widespread use of these agents and has already been considered in many of the series of Phase II and III prevention trials of AIs that have been completed, are underway, or being planned. These are reviewed in the following.

IV. PHASE II AI TRIALS

A. Letrozole Intermediate Tissue Marker Study

The primary aim of the Letrozole Intermediate Tissue Marker Study (LITMaS), that was conducted by our group at the Royal Marsden Hospital, was to investigate the effects of letrozole on the expression of the proliferation marker Ki67 in the luminal epithelial cells of the normal postmenopausal breast, the rationale being that this would indicate a likely reduction in the susceptibility of these cells to malignant transformation (11). The study recruited 32 women without active breast disease to receive 3 months of treatment with letrozole (2.5 mg/day). The women had no active disease but had a preexisting diagnosis of ductal carcinoma in situ (DCIS) or benign breast disease and a normal contralateral breast. Core-cut biopsies were taken before and at the end of treatment to allow the assessment of Ki67.

As expected, plasma estradiol levels were markedly suppressed other than in two patients who may have been noncompliant. A 30% reduction in Ki67 was found following therapy but this was not statistically significant. Therefore, we concluded that any prophylactic effect of letrozole would most likely not be dependent on antiproliferative effects on normal breast. This does not discount the possibility of letrozole having prophylactic effects by impacting on later stage events that are estrogen dependent, e.g., the promotion of subclinical carcinomas.

B. WISE Study

The Women with Increased Serum Estradiol levels (WISE) study is investigating the effects of suppressing estrogen levels with full-dose letrozole in approximately 100 women who are at increased risk of developing breast cancer because of their increased exposure to estrogen. The women are required to have a plasma estradiol level $\geq$ 12 pg/mL (~40 pmol/L), and the study is placebo-controlled. The 12 pg/ml cut-off for increased risk was selected as it defined the upper quartile of estradiol levels in the Nurses' Health Study (NHS) of epidemiology and associated breast cancer risk (12). The primary endpoint is the change in bone-mineral density. The trial is still in its recruitment stage.

C. MAP1 and MAP2

The MAP1 and 2 trials aim to randomize women with high breast density to 1 year of letrozole or placebo or 1 year of exemestane or placebo, respectively. The primary endpoint for both studies is change in breast density at 1 year. Target recruitment is 137 and 120 women, respectively. The MAP2 trial will randomize 120 patients, also at high-risk of breast cancer, to 1 year of either exemestane or placebo.

V. PHASE III AI TRIALS

A. International Breast Cancer Intervention Study II

The International Breast Cancer Intervention Study II (IBIS II) is a randomized, double-blind, double-dummy study with two strata: a preventive stratum and a DCIS stratum. The preventive stratum has a similar design to IBIS I, however anastrozole, in place of tamoxifen, is being compared with placebo and all subjects are postmenopausal. This stratum has a target enrollment of 6,000 post-menopausal women, aged 40–70 years, who are at increased risk of breast cancer. Increased risk is assessed using the factors of nulliparity, a family history, benign proliferative disease and high breast density. The primary endpoint is the development of histologically confirmed breast cancer. The second stratum of the study, recruiting 4,000 patients, will investigate the efficacy of anastrozole compared with tamoxifen in women with locally excised ductal carcinomas in situ (DICS). The efficacy endpoint is the prevention of local recurrence or a second breast cancer after completion of surgery for DCIS.

Importantly, IBIS II has a detailed bone subprotocol. It is planned that the first 1,000 women enrolled and randomized into the trial will undergo a detailed assessment of their bone parameters in addition to receiving anastrozole or placebo. This group of 1,000 patients will be subdivided into three groups. The first group will be comprised of 300 women with normal bone density (T-scores $\geq$ -1.5) who will be monitored closely. The second group, consisting of 400 women with moderate or severe osteopenia (T-scores < -1.5 but ≥ -2.5) will be randomized to receive a bisphosphonate or placebo. The third group will consist of 300 osteoporotic women (T-scores < -2.5) and will receive bisphosphonate therapy. All women in this bone substudy will be required to take vitamin D and calcium supplements.

B. MAP3

The MAP3 prevention trial, coordinated by the National Cancer Institute in Canada, will enroll 5,100 postmenopausal women with increased risk of breast cancer and randomize them to either placebo, exemestane, or exemestane plus celecoxib (a COX-II inhibitor). The study's objective is to determine if exemestane, with or without celecoxib, reduces the incidence of invasive breast cancer compared with placebo.

VI. NOVEL APPROACHES TO THE USE OF AIs IN BREAST CANCER PREVENTION

It has become clear that there is a significant relationship between high plasma estradiol levels and risk of breast cancer (see the following for a more detailed discussion). This suggests that any reduction of these levels might reduce breast cancer risk. Reducing rather than eliminating levels of estrogen in women who have high levels of estrogen could theoretically reduce the number of clinical complications associated with complete estrogen deprivation. Such reductions might be achieved by the use of low-doses of a third-generation inhibitor or conventional doses of a lower-potency second-generation compound. The latter include rogletimide, developed at the Institute of Cancer Research, London, or oral 4-hydroxyandrostenedione, both of which provide 50–80% suppression of whole body aromatase activity (13, 14).

However, it is likely that such an approach could be problematic, as it essentially involves down-titrating an individual's estrogen levels. This could prove logistically difficult, especially when attempting to make broad recommendations for treatment practice, because it would involve sequential estrogen measurements and dose adjustments based on these. A more practical approach might emulate the premenopausal prevention strategy suggested by Pike et al. (15) that suggested that a gonadotrophin-releasing hormone agonist be used to eliminate estrogen production in the ovaries of premenopausal woman, followed by treatment with low doses of hormone-replacement therapy in order to provide low level, controlled estrogen exposure.

Such an approach could also work for postmenopausal women. In this case, a full dose of AI could be used to halt estrogen production, with subsequent replacement of very low doses of estradiol following the interruption of estrogen production. Pilot studies of this approach are currently underway to establish the optimal dose and pharmaceutical preparation for such replacement. Such an up-titration approach might be more attractive compared with the equivalent down-titration method, especially with respect to dose control in individual patients. Additionally, the approach of complete aromatase inhibition with add-back estradiol has theoretical advantages because: 1) the component of estrogen in the tumor or premalignant lesion that is due to local aromatization would be ablated by this approach, and 2) only that component that is derived from the circulation would be supplemented. This would lead to lower exposure of the target tissue to estrogen than with the down-titration approach for the same level of circulating estrogen.

It may also be possible to target local breast aromatase activity while avoiding or minimizing systemic effects by delivering the AI percutaneously through the skin of the breast. Again, pilot studies are underway but much more data are required to establish the viability of this approach.

Lastly, the use of tissue-targeted aromatase suppressants may be a viable approach to estrogen deprivation in the breast. Specifically, we are currently assessing inhibition of cyclooxygenase-2 (COX-2) for its possible suppression of aromatase activity in and adjacent to breast carcinomas (16). Confirmation of this would make these particularly attractive for possible use in breast cancer prevention based on this mechanism as well as their other effects, such as reduced tumor angiogenesis.

VII. IMPROVING PREDICTION OF PREVENTABLE BREAST CANCER

The meta-analysis of breast cancer prevention trials with tamoxifen reported that only about one-third of breast carcinomas were prevented in the selected

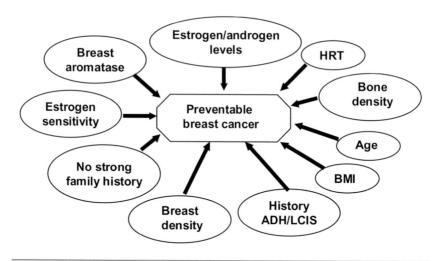

Figure 2 Possible components of an algorithm to predict hormone-dependent breast cancer risk.

populations (1). It is clear that in order to make chemoprevention a viable proposition, the identification of women at high risk for the development of breast cancer that is preventable by a particular maneuver must be improved. At the present time, because our focus is on the use of estrogen deprivation or anti-estrogenic maneuvers, the identification of women likely to develop an ER+ breast carcinoma would be highly advantageous.

At present, the most widely used model for breast cancer risk estimation is the Gail Model (17). This was used to identify high-risk women in the NSABP P1 study (3). The model uses age, first-degree relative with breast cancer, nulliparity/age at first live birth, number of breast biopsies, pathological diagnosis of atypical hyperplasia, and age at menarche. However, the majority of these criteria do not relate to the development of hormone sensitive disease. Indeed, factors such as the number of first-degree relatives with breast cancer may actually predict a greater proportion of ER− disease (18). However, there are several other factors that may influence or be associated with breast cancer risk by virtue of an estrogenic pathway (Fig. 2). Some of the key factors are considered in the following.

A. Plasma Estradiol

Over recent years there have been nine reports on the association between plasma estradiol and other hormone levels in postmenopausal women and their subsequent development of breast cancer. These have recently been subject to overview analysis (19). Plasma estradiol showed a strong and highly significant response rate (RR)

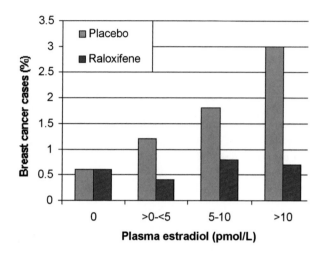

Figure 3 Risk of breast cancer in the MORE study: influence of plasma estradiol. (From Ref. 20)

for increased breast cancer risk. Testosterone (and some of the other hormones) also showed a strong relationship, but this was largely lost when adjusted for estradiol levels, although some independent predictive value was retained, even when corrected for estradiol. Of particular note, data from the MORE study suggest that high plasma estradiol levels select women at high risk of "preventable" breast cancer. In an analysis of the data by Cummings et al., the RR of breast cancer was assessed using a quartile analysis of estradiol levels in the study's patients (20). As estradiol levels increased, so too did the risk of breast cancer (Fig. 3). Raloxifene had a much greater preventive effect at these higher levels of estradiol, suggesting that what is seen is indeed the identification of "preventable" breast cancer. Thus, selection of patients on the basis of plasma estradiol—possibly together with testosterone and sex-hormone-binding globulin (SHBG)—levels could contribute to an estrogen-dependent risk algorithm. But for these to be widely acceptable, much more rugged, well-validated assays will need to be developed for these analyses in postmenopausal women than are currently available.

B. Bone Mineral Density

The correlation between bone density and incidence of breast cancer was shown in a publication by Zhang et al. (21), which suggested that the risk of breast cancer increased in the highest quartile of bone density. However, it seems likely that high estradiol levels explain much of this relationship such that limited information might be derived in addition to the measurement of plasma estradiol levels. Thus, while the possibility of bone-mineral density as an independent marker for breast cancer risk should not yet be discounted, correction of bone density for estradiol levels is needed to confirm if it has any independent predictive value. Additional factors that reduce the attractiveness of this measure as a potential component of a new algorithm are that bone-mineral density is not being routinely collected in postmenopausal women and the wide variability in performance between various instruments for assessing density.

C. Body Mass Index

Body mass index (BMI) has long been known to correlate with increased risk of breast cancer. In the overview analysis of plasma steroids and breast cancer risk, it was possible to assess the degree to which this relationship could be explained by the higher estradiol levels seen in women with higher BMI. For every increase of 5 kg/m^2 in BMI, an increase of 1.19 in the RR of breast cancer was seen (22). However, once adjusted for protein-free plasma estradiol, this increase in RR was reduced to 1.02. Thus, if estradiol and sex hormone-binding glogulin (SHBG) levels are included in the algorithm, very little predictability would be gained by adding BMI.

D. Breast Density

Breast density is a strong risk factor for breast cancer: Women with density >75% have an RR of being diagnosed with breast cancer of 5.0 (23). Breast density is readily available for the majority of postmenopausal patients because most will have mammograms taken at regular intervals during the first 10–20 years of their postmenopausal life via standard breast screening. At present, it remains unclear whether breast density is a greater risk factor for ER+ disease but its strength as a risk factor for breast cancer in general and its ready availability make it likely that breast density will be more widely included in risk algorithms in future. Even if it were not to enhance prediction of ER+ tumors specifically, it could usefully be included in an estrogen-dependent algorithm in which other factors are used to enrich for the estrogen-dependent population.

It is clear that density changes markedly with age and menopause, but the exact relationships are not well-defined. In order to make use of breast density in guiding therapy, its relationship with age and menopause needs to be characterized better, particularly in relation to how this influences breast cancer risk prediction. Interestingly Boyd et al. reported that breast density had a heritability component of up to 60% (24) such that if the genes responsible can be identified, it may eventually be better to characterize these than to quantify breast density itself.

Thus, at the present time, plasma estradiol and possibly testosterone and SHBG analysis alongside breast-density measurements are attractive to consider as components of a new estrogen-dependent breast cancer risk algorithm. Looking to the future, it is attractive to speculate that these analyses might be routinely available to women attending for breast cancer screening who might then evaluate the derived data as a way of determining whether risk-reduction strategies merit their personal consideration.

VII. CONCLUSIONS

Data from trials with tamoxifen have provided "proof-of-concept" about using preventive therapy for reducing breast cancer incidence. However, long-term therapy with agents like AIs merit study in postmenopausal women due to the possibility of decreased side-effects and improved efficacy. While newer therapies can provide improved prognosis, the future need will be to improve the identification of patients for whom preventive treatment would be most beneficial. In this respect, the next generation of aromatase trials, described herein, will provide crucial information on surrogate markers of breast cancer.

REFERENCES

1. Cuzick J, Powles T, Veronesi U, Forbes J, Edwards R, Ashley S, Boyle P. Overview of the main outcomes in breast-cancer prevention trials. Lancet 2003; 361:296–300.
2. Cuzick J, Forbes J, Edwards R, Baum M, Cawthorn S, Coates A, Hamed A, Howell A, Powles T; IBIS investigators. First results from the International Breast Cancer Intervention Study (IBIS-I): a randomised prevention trial. Lancet 2002; 360: 817–824.
3. Fisher B, Costantino JP, Wickerham DL, Redmond CK, Kavanah M, Cronin WM, Vogel V, Robidoux A, Dimitrov N, Atkins J, Daly M, Wieand S, Tan-Chiu E, Ford L, Wolmark N. Tamoxifen for prevention of breast cancer: report of the National Surgical Adjuvant Breast and Bowel Project P-1 Study. J Natl Cancer Inst 1998; 90:1371–1388.
4. Powles T, Eeles R, Ashley S, Easton D, Chang J, Dowsett M, Tidy A, Viggers J, Davey J. Interim analysis of the incidence of breast cancer in the Royal Marsden Hospital tamoxifen randomised chemoprevention trial. Lancet 1998; 352:98–101.
5. Veronesi U, Maisonneuve P, Costa A, Sacchini V, Maltoni C, Robertson C, Rotmensz N, Boyle P. Prevention of breast cancer with tamoxifen: preliminary findings from the Italian randomised trial among hysterectomised women. Italian Tamoxifen Prevention Study. Lancet 1998; 352:93–97.
6. Veronesi U, Maisonneuve P, Sacchini V, Rotmensz N, Boyle P; Italian Tamoxifen Study Group. Tamoxifen for breast cancer among hysterectomised women. Lancet 2002; 359:1122–1124.
7. Cauley JA, Norton L, Lippman ME, Eckert S, Krueger KA, Purdie DW, Farrerons J, Karasik A, Mellstrom D, Ng KW, Stepan JJ, Powles TJ, Morrow M, Costa A, Silfen

SL, Walls EL, Schmitt H, Muchmore DB, Jordan VC, Ste-Marie LG. Continued breast cancer risk reduction in postmenopausal women treated with raloxifene: 4-year results from the MORE trial. Multiple outcomes of raloxifene evaluation. Breast Cancer Res Treat 2001; 65:125–134.

8. Chlebowski RT, Col N, Winer EP, Collyar DE, Cummings SR, Vogel VG 3rd, Burstein HJ, Eisen A, Lipkus I, Pfister DG; American Society of Clinical Oncology Breast Cancer Technology Assessment Working Group. American Society of Clinical Oncology technology assessment of pharmacologic interventions for breast cancer risk reduction including tamoxifen, raloxifene, and aromatase inhibition. J Clin Oncol 2002; 20:3328–3343.

9. Early Breast Cancer Trialists' Collaborative Group. Tamoxifen for early breast cancer: an overview of the randomised trials. Lancet 1998; 351:1451–1467.

10. Baum M, Budzar AU, Cuzick J, Forbes J, Houghton JH, Klijn JG, Sahmoud T; ATAC Trialists' Group. Anastrozole alone or in combination with tamoxifen versus tamoxifen alone for adjuvant treatment of postmenopausal women with early breast cancer: first results of the ATAC randomised trial. Lancet 2002; 359:2131–2139.

11. Harper-Wynne C, Ross G, Sacks N, Salter J, Nasiri N, Iqbal J, A'Hern R, Dowsett M. Effects of the aromatase inhibitor letrozole on normal breast epithelial cell proliferation and metabolic indices in postmenopausal women: a pilot study for breast cancer prevention. Cancer Epidemiol Biomarkers Prev 2002; 11:614–621.

12. Hankinson SE, Colditz GA, Hunter DJ, Manson JE, Willett WC, Stampfer MJ, Longcope C, Speizer FE. Reproductive factors and family history of breast cancer in relation to plasma estrogen and prolactin levels in postmenopausal women in the Nurses' Health Study (United States). Cancer Causes Control 1995; 6:217–224.

13. MacNeill FA, Jones AL, Jacobs S, Lonning PE, Powles TJ, Dowsett M. The influence of aminoglutethimide and its analogue rogletimide on peripheral aromatisation in breast cancer. Br J Cancer 1992; 66:692–697.

14. MacNeill FA, Jacobs S, Dowsett M, Lonning PE, Powles TJ. The effects of oral 4-hydroxyandrostenedione on peripheral aromatisation in post-menopausal breast cancer patients. Cancer Chemother Pharmacol 1995; 36:249–254.

15. Spicer DV, Pike MC. Sex steroids and breast cancer prevention. J Natl Cancer Inst Monogr 1994; 16:139–147.

16. Simpson ER, Dowsett M. Aromatase and its inhibitors: significance for breast cancer therapy. Recent Prog Horm Res 2002; 57:317–338.

17. Gail MH, Brinton LA, Byar DP, Corle DK, Green SB, Schairer C, Mulvihill JJ. Projecting individualized probabilities of developing breast cancer for white females who are being examined annually. J Natl Cancer Inst 1989; 81:1879–1886.

18. Cummings SR, Lee J, LUI L-Y, Stone K, Ljung B-M, Rugo, HS, Cauley JA. Risk factors and endogenous sex hormones for prediction of ER+ and ER− breast cancer in older women: findings from the study of osteoporotic fractures. Proc Amer Soc Clin Oncol. 2003; 22:846.

19. Endogenous Hormones Breast Cancer Collaborative Group. Endogenous sex hormones and breast cancer in postmenopausal women: reanalysis of nine prospective studies. J Natl Cancer Inst 2002; 94:606–616.

20. Cummings SR, Duong T, Kenyon E, Cauley JA, Whitehead M, Krueger KA; Multiple Outcomes of Raloxifene Evaluation (MORE) Trial. Serum estradiol level and risk of breast cancer during treatment with raloxifene. J Am Med Assoc 2002; 287:216–220.

21. Zhang Y, Kiel DP, Kreger BE, Cupples LA, Ellison RC, Dorgan JF, Schatzkin A, Levy D, Felson DT. Bone mass and the risk of breast cancer among postmenopausal women. N Engl J Med. 1997; 336:611–617.

22. Endogenous Hormones Breast Cancer Collaborative Group. Body mass index, serum sex hormones, and breast cancer risk in postmenopausal women. J Natl Cancer Inst 2003; 95:1218–1226.

23. Yaffe MJ, Boyd NF, Byng JW, Jong RA, Fishell E, Lockwood GA, Little LE, Tritchler DL. Breast cancer risk and measured mammographic density. Eur J Cancer Prev 1998; 7 (suppl):S47–55.

24. Boyd NF, Dite GS, Stone J, Gunasekara A, English DR, McCredie MR, Giles GG, Tritchler D, Chiarelli A, Yaffe MJ, Hopper JL. Heritability of mammographic density, a risk factor for breast cancer. N Engl J Med 2002; 347:886–894.

Chemoprevention

Trevor J. Powles and Wolfgang Eiermann, *Chairmen*

Tuesday, July 8, 2003

T. Powles: I thought if we could try and structure the first part of the discussion toward the issues related to tamoxifen versus aromatase inhibitors, and questions about the trials which are underway at present and the proposed new trials. Then in the second part we can move on to risk factors.

W. Miller: I think those were tremendous talks; both are to be congratulated. I wanted to pull together the two elements that you just mentioned. It seems to me that Mitch [Dowsett] has put forward a case that hormones may be usefully manipulated in preventing breast cancer. Most of the data he puts forward for this suggest that what we are looking at are high-risk women who essentially have normal levels of hormones and, for example, the groups which comprise the top and lowest quintile still have normal levels although there is a difference in incidence. Similarly, the Judy Garber risk groups still encompass normal levels.

So the suggestion from the epidemiology would be that excess risk is accompanied with comparatively small differences in hormone levels. I know you have got to build exposure time into this equation but I am concerned that against this background we are discussing doing studies where we use endocrine agents such as aromatase inhibitors.

Therefore, I am concerned about embarking upon large studies in which the vast majority of women will not subsequently develop breast cancer. I was wondering whether Mitch [Dowsett] may share some of these concerns and that we shouldn't be treating women that have been exposed to a comparatively small excess of estrogen with regimes that are developed to treat patients with advanced or early breast cancer. Rather, one should be looking at an intermediate concept in which one reduces estrogen but not to the levels that you would achieve with the currently used clinical doses of these potent aromatase inhibitors.

M. Dowsett: As I've tried to illustrate in the talk, I very much do favor the concept of reduced estrogen levels as opposed to completely wiping out the estrogen levels. Unfortunately, those approaches still have to be developed.

P. Goss: Mitch [Dowsett] and I have shared the concept of developing better algorithms for selecting impartial reduction. I think, Bill, to some extent you may have answered your own question. That is, the whole issue about preventing breast cancer over a period of time may relate to a small and modest change in the estrogen environment for a prolonged period of time, or a substantial change for a short period of time.

What we think about the aromatase inhibitor trial is that we're moving the proof of concept that's been established by tamoxifen gradually forward. We strongly feel still that you have to do large endpoint Phase III trials and verify some of these risk profiles prospectively before you start applying them.

W. Miller: I accept what you say that it may very well be that the exposure time, if we multiply things, makes a difference. But I do have some concerns still that without pilot data you are embarking on large prevention trials with aromatase inhibitors when we do not have the long-term toxicities from patients who have been treated with breast cancer at this time. We don't even know what length of time to use these aromatase inhibitors. In the prevention studies, we have quite a long exposure time.

P. Goss: To some extent, the corollary point could be made though, Bill, in that there are about 20–30 thousand adjuvant breast cancer patients who fulfill the criteria for prevention trials in terms of age and health profile, who are already on aromatase inhibitors. This provides a vanguard body of data evolving ahead of prevention trials in healthy women.

These trials are often conceived of as a static point in time. But we have the safety net of the data coming from 30,000 women to study, on aromatase inhibitors, with a lead time of 3 to 4 years. For instance, we have 6 years of follow up in the MA.17 trial with placebo-controlled toxicity data on 5,000 patients. There is quite a body of data. Our view is that we plan to assess these risk factors, as Mitch [Dowsett] has outlined: bone-mineral density, breast density and plasma hormone levels. Similar safety studies in IBIS II will be undertaken to try to tie down how they can be incorporated into final selection of women for the next generation of prevention trials.

R. Santen: I'd just like to make a general comment and try to have us put the horse before the cart rather than vice versa. We have to look at this problem from a general perspective. If you look at the prevention of heart disease and the use of statins, this area of disease prevention is probably 10 or 15 years ahead of the status of breast cancer prevention.

What has happened in the cardiovascular area? The first thing is that the people selected for heart disease prevention have at least a 10% chance of getting heart disease in 5 years. The benefit/risk ratio from prevention therapy is going to be substantially greater in those individuals. We've had a lot of discussion about this, but I really think that if we're going to put the horse before the cart, what we've got to do is to develop these risk algorithms. We have that for heart disease. It's multi-factorial: LDL cholesterol, HDL cholesterol, and so on. First, we need to concentrate on developing powerful means to predicate who will get breast cancer. Only then can we select patients at high risk to treat with aromatase inhibitors.

I.C. Henderson: I feel like I may be somewhat of a lone voice here. My comments have to do with where we go with future trials as well as how we interpret them. I think Bernie Fisher is quoted as saying something to the effect that there aren't immature data, but only premature conclusions. I wonder if that might apply here.

I find the rationale for these trials elegant and the data very compelling. I think that the trial data thus far from the tamoxifen studies are consistent and do show that for a period of 5 years we decrease the incidence. However, I think I would take issue with Mitch's [Dowsett] final slide where he said we have proof of concept. It depends on which concept we're talking about.

We certainly do have proof of concept that we have a delay in the appearance of breast cancer. That might be a worthwhile goal in itself if that delay is sufficiently long. It's like saying we don't cure breast cancer but you live 20 years before you die of it—20 additional years. That's a worthwhile goal. Delay may be a worthwhile goal, but that wasn't our original goal when we started this. Our original goal was to prevent breast cancer, and I think it's too early to say that we have proof of concept.

However, we saw no data on mortality. I think it's too early to expect such data, but nonetheless, ultimately, [what] was the goal for most of the patients who have gone on these studies? They hope they will decrease mortality.

I think that our goals have not yet been met. This is relevant to the trial design in that I think there is still a lot of room for a wide variety of trial designs.

I would make a plea for us to keep our minds open at least. I'm very supportive of all these trials. I'm supportive of looking for surrogate markers. But I think we have to keep our analytical brains open and not overinterpret our data and not reach premature conclusions. I'm just not convinced that we do have proof of principle yet for the important endpoints, which is prevention or a reduction in mortality or, much weaker, a prolonged delay that the patients would consider humanly worthwhile.

I. Smith: One of the problems the aromatase inhibitors introduced into this area is that they are only effective in postmenopausal women. That may turn out to be effective in terms of delaying breast cancer. But it seems to me there is quite a reasonable hypothesis that the original event that you're trying to prevent may have occurred premenopausally. I have got a question [for] the aromatase-inhibitor proponents: Do you just accept this and say pragmatically there is nothing we can do about that? Or do you think that there are theoretical reasons to believe that, in fact, the initial event that you're trying to prevent occurs only in the postmenopausal environment.

P. Goss: My own view is both those possibilities are correct. I agree that there is some suggestion from the calculations and the theories about the pathway to breast cancer that many of the events may have started before the menopause. But like Craig [Henderson] said, the division between invasive breast cancer and ductal carcinoma in situ (DICS) or preinvasive cancer, is a human-made division.

With regard to preventive versus early treatment, I think substantial delay in the clinical occurrence of cancer is prevention. I am not sure it's clinically important that we have to prove that we've prevented one of the steps in the multistep pathway of breast cancer.

If we can arrest it or make the transition time between atypical ductal hyperplasea (ADH) and DCIS to invasive cancer an extra 5 or 10 years by switching off the estrogen signal, and it translates clinically into delaying the median age of invasive breast cancer in North American from 63 to 75, that's going to allow other competing causes of death to catch up. More importantly, it's going to shift breast cancer away as a major cause of mortality from the perimenopausal age when it has its greatest impact.

T. Powles: I think the point Craig [Henderson] was making is it is important that we only have reduction in incidence data at the moment. In terms of proof of principle about whether we have clinical benefit or reduction in mortality is questioned at this stage. He's not saying that we shouldn't go ahead with the trials, but that we shouldn't overplay it. I think that's the issue.

J. Bergh: I would really underline what Craig Henderson said. I think the studies should of course be carried out as planned and I think they will answer important questions. However, another issue is that the cancers which are prevented are receptor-positive breast cancers. It is possible that early-diagnosis strategies and treating those cancers would be similarly effective.

I have to quote Danish data saying that receptor-positive small tumors have an equivalent prognosis as in Danish women without breast cancer. You are actually dealing with a scenario [in which] in the current published prevention studies, although it's too early to see it, still show no survival gain whatsoever, even in the meta-analysis produced. You clearly must have concern at least for skeletal events with new strategies using aromatase inhibitors.

For the long run, I would also have concern for the lipid profile and what that will make with the cardiovascular issues. If we are looking at the risk/benefit calculation, and have a more global view on this, I'm not sure that we so far have got the right drugs, the right instruments, to try and identify the correct population [with which] to go ahead. This is my rather conservative view on this.

J.-J. Body: I would like to raise two points. First, one about the selective estrogen receptor modulators (SERMs). It is clear to me that they are not all the same. I would like to come back to the results of the MORE trial, where you had a larger effect on the reduction in breast cancer incidence than in the tamoxifen trials. You have to know that these patients included in the MORE trial were certainly not at increased risk of cancer of the breast since they could not enter the study if they had a past history of breast cancer. In other words, this was a population with an apparently low risk at baseline but with a larger preventive effect than in the tamoxifen studies.

If I may go to another point, namely the use of aromatase-inhibitors for prevention. One has alluded to the side effects. I would like to insist upon the increased risk of the fractures, notably of the hip. This has now been well demonstrated in the ATAC trial. We have to know that this is an event that carries a risk of death of about 15%, if not 20%. I would like to know your opinion, if we have the right to include patients in these long-term trials with a T-score less than −2.5 and not treat them, for example, with bisphosphonates. You have shown that the bisphosphonates even prolong survival in patients with operable breast cancer, and we have not mentioned these drugs at all.

M. Ellis: Actually this follows on. I think the concept of global health is so important in these prevention trials. I'd like to see Kaplan-Meier not only focusing on breast events but also in combination with freedom from serious side effects. That's what is so nice about the hormone replacement therapy (HRT) trials. They tried to use all these endpoints to make an informed decision as to whether HRT was globally good for health or not. I think we should take the same approach in prevention trials.

N. Wolmark: I always marvel how a group of compelling individuals with lucid and penetrating ideas can talk their way out of a perfectly good trial that not only needs to be done but must be done. These are not mutually exclusive endeavors. I mean, the trials are in essence our laboratories. We will learn a great deal more about these questions that are being asked suggesting that we may not be addressing the correct endpoint or that we should have surrogate markers that are more predictive of events. We will. I think that the most compelling catalyst for obtaining that information is from the trials themselves.

The nihilistic suggestion is that we have not demonstrated a mortality difference. Yes, we would all like to see a difference in mortality but we know very well that to demonstrate that in the same time interval we would need eight- to ten-fold the population. This clearly, a priori, was not the endpoint of these trials. You can say and hypothesize that we are only eliminating the banal tumors and allowing the virulent ones to continue. There is little evidence to support that.

In this process there certainly will be a mortality difference that we will see. We have to evolve that from the strength of the trials. We continue to do prevention. We have sera and lymphocytes on all these women. We will analyze the sera on all these women and correlate levels of hormones and other markers with events and with nonevents. We've done it for BRCA1 and 2; we're going to do it for hormones in conjunction with the Cummings and Harvard Group, as I'm sure you are as well.

I hope that we will be significantly enlightened by the information that comes from these analyses as opposed to saying that we ought to wait until the pristine model is going to be apparent. We ought not wait. That is an act of commission.

T. Powles: Norman [Wolmark], do we need to have more information than just the early incidence data? What do you feel about where we are going with these trials? If we stop the trials at the time of first incidence, will we ever learn anything about what the real ongoing clinical benefit is likely to be, even if we take as many bloods or genes or anything we like? We don't answer that fundamental question.

N. Wolmark: I think it is impractical to wait for the ultimate endpoint; that is, difference in mortality. I think that's just not feasible in our current environment, though we would like to see it. I think we have to do the next best thing.

M. Dixon: There are three points I'd like to make. First of all, I'm surprised that we're embarking on a study of one aromatase inhibitor without having comparative morbidity data of the three aromatase inhibitors and then making a decision on which aromatase inhibitor to use based on some kind of science. It seems to me that these are pharmaceutically driven as much as science driven and that does concern me. Those studies are relatively easy to do in really quite small numbers of women. Then we can identify which of the three drugs is likely to be the best buy. As it happens, we've got two studies so we might find out eventually.

Second point I'd raise is, Mitch [Dowsett], you have an interesting slide of how many people we need to treat to benefit. It would be interesting to see how long these new drugs are going to be the price they are. Cost is an important issue in the U.K. When I actually presented the ATAC data locally and we asked the audience to vote whether they wanted women to be treated with anastrozole or they wanted everybody to get better care, about 5% of the audience voted for anastrozole. There are important health financial issues that we need to consider long term.

The other point I'd make is that quality of life is very important. I'm surprised there haven't been more studies even before we embark on trying to prevent breast cancer to try to alleviate some of the side effects. What about an agent like tibolone? There are very few studies going on to try and look at some of the aromatase inhibitors. How we can actually get rid of the side effects, actually making aromatase inhibitors much more tolerable in the long term getting around the bone problems, the flushes, and a lot of the other effects and make them more widely available. I think sometimes we jump in a little bit quickly.

T. Powles: If we could just go finally for 10 minutes on the risk factors. Mike Baum wants to comment on pathology to start with.

M. Baum: Thank you. I want to go back to basics. All of our strategies on chemo prevention presupposes that we truly understand the pathogenesis of breast cancer from the precursor lesions. I want to take you back to Craig Allred's wonderful presentation, but I want to take issue with him on one particular area that I think is relevant to chemo prevention. That is, he suggested that we excise these precursor lesions. If they excise completely, they're cured. Therefore, we are underestimating the importance of these precursor lesions.

I take a completely opposite view because I think we're overestimating. The ones that are cured by excision, as Craig Henderson pointed out, may be latent pathology, which, if left unperturbed, would never realize their malignant potential. Conversely, the ones that are incompletely excised are latent lesions which have been perturbed. Surgical perturbation of an area of a latent lesion could have incredible consequences. You then have a stew, full of growth factors, steroids, and angiogenic factors.

Therefore, we need to address the issue of latency of these lesions and the role of anti-angiogenic approaches. I think it was perhaps the first talk yesterday, Steve Johnston's talk that mentioned COX-II and COX-II inhibitors. I'm, therefore, extremely attracted by NCIC MAP3, which contains the COX-II inhibitor along with an aromatase inhibitor. Is that right?

To me, that was a wonderful example of how we can take the complete understanding of pathogenesis into a chemo preventive program. We have been totally focused on the estrogen, whether it's a direct toxic effect or an indirect effect. We've been, in the last couple of hours, just focusing on that estrogenic component. I just hope we don't lose sight of the other components.

C. K. Osborne: I guess I interpreted Craig's [Allred] statements a little bit differently. The way I understood it from the studies in the past, prior to the development and use of core biopsies, many of these lesions were surgically removed. If indeed they are precursor lesions, then you might wind up 30 years later with a lower incidence of breast cancer than if they hadn't been removed, even though the risk is still substantially higher.

Secondly, I don't think he was recommending excising them to prevent the development of breast cancer, but excising them just like we do atypical ductal hyperplasia, which is diagnosed on a core biopsy because 20% of the time, at that moment, there is an invasive cancer next to it. That's the reason that you excise them. It is not to prevent breast cancer later on, but to recognize that there is an invasive cancer there that you just missed because of sampling error.

M. Ellis: I'd like to go back to talk to Mitch [Dowsett] a little bit about the Boyd data and breast density and the implications. This relates particularly to the issue of polymorphisms in genes that might be predisposed to postmenopausal breast cancer. I'd sort of been focusing on polymorphisms in genes that increase the supply of estrogen to try and explain why some women had higher levels of postmenopausal estrogen production than others.

But I think two pieces of information from the Boyd data suggest that we should be looking at genes that may produce a relatively estrogen-hypersensitive state. That is to say that there is a 60% heritability of breast density on mammograms and also it's fairly independent of estrogen levels. Perhaps Mitch [Dowsett] and Kent [Osborne] could comment on this with respect to, for example, polymorphisms in estrogen-receptor coactivators or repressors or what's known about how polymorphic these genes are. I know there is a lot about polymorphism in genes on the estrogen synthesis side, but what about the estrogen response side?

M. Dowsett: Very briefly, we showed in San Antonio last year the data on the sort of supply side, looking at polymorphisms in CYP19, CYP17, SHBG, etc. But actually the endpoint there was estrogen levels, androgen levels, etc. There were highly significant correlations. It actually explains a tiny amount of the variability in estradiol. So that in that respect, it was fairly disappointing.

It was from that same series that we're going to overlap with 1,500 women who have had repeated mammograms, looking at polymorphisms related to the sensitized estrogen receptor—the receptor itself, the coactivators, and perhaps also some of the things we talk about this afternoon, the growth factor receptors and their downstream effectors. That's in hand. I think it's a very important issue.

C. K. Osborne: With regard to the coactivators and corepressors, there is almost nothing known that I'm aware of, other than [the fact that] we know that their absolute levels are different in breast cancers than they are in normal tissue, at least in some cases. There are 30 coactivators and only a couple of them have even been studied. SRC3 or AIB1, the one that we've been working on, is overexpressed in two-thirds of breast cancer relative to normal ductal epithelium.

But what we don't know, because we haven't, until now, had the reagents, is: When do these receptor components begin to become overexpressed? Is it overexpressed in premalignant lesions? Could those lesions be particularly susceptible to malignant progression because the estrogen-response pathway is supercharged, for instance? Those are questions that we don't have the answers to. Hopefully we'll get the answers. One could imagine that patients whose tumors have a lot of coactivator relative to corepressor, the estrogen pathway is going to be supercharged. Maybe that group would be a good group to target for hormonal therapy.

T. Powles: Presumably that could give rise to phenotypic features like breast density or lack of osteoporosis?

H-J Senn: I would like to come back to breast density. Mitch [Dowsett], you have just—in a very short side sentence—mentioned this when you were showing the entrance criteria for IBIS II. You said that with digitalization of mammography this could be done very easily. Could you enlarge about the standardization of measurement or classification of breast density? It's an intriguing risk factor, no doubt, but how to implement it in an international study?

M. Dowsett: I'm not a radiologist but the study which we'll be doing with Steve Cummings will, in fact, make use of something called a "phantom," which will involve putting a block of some sort between the plates which will then allow for the exposure of the breast. This, as I understand it, is needed for getting an appropriate contrast and will allow standardization of that level.

P. Goss: Just one word on that quickly. It depends what your purpose is. If you just want to use breast density as a tool, you can do it categorically like Boyd by looking at a mammogram and seeing if there is 50% or more density on the mammogram. If you're using it as an enrollment tool in a post-menopausal woman, you need a continuous variable change in density, which can be done by digital rescreening of the film to give an actual read-out using a simple computer program. It's not a difficult tool.

On Matt's [Ellis] point, I think the answer with breast density and estrogen is [that] it could be a supply side, receptor sensitivity or a metabolism issue, but within the breast. I don't think the answer will necessarily come from the plasma. I think we need to find out.

P. Lonning: Just a question for you, Mitch, relating to the risk factor of estrogen levels and the meta-analysis. As we both are aware, in some of these studies, the mean estrogen levels vary substantially, some studies have reported estradiol levels of 70 or 80 pM per liter. As pointed out by Pentti Siterii, this is theoretically impossible. Have you considered to reanalyze some of these samples from the other studies with a standardized assay? That's the first question.

The second question is regarding a potential of a publication bias error. Are you absolutely confident that there are no negative studies that have not been published in the literature in this issue?

M. Dowsett: I will try to be brief. There was this meeting 11 days ago of this consensus group. I spoke about the need for precise assays and Steve Cummings was there as well. It's a little disappointing, from our perspective, regarding the use of these as preventive tools for developing an algorithm, that the epidemiologists were not too concerned about using assays that had these deficiencies. They have the perspective that there are variations in the assays but irrespective of this, analyzing the results together indicates that estrogen is important.

We need to know how important estrogen is in relation to testosterone and other issues. To do that, we need to be able to get better analyses. Steve Cummings has an analysis of about eight different assays comparing them for predictability and association with body mass index and bone density. I'm pleased to say that our assay comes out on top. I hope that we'll actually be collaborating with Steve [Cummings] on the P1 study and Norman's [Wolmark] samples.

T. Powles: Thank you very much. I'd like to thank you all. This has been a really important discussion. There are major decisions being made about where chemo prevention goes.

I have a sense of cautious enthusiasm to continue the prevention trials. I hope that's correct. I think that we must never forget that we are talking about very large numbers of healthy women, that there are only a few events that occur. It takes us a long time to get there. What's worse is that there is always the potential that an unexpected toxicity will occur, in spite of what Paul [Goss] said. A 4-year lead time is not sufficient for these trials which take many years to complete. There is always the potential that we could have a very large number of healthy women where a problem arises that could be a major iatrogenic problem.

Having said that, because as the discussions have gone today, clearly everybody is aware of those risks and everybody wants to do the best. We do have an opportunity of preventing a major disease. Number one, it is going to be important that the interventions are safe. And number two, it's clinically clearly important from the talks we've had today that we identify the risk groups where we're likely to have maximum benefit from endocrine intervention. I think I am right in saying that we should be progressing along the path that's been proposed with the trials that we have, but we have to be very, very careful.

Thank you very much.

14

Crosstalk Between Estrogen-Receptor and Growth-Factor-Receptor Pathways as a Mechanism of Endocrine Therapy Resistance

C. Kent Osborne and Rachel Schiff

Baylor College of Medicine and The Methodist Hospital,
Houston, Texas, U.S.A.

I. INTRODUCTION

Endocrine therapy of breast cancer remains the most important treatment modality for those tumors that demonstrate dependence on the female hormone estrogen. Currently these tumors are defined in part by their expression of estrogen receptors-alpha/-beta (ER), predominantly nuclear transcription factors that mediate the genomic effects of estrogen on target genes. All endocrine therapies, in one way or another, target the ERs. Although there are two ERs (ERalpha and ERbeta) that are products of different genes, this chapter focuses on ERalpha since the importance of ERbeta in breast cancer development and progression is not yet understood.

Endocrine therapies for breast cancer can be divided into four classes. The first class includes those agents or techniques that lower the level of estrogen available to bind to ER. Ovarian ablation, the luteinezing hormone-releasing hormone LHRH agonists to suppress ovarian function, aromatase inhibitors (AIs), and the older forms of surgical ablative procedures are members of this class. The second class includes selective estrogen-receptor modulators (SERMs), such as tamoxifen and toremifene. These drugs bind to ER and prevent the binding of estrogen. Although these drugs are normally thought of as anti-estrogens, conceptually, it is better to think of them as weak estrogens. The degree of estrogenic activity generated when these drugs bind ER is partly dependent upon the species, tissue, cell, and gene-promoter context. In some tissues and on some genes, the estrogen agonist activity predominates, whereas in others only a weak estrogenic signal is observed and the drugs are able to antagonize the more potent effects of endogenous estrogen by displacing it from ER. The third class of endocrine agents is the pure anti-estrogens, which bind and block ER and induce its degradation. Pure anti-estrogens have little or no estrogen agonist activity. The new agent fulvestrant is an example of this class. The fourth class includes pharmacologic doses of estrogens, androgens, and progestins. The mechanisms by which these agents induce tumor regression remain obscure. Because each of these classes of endocrine therapy works by a slightly different mechanism of action, they frequently demonstrate non–cross-resistance and, therefore, are often used sequentially in patients with metastatic breast cancer who develop resistance to one class of agents.

De novo and acquired resistance to these various therapies remain a major problem. Understanding the mechanisms by which breast tumors become resistant to endocrine therapy would reveal new strategies to predict resistance or to reverse it in the clinic. Although there are many possible mechanisms for the development of resistance, one mechanism for which there is now considerable supporting data is bidirectional crosstalk between ER and growth factor receptor (GFR) signaling pathways.

II. ER STRUCTURE AND FUNCTION

ER-alpha in contrast to ER-beta has been studied in great detail and it serves as a clinically useful predictive marker and treatment target. Although ER has classically been considered a transcription factor regulating the expression of estrogen target genes in the nucleus, new data suggest that ER can also affect cells via nonclassical or membrane affects and by modifying the activity of other transcriptional factors through protein:protein interactions.

A. Classical Mechanism of ER Action

The ER proteins contain several important functional domains (1). The hormone-binding domain in region E of the ER also contains an estrogen-inducible transcription-activating function called AF-2. A second, constitutively active transcription-activating function (AF-1) is located in the A/B region of the receptor. The DNA-binding domain and the hinge region reside between the two transcription-activating functions. Several mutant and variant ERs have also been identified, and one of these, K303R ERα, may be very important in clinical breast cancer (2).

In the absence of ligand, ERs exist as monomers bound by heat-shock proteins (3). Ligand binding activates the receptor, dissociates the heat-shock proteins, and alters receptor conformation in a specific way. Estrogen binding also induces phosphorylation of ER in several distinct serine/threonine residues (4). These activated receptors then homodimerize and become complex with a variety of coregulatory molecules, and the complex then binds to an ER response element in the promoter region of target genes (ERE) to alter gene transcription (5). The coregulatory molecules, many of which have now been identified and studied, modulate this classical pathway for ER transcriptional activation (6). Some function as coactivators to amplify ER-mediated gene transcription by interacting with the basal transcription machinery and by altering chromatin structure via their histone acetylase activity. Others function as corepressors to inhibit this function by preventing chromatin unwinding via their deacetylase activity. The corepressor proteins may be important for those genes whose transcription is normally blocked by estrogen, and they may also be important for the anti-estrogenic activities of certain ligands. The coactivator AIB1 (SRC-3), which is often overexpressed and sometimes amplified in breast cancer, may be important in tamoxifen resistance by enhancing its estrogen agonist activity when it is present at high levels in the cell (7, 8). These nuclear functions of ER that regulate gene transcription via specific response elements in the promoter of target genes have been labeled the classical functions of ER.

Various ligands modify the receptor in different ways. Selective estrogen receptor modulators (SERMs) such as tamoxifen also bind ER, dissociate heat-shock proteins from the receptor, and induce receptor dimerization and binding to ER-response elements on target genes (9). However, the conformation of the receptor is different when bound by tamoxifen, and tamoxifen-bound receptor associates with a different set of coregulatory molecules and corepressors (10). Tamoxifen has long been known to exert both agonist and antagonist effects, depending somewhat on the species, tissue, or gene. It is predominately an agonist in bone and in endometrium, whereas it is an antagonist, at least on genes important for cell proliferation and survival, in the breast. The agonist/antagonist profile of tamoxifen and other SERMs may in part be related to the particular milieu of coactivators and corepressors in a cell. Different response elements in the promoter of target genes may also contribute to the agonist/antagonist properties of these drugs. Experimental manipulation of coactivators and corepressors can greatly influence transcriptional activity from tamoxifen-bound receptor (8, 11). An abundance of coactivators like AIB1 leads to greater agonist activity, whereas a reduction in coactivators or an increase in corepressors enhances tamoxifen's antagonist activity. These studies have led to the hypothesis, not yet proved, that altered expression of coactivators and corepressors may contribute to endocrine therapy resistance in patients (7).

Steroidal anti-estrogens, such as fulvestrant, also bind the ER (12). However, this class of agents has an entirely different effect. These drugs inhibit ER dimerization and binding to DNA (13). Furthermore, they antagonize both the AF-1 and AF-2 transcription-activating functions of ER, whereas the SERMs only inhibit AF-2 (14). Finally, the steroidal anti-estrogens induce ER degradation and ER loss from the cell (13). Because inhibiting ER function is the therapeutic goal, these drugs theoretically offer the optimal approach to endocrine therapy by eliminating the cellular target.

Estrogen deprivation therapies, such as the AIs, lower estrogen in the tumor to very low levels (15). ER is not active in the absence of ligand and it cannot dimerize or bind to the promoters of target genes. As a result, there is a profound reduction in ER-mediated transcriptional activity and suppression of estrogen-induced tumor growth.

ER transcriptional activity thus is governed by the particular ensemble of ligand, receptor subtype, receptor phosphorylation, the milieu of coregulatory proteins and their phosphorylation status, and the promoter sequences in specific genes. This complexity of ER structure and function may offer new diagnostic and treatment strategies. Just as ER is necessary for response to endocrine therapy, it is possible that the levels of coactivators and corepressors are just as important, and studies are under way to measure these factors in clinical samples. The blockade of coactivator function or drugs mimicking corepressor function might even offer new treatment approaches. Finally, it is theoretically possible to develop new SERMs that modulate the receptor in specific ways, thereby achieving many of the desirable estrogen agonist activities in specific tissues while avoiding undesirable estrogenic effects in others.

The mechanisms by which estrogen increases breast-tumor growth are multiple. Several estrogen regulated genes are important for cell proliferation and survival. Although there are probably many such genes that have not yet been identified and characterized, estrogen does increase the expression of transforming GFR-alpha which, through an autocrine fashion can activate signaling through the epidermal growth factor recptor (EGFR) (16). Several key signaling molecules in the insulin growth factor (IGF) pathway are regulated by estrogen. These include the levels of insulin receptor substrates (IRS1 and IRS2), the levels of IGF2 secreted by the tumor itself or its stroma, and the levels of the IGF1 receptor (17–19). Cyclin-D1 and the anti-apoptosis protein, Bcl-2, are also induced by estrogen (20, 21). The net effect of these classical effects of estrogen is to enhance tumor cell proliferation and survival of the cells.

B. Nonclassical and Membrane Effects of ER

A growing body of evidence also suggests that ER can regulate cellular function through nonclassical mechanisms of action. Recent studies indicate that ER not only resides in the nucleus, but may reside in the cytoplasm or in or near the plasma membrane (22–24). Although ER is present in these subcellular locations, its concentration is probably low, and its detection requires more sophisticated molecular and imaging studies. This nonnuclear ER is important in breast cancer because it may directly and indirectly activate several growth-factor-signaling pathways. The binding of estrogen and even SERMs like tamoxifen to the membrane ER can activate the PI3K/AKT cell survival pathway and it can also activate the EGF family of receptors. The molecular mechanisms for this activation by ER is still being clarified, but activation of G proteins—which then activate SRC followed by activation of metalloproteinases and the cleavage of membrane-bound heparin-binding EGF—may be one such mechanism (23). The heparin-binding EGF released from the cell can then activate the EGF receptor family of tyrosine kinases in an autocrine mechanism. These data suggest the possibility that, in cells that have abundant EGFR and/or HER-2 in addition to ER, the administration of tamoxifen, like estrogen, might stimulate cell proliferation and cell survival through these alternative pathways. This membrane ER could then play a part in de novo or acquired resistance to tamoxifen.

Data also suggest that ER through protein:protein interaction with other transcription factors can itself function as a coactivator for these alternative pathways (25). ER has been reported to bind to fos/jun complexes bound to their specific response elements in the promoter of AP-1 responsive genes, and, thereby, augment transcription of these genes that are not normally thought to be estrogen targets.

C. Ligand-Independent Activation of ER by Growth-Factor-Mediated Phosphorylation

Although the data just described indicate that ER can activate growth factor signaling via its classical and its membrane effects, growth factor signaling can, in turn, functionally activate ER and its coregulatory proteins. Several different pathways, including cell-proliferation pathways, survival pathways, and even stress/cytokine-signaling pathways, can activate ER.

The PI3K pathway mediates cell survival and proliferation signals coming from a variety of growth factors including insulin, the insulin-like growth factors, and members of the EGF family (26). PI3K is activated by the binding of these growth factors to their respective membrane receptors. The tumor suppressor gene PTEN inhibits PI3K, and loss of its function constitutively activates this pathway contributing to the development and progression of cancer. Activation of PI3K results in the inactivation of several apoptosis mediators including FKHR, Bad, GSK-3, and caspases (26, 27). PI3K activates AKT which in turn activates cyclin-D1 (26).

The PI3K/AKT pathway can also modulate ER. AKT phosphorylates ER at serine 167, and thereby enhances transcriptional activation (28). Interestingly, recent data demonstrate that FKHR, which is inactivated by AKT, can interact with the ER and repress its transcription activating function (29). Loss of FKHR function would, therefore, have important effects in breast ductal epithelium by enhancing cell survival and augmenting ER mediated events. This crosstalk between ER and the PI3K pathway may explain the previous observations of additive or synergistic effects on cultured breast cancer cells treated with estrogen and IGFs (17, 18).

GFR pathways consist of a protein kinase cascade that links growth factor signals at the membrane with activation of transcription factors in the nucleus (30). Among several growth factors, the IGF and EGF families can activate the tyrosine kinase activity of their respective receptors which then activate ras. Ras then activates other signaling intermediates eventuating in the phosphorylation and activation of ERK1,2 mitogen activated protein kinase (MAPK). ERK1,2 can then activate other kinases such as P90RSK and MSK, and also activate transcription factors such as Myc and Elk 1 (31, 32). These pathways activate cell proliferation and have transforming capabilities.

This signaling pathway also interacts with the ER at several levels. ER can increase expression of several growth factors and their receptors to amplify signals generated through these pathways as just described, whereas ERKs can phosphorylate the ER at serine 118 to functionally activate the receptor (33). ERKs also phosphorylate P90RSK, which can also phosphorylate ER (34). Finally, phosphorylation of ER coactivators and corepressors is also important for ER function. Phosphorylation of ER coactivators such as AIB1/SRC3 augments their interaction with the receptor and their ability to activate the transcriptional effects of ER, whereas phosphorylation of corepressors such as N-CoR inhibits the interaction with ER (35, 36). AIB1 is phosphorylated by ERKs and other kinases in the growth factor/stress/cytokine pathways (36).

The SAPK/JNK pathway and the p38 MAPKs are activated by distinct extracellular stimuli, including inflammatory cytokines and various cellular stresses such as hypoxia or oxidative stress (37). The phosphorylation cascade resulting from these pathways activates a variety of transcription factors, which can affect many cellular functions including cell proliferation. JNK and p38 MAPK can phosphorylate ER and/or its coactivator proteins, thereby further augmenting ER-mediated gene transcriptional activity (38, 39).

Thus, there is considerable crosstalk between ER pathways and pathways mediating a variety of other important cellular functions. Experimental and clinical data also suggest that this crosstalk can be important for resistance to specific endocrine therapies. Breast tumors that overexpress members of the EGF receptor family may be less responsive to anti-estrogens such as tamoxifen (40–42). Blockade of these receptor pathways restores growth inhibition by anti-estrogens in model systems (43). It is intriguing to speculate that phosphorylation of ER and its coactivators by growth-factor signaling explains, in part, de novo,

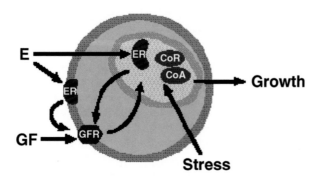

Figure 1 Interaction between estrogen receptor (ER), growth factor receptor (GFR) and stress-response pathways. E = estrogen; GF = growth factor; COA = ER coactivator; CoR = ER corepressor.

and, perhaps, acquired tamoxifen resistance, and that simultaneous treatment with inhibitors of these growth-factor pathways and tamoxifen may overcome or prevent the development of this form of resistance. It is also likely that some of the many proteins now known to modulate ER activity may eventually prove to be clinically useful predictive markers for initial response to endocrine therapy. In the future, molecular profiling of these many signaling pathways in a tumor from an individual patient may enhance our ability to predict response, select the particular class of endocrine therapy to use at a given point in time, and select the appropriate signaling pathway to block or overcome resistance to that endocrine therapy.

Thus estrogen-regulated growth of breast cancer is more complex than originally thought (Fig. 1). We can no longer think of ER as simply a nuclear protein regulating transcription of estrogen target genes. ER has both genomic and nongenomic effects that can contribute to cell proliferation and cell survival. Estrogen's effects are further modified by signaling coming from growth factor, cytokine, and stress-response pathways, which can functionally activate ER and its coregulatory proteins. ER through its nongenomic and genomic effects can, in turn, activate growth-factor pathways. This bidirectional crosstalk, if operative in a breast cancer, could contribute to resistance to a variety of different endocrine therapies.

III. CLINICAL VALIDATION OF RECEPTOR CROSSTALK

Recent clinical data support the idea that crosstalk between ER and growth factor pathways contributes to tamoxifen resistance in patients with breast cancer (40). AIB1, also called SRC-3, RAC3, ACTR, and p/CIP, is an ER coactivator that is thought to be important in breast cancer. AIB1 is overexpressed in breast cancer cells compared with normal duct epithelial cells and is amplified in a small proportion of breast tumors (44–46). AIB1 is highly expressed in cultured MCF-7 human breast cancer cells, and its activity is essential for the growth of these cells both in vitro and in vivo (47). AIB1, like the ER itself, is phosphorylated and, thereby, functionally activated by MAPKs (36); therefore, high levels of activated AIB1 could reduce the antagonist effects of tamoxifen, especially in tumors that also overexpress the HER-2 receptor, a member of the EGF-receptor family that activates MAPKs.

Laboratory studies suggest that ER+ breast cancers that overexpress HER-2 may be less responsive to tamoxifen than breast cancers with low HER-2 expression (48). The mechanisms for this resistance are not yet clear; however, ligand-independent activation of the ER by MAPKs, which themselves are phosphorylated and, thereby, activated by HER-2 signaling in such tumors, may contribute to it. High HER-2 expression has also been shown to be associated with tamoxifen resistance in some clinical studies, but this association is not strong and other studies have failed to confirm it (41).

The cumulative data from laboratory studies suggest the hypothesis that tumors expressing high levels of AIB1 might be relatively resistant to tamoxifen due to loss of its antagonist qualities (7). In addition, those breast tumors expressing high levels of AIB1 together with high levels of HER-2, which can activate AIB1, should be even more resistant to tamoxifen therapy.

To explore these hypotheses, AIB1 protein levels and HER-2 levels were measured in extracts from frozen tumors from 316 patients with long-term clinical follow-up (7). Nearly all these tumors were ER+. AIB1 protein expression did not correlate with the quantity of ER, but it was inversely correlated with PR expression. AIB1 was also positively correlated with higher S-phase fraction and higher HER-2 expression. There were no significant correlations with p53 status, age, tumor size, Bcl-2 expression or lymph node status. Despite the correlation of AIB1 with S-phase and HER-2 (both markers of a more aggressive tumor phenotype), high AIB1 in tumors from patients who were treated with surgery alone without adjuvant therapy was a good prognostic factor (Fig. 2). When AIB1expression was considered in a Cox multivariable analysis of disease free survival in which ER, PR, S-phase fraction, HER-2, number of positive lymph nodes, and tumor size were all considered together, the number of lymph nodes, ER status, AIB1 expression, and HER-2 expression were statistically significant.

Although high AIB1 expression was associated with better disease-free survival in untreated patients, in those patients receiving tamoxifen adjuvant therapy, high AIB1 expression was associated with worse disease-free survival, as one

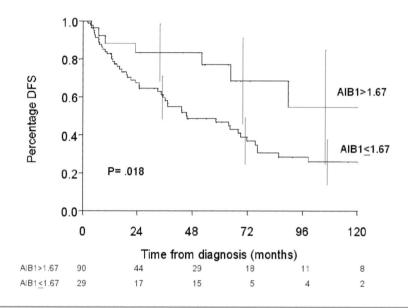

Figure 2 Kaplan-Meier estimates of disease-free survival (DFS). DFS according to AIB1 expression for patients who did not receive adjuvant therapy ($n = 119$). Patients with high AIB1 expression (top quartile: AIB1>1.67 densitometric units) were compared with patients with lower AIB1 expression ($\leq$1.67 densitometric units).

would predict from the preclinical data (7). In a multivariable analysis that included the same biomarkers described above, only the number of positive lymph nodes and AIB1 status were statistically significant predictors of outcome, consistent with the hypothesis that high AIB1 expression reduces tamoxifen's antagonist activity. When AIB1 expression was considered together with HER-2 expression, even more impressive results were obtained (Fig. 3) (7). Only those patients whose tumors expressed high AIB1 and high HER-2 had adverse disease-free survival with tamoxifen. Patients with low expression of one or both of these proteins had significantly better disease-free survival with tamoxifen adjuvant therapy. These data are consistent with the receptor crosstalk described earlier. Phosphorylation of AIB1, by the HER-2 tyrosine kinase signaling cascade functionally activates AIB1, which then increases the relative agonist activity of tamoxifen-bound ER. In the absence of significant GFR signaling, AIB1, despite being expressed at a high level, is not as functionally active and tamoxifen remains a more potent antagonist.

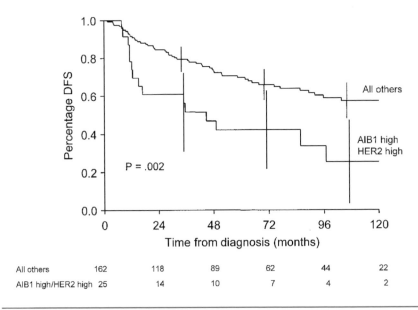

All others	162	118	89	62	44	22
AIB1 high/HER2 high	25	14	10	7	4	2

Figure 3 DFS for patients who received adjuvant tamoxifen therapy ($n = 187$). Patients with high AIB1 expression (top quartile) and high HER-2 expression were compared with patients with high expression of AIB1 and low expression of HER-2, low expression of both AIB1 and HER-2, or low AIB1 expression and high HER-2 expression. All p values refer to two-sided log-rank tests. Numbers below each graph indicate the number of patients remaining at risk in each group. Vertical lines are the 95% confidence intervals at selected time points.

IV. CONCLUSIONS AND CLINICAL IMPLICATIONS

Ample biological evidence, and now preliminary clinical evidence, support the idea that cross-talk between GFR and ER pathways is important in the regulation of breast cancer cell proliferation. Enhanced signaling through the growth-factor pathway in a cell with an abundance of ER coactivators can modulate the signal generated by tamoxifen-bound ER, increasing its agonist properties at the expense of its antagonist activity. If these preliminary studies can be confirmed in other patients, then we must consider several clinical implications. First, AIB1 together with ER, and HER-2, would be useful clinical predictive markers to determine which patients should or should not receive tamoxifen therapy for breast cancer. Confirmatory studies are now in progress. Second, if activation of AIB1 by the HER-2 signaling pathway is the major mechanism for this interaction, then inhibition or blockade of the growth-factor-signaling pathway should restore tamoxifen's antagonist activity and overcome tamoxifen resistance in patients. Although this strategy is only now being tested in humans, data from experimental models in several laboratories suggest that this hypothesis deserves additional testing (43, 49–52). Receptor tyrosine kinase inhibitors, MAPK inhibitors, and receptor-blocking antibodies such as Herceptin® have all been shown to restore tamoxifen's growth-inhibitory properties in human breast cancer cells expressing high levels of HER-2 growing in athymic nude mice. Unfortunately, there are several redundant pathways all leading to phosphorylation and functional activation of ER and its coactivators. This pathway redundancy might then necessitate multiple pathway inhibitors or an inhibitor of the interaction of AIB1 with the ER. These data also provide rationale to study other ER coactivators and corepressors, which can also modulate ER activity.

Clinical trials are now starting to evaluate combinations of endocrine therapy with growth factor inhibitors to overcome de novo resistance and delay acquired resistance. The neoadjuvant setting in locally advanced breast cancer represents an ideal setting to test this concept because of the accessibility of tissue for biomarker studies. A Phase II study combining the receptor tyrosine kinase inhibitor gefitinib with tamoxifen will address the issue of de novo resistance in HER-2 overexpressing tumors. A randomized trial of tamoxifen with/without gefitinib in patients with metastatic disease will also be initiated in the near future to examine the ability of the receptor tyrosine kinase inhibitor to overcome de novo and delay acquired resistance. Finally, studies of AIs and the pure anti-estrogen fulvestrant combined with the GFR tyrosine kinase inhibitors are also in the planning stage.

REFERENCES

1. Schiff R, Saw F. The importance of the estrogen receptor in breast cancer. In: Pasqualini, Jr, ed. Breast Cancer: Prognosis, Treatment, and Prevention. New York: Marcel Dekker, 2002; pp.149–186.
2. Fuqua SA, Wiltschke C, Zhang QX, Borg A, Castles CG, Friedrichs WE, Hopp T, Hilsenback S, Mohsin S, O'Connell P, Allred DC. A hypersensitive estrogen receptor-alpha mutation in premalignant breast lesions. Cancer Res 2000; 60:4026–4029.
3. Jensen EV. Overview of the nuclear receptor family. In Parker MG, ed. Nuclear Hormone Receptors: Molecular Mechanisms, Cellular Functions, Clinical Abnormalities. London: Academic Press, 1991; pp. 1–13.
4. Le Goff P, Montano MM, Schodin DJ, Katzenellenbogen BS. Phosphorylation of the human estrogen receptor identification of hormone-regulated sites and examination of their influence on transcriptional activity. J Biol Chem 1994; 269:4458–4466.
5. Kumar V, Chambon P. The estrogen receptor binds tightly to its responsive element as a ligand-induced homodimer. Cell 1988; 55:145–156.
6. McKenna NJ, Lanz RB, O'Malley BW. Nuclear receptor coregulators: cellular and molecular biology. Endocr Rev 1999; 20:321–344.
7. Osborne CK, Bardou V, Hopp TA, Chamness GC, Hilsenbeck SG, Fuqua SA, Wong J, Allred DC, Clark GM, Schiff R. Role of the estrogen receptor coactivator AIB1

(SRC-3) and HER-2/neu in tamoxifen resistance in breast cancer. J Natl Cancer Inst 2003; 95:35361.

8. Smith CL, Nawaz Z, O'Malley BW. Coactivator and corepressor regulation of the agonist/antagonist activity of the mixed antiestrogen, 4-hydroxytamoxifen. Mol Endocrinol 1997; 11:657–666.

9. Osborne CK, Zhao H, Fuqua SA. Selective estrogen receptor modulators: structure, function, and clinical use. J Clin Oncol 2000; 18:3172–186.

10. Shang Y, Hu X, DiRenzo J, Lazar MA, Brown M. Cofactor dynamics and sufficiency in estrogen receptor-regulated transcription. Cell 2000; 103:843–852.

11. Jackson TA, Richer JK, Bain DL, Takimoto GS, Tung L, Horwitz KB. The partial agonist activity of antagonist-occupied steroid receptors is controlled by a novel hinge domain-binding coactivator L7/SPA and the corepressors N-CoR or SMRT. Mol Endocrinol 1997; 11:693–705.

12. Wakeling AE. Use of pure antioestrogens to elucidate the mode of action of oestrogens. Biochem Pharmacol 1995; 49:1545–1549.

13. Howell A, Osborne CK, Morris C, Wakeling AE. ICI 182,780 (Faslodex): development of a novel, "pure" antiestrogen. Cancer 2000; 89:817–825.

14. Jordan VC. Selective estrogen receptor modulation: a personal perspective. Cancer Res 2001; 61:5683–5687.

15. Smith IE, Dowsett M. Aromatase inhibitors in breast cancer. N Engl J Med 2003; 348:2431–2442.

16. Reddy KB, Yee D, Hilsenbeck SG, Coffey RJ, Osborne CK. Inhibition of estrogen-induced breast cancer cell proliferation by reduction in autocrine transforming growth factor alpha expression. Cell Growth Differ 1994; 5:1275–1282.

17. Lee AV, Cui X, Oesterreich S. Cross-talk among estrogen receptor, epidermal growth factor, and insulin-like growth factor signaling in breast cancer. Clin Cancer Res 2001; 7:4429s–4435s; discussion 11s–12s.

18. Osborne CK, Coronado EB, Kitten LJ, Arteaga CI, Fuqua SA, Ramasharma K, Marshall M, Li CH. Insulin-like growth factor-II (IGF-II): a potential autocrine/paracrine growth factor for human breast cancer acting via the IGF-I receptor. Mol Endocrinol 1989; 3:1701–1709.

19. Lee AV, Jackson JG, Gooch JL, Hilsenbeck SG, Coronado-Heinsohn E, Osborne CK, Yee D. Enhancement of insulin-like growth factor signaling in human breast cancer: estrogen regulation of insulin receptor substrate-1 expression in vitro and in vivo. Mol Endocrinol 1999; 13:787–796.

20. Liu MM, Albanese C, Anderson CM, Hilty K, Webb P, Uht RM, Price Jr. RH, Pestell RG, Kushner PJ. Opposing action of estrogen receptors alpha and beta on cyclin D1 gene expression. J Biol Chem 2002; 277:24353–24360.

21. Perillo B, Sasso A, Abbondanza C, Palumbo G. 17-beta-estradiol inhibits apoptosis in MCF-7 cells, inducing bcl-2 expression via two estrogen-responsive elements present in the coding sequence. Mol Cell Biol 2000; 20:2890–2901.

22. Haynes MP, Sinha D, Russell KS, Collinge M, Fulton D, Morales-Ruiz M, Sessa WC, Bender JR. Membrane estrogen receptor engagement activates endothelial nitric oxide synthase via the PI3-kinase-Akt pathway in human endothelial cells. Circ Res 2000; 87:677–682.

23. Razandi M, Pedram A, Park ST, Levin ER. Proximal events in signaling by plasma membrane estrogen receptors. J Biol Chem 2003; 278:2701–2712.

24. Levin ER. Bidirectional signaling between the estrogen receptor and the epidermal growth factor receptor. Mol Endocrinol 2003; 17:309–317.

25. Kushner PJ, Agard DA, Greene GL, Scanlan TS, Shiau AK, Uht RM, Webb P. Estrogen receptor pathways to AP-1. J Steroid Biochem Mol Biol 2000; 74:311–317.

26. Cantley LC. The phosphoinositide 3-kinase pathway. Science 2002; 296:1655–1657.

27. Vanhaesebroeck B, Alessi DR. The PI3K-PDK1 connection: more than just a road to PKB. Biochem J 2000; 346:561–576.

28. Campbell RA, Bhat-Nakshatri P, Patel NM, Constantinidou D, Ali S, Nakshatri H. Phosphatidylinositol 3-kinase/AKT-mediated activation of estrogen receptor alpha: a new model for anti-estrogen resistance. J Biol Chem 2001; 276:9817–9824.

29. Zhao HH, Herrera RE, Coronado-Heinsohn E, Yang MC, Ludes-Meyers JH, Seybold-Tilson KJ, Nawaz Z, Yee D, Barr FG, Diab SG, Brown PH, Fuqua SA, Osborne CK. Forkhead homologue in rhabdomyosarcoma functions as a bifunctional nuclear receptor-interacting protein with both coactivator and corepressor functions. J Biol Chem 2001; 276:27907–27912.

30. Cobb MH. MAP kinase pathways. Prog Biophys Mol Biol 1999; 71:479–500.

31. Frodin M, Gammeltoft S. Role and regulation of 90 kDa ribosomal S6 kinase (RSK) in signal transduction. Mol Cell Endocrinol 1999; 151:65–77.

32. Davis RJ. Transcriptional regulation by MAP kinases. Mol Reprod Dev 1995; 42:459–467.

33. Kato S, Endoh H, Masuhiro Y, Kitamoto T, Uchiyama S, Sasaki H, Masushige S, Gotoh Y, Nishida E, Kawashima H. Activation of the estrogen receptor through phosphorylation by mitogen-activated protein kinase. Science 1995; 270:1491–1494.

34. Joel PB, Smith J, Sturgill TW, Fisher TL, Blenis J, Lannigan DA. pp90rsk1 regulates estrogen receptor-mediated transcription through phosphorylation of Ser-167. Mol Cell Biol 1998; 18:1978–1984.

35. Lavinsky RM, Jepsen K, Heinzel T, Torchia J, Mullen TM, Schiff R, Del-Rio AL, Ricote M, Ngo S, Gemsch J, Hilsenbeck SG, Osborne CK, Glass CK, Rosenfeld MG, Rose DW. Diverse signaling pathways modulate nuclear receptor recruitment of N-CoR and SMRT complexes. Proc Natl Acad Sci U S A 1998; 95:2920–2925.

36. Font de Mora J, Brown M. AIB1 is a conduit for kinase-mediated growth factor signaling to the estrogen receptor. Mol Cell Biol 2000; 20:5041–5047.

37. Kyriakis JM, Avruch J. Mammalian mitogen-activated protein kinase signal transduction pathways activated by stress and inflammation. Physiol Rev 2001; 81:807–869.

38. Feng W, Webb P, Nguyen P, Liu X, Li J, Karin M, Kushner PJ. Potentiation of estrogen receptor activation function 1 (AF-1) by Src/JNK through a serine 118-independent pathway. Mol Endocrinol 2001; 15:32–45.

39. Lee H, Bai W. Regulation of estrogen receptor nuclear export by ligand-induced and p38-mediated receptor phosphorylation. Mol Cell Biol 2002; 22:5835–5845.

40. Dowsett M. Overexpression of HER-2 as a resistance mechanism to hormonal therapy for breast cancer. Endocr Relat Cancer 2001; 8:191–195.

41. Piccart M, Lohrisch C, Di Leo A, Larsimont D. The predictive value of HER2 in breast cancer. Oncology 2001; 61:73–82.

42. Mass R. The role of HER-2 expression in predicting response to therapy in breast cancer. Semin Oncol 2000; 27:46–52; discussion 92–100.

43. Kurokawa H, Lenferink AE, Simpson JF, Pisacane PI, Sliwkowski MX, Forbes JT, Arteaga CL. Inhibition of HER2/neu (erbB-2) and mitogen-activated protein kinases enhances tamoxifen action against HER2-overexpressing, tamoxifen-resistant breast cancer cells. Cancer Res 2000; 60:5887–5894.

44. Anzick SL, Kononen J, Walker RL, Azorsa DO, Tanner MM, Guan XY, Sauter G, Kallioniemi OP, Trent JM, Meltzer PS. AIB1, a steroid receptor coactivator amplified in breast and ovarian cancer. Science 1997; 277:965–968.

45. Murphy LC, Simon SL, Parkes A, Leygue E, Dotzlaw H, Snell L, Troup S, Adeyinka A, Watson PH. Altered expression of estrogen receptor coregulators during human breast tumorigenesis. Cancer Res 2000; 60:6266–6271.

46. List HJ, Reiter R, Singh B, Wellstein A, Riegel AT. Expression of the nuclear coactivator AIB1 in normal and malignant breast tissue. Breast Cancer Res Treat 2001; 68:21–28.

47. List HJ, Lauritsen KJ, Reiter R, Powers C, Wellstein A, Riegel AT. Ribozyme targeting demonstrates that the nuclear receptor coactivator AIB1 is a rate-limiting factor for estrogen-dependent growth of human MCF-7 breast cancer cells. J Biol Chem 2001; 276:23763–23768.

48. Benz CC, Scott GK, Sarup JC, Johnson RM, Tripathy D, Coronado E, Shepard HM, Osborne CK. Estrogen-dependent, tamoxifen-resistant tumorigenic growth of MCF-7 cells transfected with HER2/neu. Breast Cancer Res Treat 1993; 24:85–95.

49. Witters L, Engle L, Lipton A. Restoration of estrogen responsiveness by blocking the HER-2/neu pathway. Oncol Rep 2002; 9:1163–1166.

50. Knowlden JM, Hutcheson IR, Jones HE, Madden T, Gee JM, Harper ME, Barrow D, Wakeling AE, Nicholson RI. Elevated levels of epidermal growth factor receptor/c-erbB2 heterodimers mediate an autocrine growth regulatory pathway in tamoxifen-resistant MCF-7 cells. Endocrinology 2003; 144:1032–1044.

51. Massarweh S, Shou J, Mohsin SK, Ge M, Wakeling AE, Osborne CK, et al. Inhibition of epidermal growth factor/HER-2 receptor signaling using ZD1839 ("Iressa") restores tamoxifen sensitivity and delays resistance to estrogen deprivation in HER2-overexpressing breast tumors. Program/Proceedings American Society of Clinical Oncology 2002; 21:33a.

52. Nicholson RI, McClelland RA, Robertson JF, Gee JM. Involvement of steroid hormone and growth factor cross-talk in endocrine response in breast cancer. Endocr Relat Cancer 1999; 6:373–387.

15

erbB2/HER-2 and Other Molecular Pathways in Estrogen-Receptor-Positive Breast Cancer: Impact on Endocrine Resistance and Clinical Outcome

Christopher C. Benz

Buck Institute for Age Research
Novato, California, U.S.A.

I. OVERVIEW

Levels of estrogen receptor (ER) overexpression as well as the co-expression of ER-associated gene products (e.g., PR, pS2) have long been recognized as markers of breast cancer prognosis and, more importantly, predictors of response to endocrine therapy and clinical outcome. Several emerging lines of evidence support the fact that ER+ breast cancers can be divided into clinically relevant subsets with extremely different outcomes, ranging from tumors with good clinical prognosis and endocrine responsiveness, to others with de novo or acquired endocrine resistance and risk for early metastatic relapse. Design of novel therapeutic strategies that target the erbB/HER family of growth factor receptors (GFR) in conjunction with endocrine therapies [selective estrogen receptor modulators (SERMs), aromatase inhibitors (AIs)] is being driven by: 1) improved understanding of the age-dependence of breast cancer biology, its receptor-activated pathways, crosstalk signaling between these pathways, and the co-expression of other biomarkers (e.g., abnormal p53) as well as unique gene expression signatures in SERM-resistant ER+ breast cancers; and 2) increasing clinical availability of new erbB/HER-targeted therapies [e.g., trastuzumab, tyrosine kinase inhibitors (TKI)] that appear promising in preclinical models for their ability to reverse or prevent some forms of endocrine resistance.

II. AGE DEPENDENCE OF ER+ BREAST CANCERS, THEIR CLINICAL BEHAVIOR, AND CO-EXPRESSED BIOMARKERS

Primary breast cancers arising before age 40 are far more aggressive and likelier to metastasize and reduce patient survival than those arising in older patients, regardless of hormone receptor [ER, progesterone receptor (PR)]) status; yet, there has been little progress to date in defining biomarker profiles capable of distinguishing these from less aggressive breast cancers arising later in life, especially among the group of receptor-positive tumors that are candidates for endocrine therapy. As summarized from a recent comprehensive analysis of age-associated breast cancer biomarker profiles (1), Figure 1 shows the different age variations for several well-studied breast cancer biomarkers that may also be considered credentialed (ER, erbB2/HER-2), emerging (EGFR/erbB1/HER-1), or putative (abnormal p53) predictive markers for a new generation of targeted breast cancer therapeutics. Additional studies are needed to understand why such different age variations are observed, with some biomarkers appearing less frequent after age 50 (e.g., p53 abnormalities), others exhibiting a continuous decline with aging (e.g., erbB2/HER-2 and EGFR overexpression), and with ER overexpression showing an inverse and ever-increasing prevalence with age (1).

Only 40% of breast tumors arising before age 45 overexpress ER, but these ER+ younger age tumors appear more proliferative and genetically unstable (higher nuclear grade, more frequent p53 abnormalities) than the more prevalent ER+ tumors arising later in life. The ER+ tumors arising with older age tend to exhibit slower proliferative rates, are much less likely to overexpress erbB/HER family receptors, and are thought by some investigators to be promoted by the paracrine effects of adjacent senescent stromal tissue (2). These ER+ older breast cancers also show differences in their activated intracellular signaling pathways (e.g., increased phospho-Erk5) and possess oxidatively damaged and functionally impaired regulatory proteins (e.g., the G:C box-binding transcription factor, Sp1), predisposing toward acquisition of more epigenetic rather than genetic changes during tumor progression (e.g., silencing of tumor suppressor genes by promoter methylation) (3). While younger age breast tumors that are ER+ are somewhat more likely to co-express PR (3)—a generally favorable predictor of response to endocrine therapy—paradoxically, they are also more likely to overexpress members of the erbB/HER family of membrane receptor tyrosine kinases (1), unfavorable biomarkers associated with resistance to endocrine therapy. Other amplified and overexpressed markers recently found

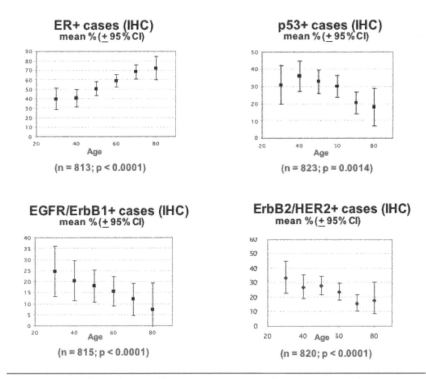

Figure 1   Age dependency of breast cancer poor-risk prognostic markers: ER, p53, EGFR/erbB1 and erbB2/HER2 overexpression. Excerpted data from our recent report (1) describing immunohistochemical results and decade-by-decade analysis of the frequency (mean % tumors ± 95% confidence intervals, CI) of primary breast cancers overexpressing each of the indicated biomarkers (n = case numbers analyzed, p-values determined for linear regression fit to scatter plot of all values against age as a continuous variable). (From Ref. 1)

associated with ER+, erbB2/HER-2+, and SERM (tamoxifen)-resistant breast cancers include the ER-coactivator, AIB1 (also phosphorylated by erbB2/HER2) (4), and the estrogen interconverting enzyme, 17β-HSD (encoded within the extended *ERBB2* amplicon) (5).

III.   CLINICAL EVIDENCE FOR ENDOCRINE RESISTANCE OF BREAST CANCERS OVEREXPRESSING ER AND erbB2/HER-2

Numerous hypotheses have been put forth to explain the clinically observed and age-adjusted inverse proportion of breast cancers that overexpress ER and erbB/HER family members (6, 7). In particular, the existence of multiple cross-talk mechanisms between activated receptor tyrosine kinases and ER signaling pathways are increasingly being appreciated and are now commonly implicated as mechanisms accounting for the endocrine resistance of some ER+ breast cancers (8, 9). However, not only are endocrine resistance mechanisms still poorly understood in general (9), how crosstalk signaling between ER and activated erbB2/HER-2 receptors leads to the profound reductions in both ER and PR tumor content associated with this endocrine resistance remains a mystery. Perhaps better understood is the mechanism by which ER overexpression down-regulates both erbB2/HER-2 and EGFR levels, via ER binding to transcriptional repression elements within these GFR-encoding genes (10–12).

We evaluated >3000 unselected primary breast tumors by quantitative enzyme-immunoassays (EIAs) and definitively showed that erbB2/HER-2 over-expressing breast cancers express much lower levels of both ER and PR protein as compared to breast tumors lacking erbB2/HER-2 overexpression (13). When dichotymized only by erbB2/HER-2 overexpression status, the breast tumor cohorts show significant differences in steroid receptor content, with overall six-fold lower mean ER and seven-fold lower mean PR levels in erbB2/HER-2+ tumors as compared to erbB2/HER-2– breast tumors (Fig. 2). These results were recently confirmed by Konecny et al. and extended to include approximately 900 breast cancer cases in which erbB2/HER-2 gene copy number (amplification status) was determined by fluorescence in situ hybridization (FISH), and to a comparative panel of human breast cancer cell lines with either normal or elevated erbB2/HER-2 gene copy number, from either endogenous gene amplification or recombinant engineering (14). Marked reductions in both ER and PR levels were observed in both the amplified tumors and engineered cell lines (14). As summarized in Figure 2, of those cases (21%) positive by FISH for erbB2/HER-2 gene amplification, 53% were also ER+ and 65% were either ER+ or PR+ (vs. 75% and 81%, respectively, in the non-amplified cohort), suggesting that a significant number of breast cancer cases eligible for treatment with an erbB2/HER-2-targeted agent like trastuzumab are also candidates for some form of endocrine therapy. While there has been no proven mechanism to explain how steroid receptor downregulation is induced by constitutively activated erbB2/HER-2-receptor tyrosine kinase, the results of the above studies suggest that the magnitude of reductions in both ER and PR levels may in part explain the apparent clinical resistance of these tumors to SERMs like tamoxifen (13, 14).

With many different assays being used to score breast cancers as positive for ER/PR and erbB2/HER-2 expression, it is difficult to state precisely what fraction of breast tumors overexpress both sets of these receptors. The Konecny et al. study (14) found that 14–18% of ER+ and/or PR+ tumors also show amplification or overexpression of erbB2/HER-2 (summarized in Fig. 2). In one retrospective cooperative group study (CALGB 8541) in which > 600 ER+ cases were treated with or without tamoxifen adjuvant therapy and subsetted according to erbB2/HER-2-positivity measured by three different techniques [immunohisto-

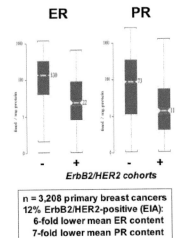

- Eppenberger-Castori et al. (JCO, 2001)
- Konecny et al. (JNCI, 2003)

ErbB2/HER2-positive cohorts

A. 17% overexpressing (n = 665; ELISA)
   63% ER &/or PR-positive
   (81% if ErbB2/HER2-negative
B. 21% amplified (n = 894; FISH)
   65% ER &/or PR-positive
   (81% if ErbB2/HER2-negative)

ER &/or PR-positive cohorts

A. 14% ErbB2/HER2-positive (ELISA)
B. 18% ErbB2/HER2-positive (FISH)

ErbB2/HER2 cohorts

n = 3,208 primary breast cancers
12% ErbB2/HER2-positive (EIA):
   6-fold lower mean ER content
   7-fold lower mean PR content

ER+ cell lines +/- ErbB2/HER2

(fold decline in)	ER:	PR:
MCF-7	5-fold	20-fold
ZR-75-1	2-fold	>300-fold
T-47D	4-fold	2-fold

Figure 2 Summary data from two reports showing dramatic reductions in tumor ER and PR content associated with amplification and/or overexpression of erbB2/HER-2. The study by Eppenberger-Castori et al. (13) dichotymized tumors by erbB2/HER-2 overexpression status (+ vs. − cohorts, determined by EIA for $n = 3,208$ cases) and evaluated the distribution of their ER and PR values (fmol/mg protein cytosol); the resulting notch box-plots demonstrate the six-fold and seven-fold lower tumor ER and PR content, respectively, in the erbB2/HER-2-+ cohort. The Konecny et al. study (14) dichotymized (+ vs. − cohorts) two separate groups of primary breast tumors according to either ErbB2/HER-2 amplification (FISH, $n = 894$ cases) or overexpression (ELISA, $n = 665$ cases) status. They determined the frequency of ER+ and ER− and/or PR+ tumors in each cohort and described the frequency of erbB2/HER-2-positivity (amplification, overexpression) among their two separate groups of ER− and/or PR+ breast cancers. Included in this study was a comparison of reductions induced in the ER and PR protein levels of several breast cancer cell lines following stable introduction and overexpression of erbB-2. (From Ref.14)

chemistry (IHC), FISH, polymerase chain reaction (PCR)], the fraction of ER+ and erbB2/HER-2+ cases was reported to range between 12% and 28% (15). That same CALGB study observed no significant difference in clinical benefit (improved disease-free and overall survival) with tamoxifen adjuvant therapy according to tumor erbB2/HER-2 status (15). However, a more recent retrospective analysis of another randomized adjuvant study (Naples GUN) involving > 400 patients concluded that patients with tumors overexpressing erbB2/HER-2 receive no benefit from adjuvant tamoxifen therapy (16). As recently reviewed by

Ring and Dowsett (17), and in addition to the above two conflicting adjuvant trial results, there have been four other retrospective adjuvant tamoxifen analyses and at least nine additional metastatic disease studies (six with tamoxifen, the others with AIs and/or other endocrine agents), most but not all indicating that erbB2/HER-2 overexpression predicts for some degree of endocrine resistance. A preliminary meta-analysis of the metastatic disease studies reported between 1992 and 1999 yielded an overall pooled odds ratio (OR) of 2.5 (95% CI: 1.8–3.3), confirming a statistically significant relationship between endocrine treatment failure and erbB2/HER-2 positivity (18).

Nonetheless, because of lack of prospective clinical evidence and inconsistent retrospective results addressing this issue, no definitive clinical recommendation can yet be made regarding erbB2/HER-2 status and resistance to any form of endocrine therapy, be it a SERM or an AI. Accordingly, panelists from the 2003 St. Gallen Breast Cancer Conference, like those from its preceding 2001 concensus conference, have recommended against using erbB2/HER-2 status to guide in the routine choice of adjuvant endocrine therapy. The last National Institutes of Health Concensus Conference cautioned against using erbB2/HER-2 status as a factor in making decisions about all forms of adjuvant therapy (19); and a more recent American Society of Clinical Oncology panel concurred with that recommendation, specifically regarding to adjuvant endocrine therapy (20). Because of the weight of existing preclinical evidence, a developing understanding of crosstalk mechanisms linking erbB2/HER-2 and ER pathways, and the widespread clinical perception that erbB2/HER-2+ tumors are less responsive than erbB2/HER-2– tumors to endocrine therapy (particularly SERMs like tamoxifen), an increasing number of clinicians in both the United States and Europe are currently using erbB2/HER-2 status to assist in deciding if patients should be treated with endocrine therapeutics alone or a combination of endocrine therapy with cytotoxic chemotherapy.

IV. PROPOSED MECHANISMS AND PRECLINICAL EVIDENCE FOR ENDOCRINE RESISTANCE INDUCED BY ACTIVATED erbB2/HER-2

A decade ago in collaboration with Genentech investigators (who created the sublines), we first demonstrated that responsiveness of estrogen-dependent, ER+/PR+ MCF-7 human breast cancer cells to the mixed ER agonist/antagonist, tamoxifen, could be dramatically altered by stable introduction and overexpression of otherwise normal erbB2/HER-2 gene copies (21). We first characterized a number of transfected and clonally selected MCF-7 sublines for their x-fold overexpression of erbB/HER-2 (vs. control MCF-7/neo transfectants) and these included: MCF/HER-2–18 (45-fold); MCF/HER-2–19 (25-fold); MCF/HER-2–29 (7-fold); and MCF/HER-2–30 (3-fold). While graded changes in erbB2/HER-2 modulated intracellular messengers, lipid kinases, and phosphokinase products (InsP pools, PI3K, and a p56 protein since identified as p-Shc) were observed in all of erbB2/HER-2 overexpressing sublines, only the 25-fold and 45-fold overexpressing MCF/HER-2–19 and MCF/HER-2–18 sublines exhibited any detectable differences in their in vitro and/or in vivo phenotypes, with the latter showing increased resistance in vitro to the growth inhibiting effects of tamoxifen and also to one (cisplatin) but not other chemotherapy agents. All sublines retained their ER positivity and their essential dependency on estrogen for tumorigenic in vivo growth upon implantation into athymic nude mice (21). As shown in Fig. 3A, the MCF/HER-2–18 subline not only exhibited complete in vivo resistance to tumoristatic doses of tamoxifen, it provided the first demonstration that under the influence of the constitutively activated erbB2/HER-2 receptor system tamoxifen can act as a pure agonistic ER ligand, unlike its primarily antagonistic effects observed in parental MCF-7 cells and tumors. Subsequent studies have shown that the metabolism of tamoxifen is not altered in this MCF/HER-2–18 subline and that the structure and apparent DNA-binding and transcriptional activities of the intracellular ER are intact. Importantly, in vivo tumorigenic growth of MCF/HER-2–18 revealed a more complete spectrum of phenotypic changes induced by overexpression of erbB2/HER-2. These changes include the emergence of in vivo resistance to chemotherapy agents not previously observed in vitro (e.g. doxorubicin), as well as complete loss of any tumoristatic effect by tamoxifen. Indeed, the more rapid tumorigenic growth of MCF/HER-2–18 cells in vivo relative to parental (MCF-7) or control (MCF/neo-3) cells actually reflected tamoxifen's agonistic induction of tumor growth dependent on an intact intracellular ER mechanism (21). This preclinical observation not only provided the first mechanistic rationale for tamoxifen resistance associated with erbB2/HER-2 overexpression, but it also allowed for the prediction that estrogen ablation (e.g., by AIs), or even ER ablation (e.g., by the selective ER downmodulator, ICI-182780/fulvestrant), might be clinically more effective than SERMs like tamoxifen when treating breast cancers that overexpress both ER and erbB2/HER-2. At least one randomized clinical trial supports this prediction with compelling evidence that the AI, letrozole, is significantly more effective than tamoxifen in inducing regressions of ER+ and erbB2/HER-2 (or EGFR) overexpressing primary breast cancers (22). In addition to avoiding the agonistic properties of tamoxifen, AIs like letrozole may be more effective at inhibiting growth of low ER-expressing breast tumors, as was also suggested by this study (22).

To illustrate the extent of changes induced in the profile of genes expressed within MCF-7 cells upon 45-fold overexpression of erbB2/HER-2, as well as potential gene expression differences between MCF-7 and MCF/HER-2–18 cells grown in vitro vs. in vivo, replicate pairs of MCF/neo-3 and MCF/HER-2–18 samples grown in culture or as tumors in nude mice were isolated, their total RNA extracted, and 32P-labeled RNA hybridized to low-density membrane arrays con-

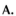

A.

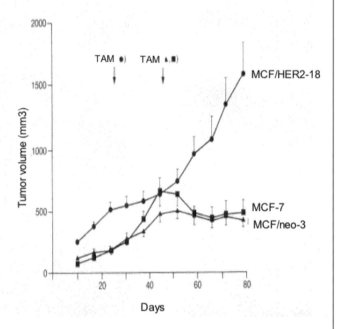

B.

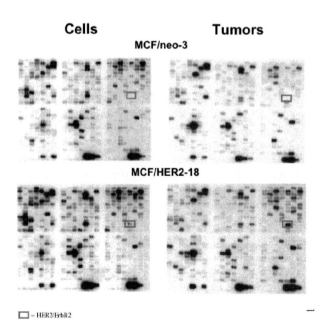

taining 597 different and functionally grouped genes (Clonetech Atlas Human Cancer kit 1.0 cDNA arrays). Principal components analysis (not shown) demonstrated consistent results between replicates but, as shown in Figure 3B, markedly dissimilar expression patterns between sample pairs and the two sets of experimental conditions. As might be expected, the majority of the arrayed and expressed genes are not affected by erbB2/HER-2 overexpression; more surprisingly, the subset of genes commonly affected by erbB2/HER-2 overexpression in both systems appear to be nonrandomly distributed ($p < 0.003$, contingency analysis) into three up-regulated gene groups (oncogenes, other receptors, cell fate/development regulators) and three down-regulated gene groups (tumor suppressors, apoptosis, intermediate filaments), lending support to the hypothesis that only a limited number of relevant gene programs are associated with erbB2/HER-2 overexpression in the absence of additional genetic changes (e.g., the chromosomal gains and losses commonly found in association with endogenously amplified *ERBB2*). ImageQuant analyses of these low-density arrays identified the 25% most highly up- or down-regulated genes induced by erbB2/HER-2 expression in both cells and tumors. When these were compared between in vitro and in vivo experimental conditions, the same MCF/HER-2–18 subline exhibited only 35 commonly erbB2/HER-2 up-regulated genes and 14 commonly down-reg-

---

Figure 3A More rapid and tamoxifen-stimulated tumorigenic growth of MCF/HER-2–18 cells in vivo relative to tumoristatic effects of tamoxifen on parental (MCF-7) or control (MCF/neo-3) cells. As originally reported (21), ovariectomized nude mice subcutaneously implanted with slow release estradiol (E) pellets were inoculated with cells at day 0. Tumor volumes (mm³) were determined on days shown (mean ± SEM), and E removed and daily tamoxifen (TAM) injections begun on day 26 for the MCF/HER-2–18 and on day 46 for the MCF-7 and MCF/neo-3 implanted mice, when E-stimulated tumors in each group reached mean tumor volumes of 500 mm³. **B** Gene expression changes induced by overexpression of erbB2/HER-2 in the cultured or xenografted sublines of MCF-7. MCF/neo-3 and MCF/HER2–18 sublines grown either in culture (50–70% confluency) or as xenografted tumors in nude mice (same tumor size) under E-stimulated conditions were harvested, their total RNA purified, 32P-labeled and hybridized to commercial low-density cDNA arrays (Clontech Atlas Human Cancer kit 1.0). As visualized (and quantified by ImageQuant), the paired dots of 597 known genes are ordered into 16 groups that include 9 different housekeeping genes, 9 negative DNA controls, and 14 different gene programs (each representing 4% to 17% of the total arrayed genes). Shown boxed is expression of erbB2/HER-2, detectable at this magnification only in the arrays from the MCF/HER2–18 samples. Vertical comparison of the arrays from each growth condition (i.e., MCF/neo-3 vs. MCF/HER-2–18 samples) shows gene expression differences induced by the overexpression of erbB2/HER-2. Horizontal comparison of the arrays for each subline shows the profoundly different influences of in vitro vs. in vivo growth conditions on both basal and erbB-2-induced gene expression profiles.

237

ulated genes. Thus, these results also illustrate the profound impact of tumor physiology and cell environment on erbB2/HER-2-inducible gene expression profiles.

Other investigators have since used this MCF/HER-2–18 model, which is appealing for its lack of other endogenous and confounding erbB/HER-receptor changes (e.g., altered levels of EGFR, erbB3/HER-3 or erbB4/HER-2), to show that tamoxifen's agonistic effects on ER-inducible gene expression and in vivo tumorigenic growth can be blocked, restoring tamoxifen's antiestrogenic activity and even delaying its emergence, through pharmacologic agents that inhibit erbB2/HER-2 receptor-activation directly (e.g., the small molecule kinase inhibitor, ZD-1839/Iressa), or through other agents and genetic constructs that target erbB/HER-activated downstream MAPK and PI3K/AKT signaling pathways (23, 24). Similar therapeutic strategies emerging from studies with the MCF/HER-2–18 model have also been successfully applied to other breast cancer models exhibiting anti-estrogen resistance in association with endogenous overexpression of both ER and erbB2/HER-2 (25). Presently, there is increasing experimental evidence that signaling pathways downstream of activated erbB/HER family receptor tyrosine kinases not only play a causal role in inducing some degree of SERM resistance, but that these pathways should now be considered promising targets for therapeutic intervention in combination with endocrine agents to treat ER+ breast cancers clinically resistant to endocrine agents alone (9, 17, 26–28).

Shown schematically in Figure 4 are some of the ligand-dependent and ligand-independent signaling influences on ER structure and its transcriptional activity, caused by cross-talk with erbB/HER and other constitutively activated membrane receptors expressed in breast cancer, and mediated primarily by activated MAPK and PI3K/AKT pathways downstream of these receptors (9, 17, 26, 28). Also shown in Figure 4 are the various ER and erbB/HER receptor-targeted interventions potentially affected by this crosstalk between receptor systems. Apart from the more recently described MAPK- and PI3K/AKT-activating nongenotropic effects of membrane-bound ER (29, 30), thought to directly involve ligand-activated heterodimeric erbB/HER receptors, there are two basic genotropic models of ligand-dependent ER transcriptional activation. These genotropic models include: 1) "classical" gene regulation in which an estrogen agonist (or mixed agonist/antagonist like tamoxifen) binds and activates ER, resulting in direct DNA binding of this ER complex to an estrogen responsive promoter element (ERE) on ERE-containing gene promoters; and 2) "non-classical" gene activation in which the ligand-bound ER complex interacts with other transcription factors like AP-1 (Jun/Fos, Jun/ATF), Sp1, C/EBP or CREB that are directly bound to their respective DNA response elements to regulate transcription off genes that lack EREs. In both classical and non-classical genotropic models, ligand binding first dissociates chaperone proteins off monomeric ER, facilitating ER dimerization, allowing the nuclear ERE-bound or DNA-tethered

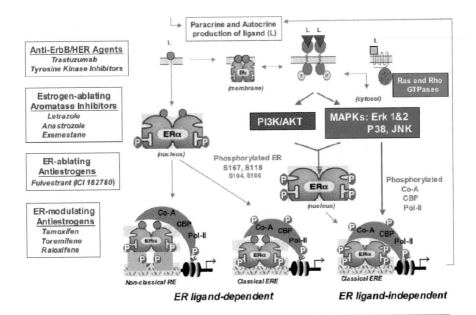

Figure 4 Schematic of signal transduction pathways and crosstalk mechanisms between ER and GFR systems co-activated and experimentally shown to be associated with the development of endocrine resistance in ER+ breast cancer models. As discussed in the text, GFR systems may be activated by their own ligands or other membrane-coupled receptor systems, including ER. ER activation of gene transcription may occur by ER dimers binding directly to classical ERE or tethered to non-classical response elements by protein–protein interactions with other DNA-binding transcription factors (e.g., Sp1, AP-1). MAPK and PI3K activated signaling leads to ER phosphorylation at several serine residues in its AF-1 domain (S167, S118, S104, S106). This can activate gene expression in the absence of available ER ligand, or further stimulate ER ligand-dependent gene enhancement at both classical and non-classical promoter response elements. These signaling pathways can also phosphorylate co-activators (Co-A) and co-activator binding proteins (CBP) needed to recruit and initiate the basic transcriptional machinery including RNA polymerase-II (Pol-II). Clinical studies are underway to determine if combination therapy with anti-GFR antibodies or kinase inhibitors and SERMs, estrogen-ablating AIs, or an ER-ablating anti-estrogen are more efficacious than single agent therapies against endocrine-resistant ER+ breast cancers.

ER to recruit in a ligand-determined manner various co-regulatory proteins (co-activators and co-repressors, whose availability and function are often dependent on phosphorylation and acetylation) at its exposed N-terminal AF-1 and C-terminal AF-2 transactivating domains (31). In addition to many other modulating and cell-specific factors, it is thought that the type and balance of co-regulators assembled at any promoter-bound ER complex is determined largely by different conformational changes in ER structure induced by liganding to different functional classes of SERMs: agonist, antagonist, or mixed agonist/antagonist (32).

The relationship of these two ligand-dependent genotropic ER models to the so-called nongenotropic signaling effects of ligand-bound ER (also seen with other sex steroid receptors) remains poorly understood. Likewise, it is still unclear how ligand-activated non-genotropic ER signaling effects are related to the better documented ligand-independent genotropic effects of ER (Fig. 4), mediated by the overexpression of erbB/HER family members (or their autocrine and paracrine produced growth factor ligands like Heregulin®), and resulting from MAPK and PI3K/AKT induced phosphorylation of nuclear ER on its AF-1 serine residues (S167 and S118, also S104 and S106). Of note, it has recently been shown that membrane-localized and ligand-bound ER can physically interact with growth factor activated erbB2/HER-2 heterodimers to stimulate MAPK and PI3K/AKT signaling, with resulting phosphorylation of nuclear ER that then stimulates transcription of both PR and pS2 but represses synthesis of new ER (33). This cell line observation showing early (6 hr) feedback inhibition of new ER production upon brief exposure to agonistic ER ligand or Heregulin stimulation of erbB2/HER-2 GFRs might explain the reduced ER content found in clinical samples of erbB2/HER-2 overexpressing breast cancers; however, this study also observed upregulated expession of PR immediately after erbB2/HER-2 stimulation and during feedback inhibiton of ER when, in fact, clinical evidence indicates that constitutive erbB2/HER-2 activation is associated with profound reductions in PR expression (see Fig. 2). One other recent study using another breast cancer cell line observed that Heregulin similarly activates PR via erbB2/HER-2 and MAPK signaling, but in this case the signaling resulted in rapid downregulation of PR levels (34), suggesting that growth factor ligand-induced signaling and cross-talk not only affects multiple members of the steroid receptor family but may lead to different receptor consequences in a rather cell-specific manner. In addition to these contradictory observations, other critical mechanistic questions that must still be addressed include: 1) the relative importance of erbB2/HER-2-induced phosphorylation of nuclear ER vs. phosphorylation of ER co-activators (Co-A) like AIB1 and/or various co-activator binding proteins (CBP) and components of the basal transcription machinery in determining crosstalk induced endocrine resistance; and 2) the relative dependence on ER ligands vs. other cell-specific factors (e.g., Co-As and CBPs) and post-translational ER modifications in addition to phosphorylation (e.g., acetylation) in determining ER membrane localization and its non-genotropic contributions to endocrine resistance.

Current in vitro and in vivo breast tumor models showing crosstalk between the proliferation- and survival-stimulating ER and erbB2/HER-2 signaling pathways also predict both estrogen antagonism of erbB2/HER-2-targeted therapeutics like trastuzumab (35) as well as resistance to various SERMs when both receptor systems are overexpressed (33). In all, the bi-directional cross-signaling observed between constitutively activated ER and erbB/HER receptor pathways in various preclinical models would appear to provide strong rationale for the clinical assessment of endocrine agents in combination with various erbB/HER-targeted therapeutics. It is worth commenting that while many promising erbB/HER tyrosine kinase inhibiting agents are currently under clinical development (e.g., ZD-1839/Iressa, AstraZeneca; OSI-774/Tarceva, Genentech; CI-1033, Pfizer; GW-572016, GlaxoSmithKline; EKB-569, Wyeth-Ayerst; AEE-788, Novartis), most breast and other tumors overexpressing the targeted erbB/HER receptors can be expected to appear clinically refractory to these inhibitors when given as single agents, and despite their general in vivo ability to inhibit the tumor's erbB/HER kinase activity and downstream signaling (36). Because reversal or prevention of endocrine resistance by these agents would seem to be dependent on their ability to inhibit erbB/HER receptor signaling, the utility of these agents in combination with endocrine agents should be assessed independent of their single agent tumor growth inhibiting potential.

V. OTHER MOLECULAR PATHWAYS DEFINING POOR-RISK AND ENDOCRINE-RESISTANT ER+ BREAST CANCER

Independent of the erbB/HER family of biomarkers, there appear to exist other less well defined molecular pathways that associate with subsets of ER+ breast cancer at risk for clinical resistance and/or early metastatic disease. This is illustrated in the following retrospective analysis from a database of > 800 primary breast cancer cases characterized by up to 20 different prognostic biomarkers and associated with 18+ years of clinical follow-up.* From 360 node-negative cases, two cohorts of ER+ cases were chosen for outcome comparison based on extreme differences in their ages at diagnosis: $n = 62$ older ($\geq$ age 70) vs. $n = 21$ younger (< age 45) cases. There were no significant differences between the age cohorts with respect to tumor size (cm), primary treatment (22% lumpectomy/radiation, 2% adjuvant chemotherapy, 2% adjuvant endocrine therapy), type of recurrences (90% distant), or several other biomarkers including apoptotic index, frequency of p53 overexpression, PR or pS2 positivity, erbB2/HER-2 or EGFR/erbB1 over-expression. The only tumor markers showing significant differences between these two age cohorts were tumor grade (45% of younger vs. 20% of older with SBR grade 3, $p = 0.03$) and proliferative status (e.g., mitotic index; and mean Ki-67/MIB-1 $= 25\%$ for younger vs. 12% for older, $p < 0.0001$). Surprisingly, however, a dramatic long-term outcome difference (disease-free survival DFS) was observed between these two ER+, node-negative cohorts, with DFS plateauing at

*Reported by Thor AD.

10 years for <30% of the younger vs. > 70% of the older cases ($p = 0.0004$). The significant differences in the observed (O) Kaplan-Meier DFS curves for these two cohorts are shown in Figure 5. Adjusting these curves to account for the only known cohort imbalances (the covariates tumor grade and proliferative index) results in a set of expected (E) DFS curves that still show significant outcome differences that cannot be accounted for by any known differences in primary tumor characteristics or biomarkers (Fig. 5).

Most interestingly, Cox proportional hazards and extensive multivariate analyses indicate that each cohort has different predictors of metastatic recur-

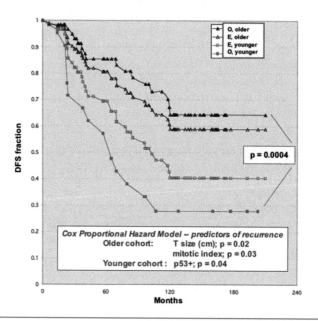

Figure 5 Observed (O) and expected (E) pairs of Kaplan-Meier disease-free survival (DFS) curves comparing older (patient age ≥70) vs. younger (patient age <45) cohorts of early-stage (node-negative) ER+ primary breast cancers ($n = 83$). As described in the text, these two cohorts were well-matched for numerous tumor biomarkers including erbB2/HER-2 and EGFR/erbB1 overexpression as well as tumor proportions overexpressing p53, and differed only in their mean tumor proliferative rates and proportions with high grade tumors. The dramatic outcome differences seen in the observed DFS curves ($p = 0.0004$) for the two cohorts could not be eliminated by adjusting for the extent of differences in their proliferative rates and tumor grade, as shown in the statistically adjusted (expected) Kaplan-Meier DFS curves. Using Cox proportional hazard modeling, tumor size (T, cm) and proliferative rate (mitotic index) were significant predictors of metastatic relapse for the older cohort of ER+ breast cancers; in contrast, only p53 overexpression (+) emerged as a predictor of metastatic relapse for the younger cohort of ER+ breast cancers.

rence, with T size ($p = 0.02$) and proliferative index ($p = 0.03$) predicting recurrence within the older cohort, and p53 overexpression ($p = 0.04$) predicting recurrence within the younger cohort. Thus, while these two ER+ cohorts did not differ significantly in their overall frequency of p53 overexpression (13/62 in older vs. 6/21 in younger), the p53 overexpressing older cases had only a 23% RR while the younger cases had an 83% RR (RR $= 3.6; p = 0.02$). This suggests that the underlying ER-associated tumorigenic mechanisms resulting in or interacting with p53 overexpression are different and of greater metastatic potential in the younger cases. Notably, p53 abnormalities and mutation types have not been well studied in ER+ breast cancers or according to age at diagnosis, despite provocative preliminary evidence that certain classes of p53 mutations are preferentially found in early-age breast tumors (e.g., G:C to T:A transversions) while others are found in later-age breast tumors (e.g., small deletions) (37, 38).

In the last half decade, high-density gene expression arrays have emerged as a powerful oncodiagnostic approach that can potentially identify additional ER-associated pathways linked to endocrine responsiveness and clinical outcome (39). With bioengineering advances enabling a single investigator to probe multiple breast tumor RNA samples and simultaneously determine the gene signature of each on microscopic arrays containing all known human genes (approximately 30,000), it is already apparent that informative groups of as few as 70 different genes may be able to identify clinically distinct subsets of ER+ breast cancers (40). Scores of previously uninteresting genes are being shown to cluster in their expression patterns with overexpression of our clinically important breast cancer biomarkers like ER and erbB2/HER-2 (40, 41). One landmark breast cancer expression array study using unsupervised clustering analysis identified at least two ER+ breast cancer subsets (A and B), each with different keratin-specific luminal gene expression patterns and very different clinical outcomes (40). Stage-matched survival analyses indicated that the ER+ subset A tumors were associated with significantly better patient survival than the ER+ subset B tumors, in which poor clinical outcome approached that of patients with ER–, erbB2/HER-2+ cancers (40).

In comparison with our earlier described biomarker findings showing the poor-risk impact of abnormal p53 status in a young age cohort of ER+ breast cancers not treated with adjuvant tamoxifen, the expression array-determined poor-risk subset B ER+ breast tumors were treated with adjuvant tamoxifen and were found to harbor a high frequency of p53 mutations (comparable to that found in the ER–, erbB2/HER-2+ subset) (40). Taken together, these studies suggest that abnormal p53 not only represents a poor-risk prognostic biomarker within subsets of ER+ breast cancer, but it also appears to be linked to an as yet undefined pathway of endocrine resistance. In support of this hypothesis, conversion of tamoxifen from a tumor-arresting ER antagonist to a tumor-stimulating ER agonist has been reported to occur more rapidly and more extensively in vivo with an

ER+ breast cancer line (T47D) bearing mutated p53 than with another (MCF-7) bearing intact p53 (42).

Once the reproducibility and predictive accuracy of high-density expression arrays and their resulting gene signatures are clinically validated by other groups (39), future challenges will face both basic and clinical investigators who must decipher the biologic roles played by individual genes within these expression signatures, according to their specific protein functions and known networks of interacting tumorigenic pathways. Besides leading to an improved understanding of the many different endocrine-dependent breast tumorigenic pathways, this wealth of biomarker data will obviously also offer new insights into the design of more effective endocrine treatment strategies.

REFERENCES

1. Eppenberger-Castori S, Moore DH, Thor AD, Edgerton SM, Kueng W, Eppenberger U, Benz CC. Age-associated biomarker profiles of human breast cancer. Int J Biochem Cell Biol 2002; 34:1318–1330.
2. Krtolica A, Parrinello S, Lockett S, Desprez P, Campisi J. Senescent fibroblasts promote epithelial cell growth and tumorigenesis: a link between cancer and aging. Proc Natl Acad Sci USA 2001;12072–12077.
3. Quong J, Eppenberger-Castori S, Moore II D, Scott GK, Birrir MJ, Kueng W, Eppenberger U, Benz CC. Age-dependent changes in breast cancer hormone receptors and oxidant stress markers. Breast Cancer Res Treat 2002; 76:221–236.
4. Osborne CK, Bardou V, Hopp TA, Chamness GC, Hilsenbeck SG, Fuqua SAW, Wong J, Allred DC, Clark GM, Schiff R. Role of the estrogen receptor coactivator AIB1 (SRC-3) and HER2/neu in tamoxifen resistance in breast cancer. J Natl Cancer Inst 2003; 95: 353–361.
5. Gunnarsson C, Ahnstrom M, Kirschner K, Olsson B, Nordenskjold B, Rutqvist LE, Skoog L, Stal O. Amplification of HSD17B1 and ERBB2 in primary breast cancer. Oncogene 2003; 22:34–40.
6. Tripathy D, Benz C. Growth factors and their receptors. In:Shapiro CL, Henderson IC, eds. New Directions in Breast Cancer Research and Therapeutics. Hematology/Oncology Clinics of North America. Philadelphia: WB Saunders, 1994; pp. 29–50.
7. Benz C, Tripathy D. ErbB2 overexpression in breast cancer: biology and clinical translation. J Womens Cancer 2000; 2:33–40.
8. Smith CL. Cross-talk between peptide growth factor and estrogen receptor signaling pathways. Biol Reprod 1998; 58:627–632.
9. Sommer S, Fuqua SAW. Estrogen receptor and breast cancer. Cancer Biol 2001; 11: 339–352.
10. Ressell KS, Hung M-C. Transcriptional repression of the neu protooncogene by estrogen stimulated estrogen receptor. Cancer Res 1992; 52:6624–6629.
11. DeFazio A, Chiew YE, McEvoy M, Watts CK, Sutherland RL. Antisense estrogen receptor RNA expression increases epidermal growth factor receptor gene expression in breast cancer cells. Cell Growth Differ 1997; 8:903–911.

12. Newman SP, Bates NP, Vernimmen D, Parker MG, Hurst HC. Cofactor competition between the ligand-bound oestrogen receptor and an intron 1 enhancer leads to oestrogen repression of ERBB2 expression in breast cancer. Oncogene 2000; 19:490–497.

13. Eppenberger-Castori S, Kueng W, Benz CC, Paris K, Caduff R, Bannwart F, Fink D, Dieterich H, Braschler C, von Castelberg B, Muller H, Eppenberger U. Prognostic and predictive significance of ErbB2 breast tumor levels measured by enzyme-immunoassay (EIA). J Clin Oncol 2001; 19:645–656.

14. Konecny G, Pauletti G, Pegram M, Untch M, Dandekar S, Aguilar Z, Wilson C, Rong H-M, Bauerfeind I, Felber M, Wang H-J, Beryt M, Seshadri R, Hepp H, Slamon DJ. Quantitative association between HER2/neu and steroid hormone receptors in hormone receptor-positive primary breast cancer. J Natl Cancer Inst 2003; 95:142–153.

15. Berry DA, Muss HB, Thor AD, Dressler L, Liu ET, Broadwater G, Budman DR, Henderson IC, Barcos M, Hayes D, and Norton L. HER2/neu and p53 expression versus tamoxifen resistance in estrogen receptor-positive, node-positive breast cancer. J Clin Oncol 2000; 18:3471–3479.

16. DePlacido S, DeLaurentiis M, Carlomagno C, Gallo C, Perrone F, Pepe S, Ruggiero A, Marinelli A, Pagliarulo C, Panico L, Pettinato G, Petrella G, Bianco AR. Twenty-year results of the Naples GUN randomized trial: predictive factors of adjuvant tamoxifen efficacy in early breast cancer. Clin Cancer Res 2003; 9:1039–1046.

17. Ring A, Dowsett M. Human epidermal growth factor receptor-2 and hormonal therapies: clinical implications. Clin Breast Cancer 2003; 4(suppl 1):S34–S41.

18. DeLaurentiis M, Arpino G, Massarelli E, Carlomagno C, Ciardiello F, Tortora G, Bianco AR, DePlacido S. A meta-analysis of the interaction between HER2 and the response to endocrine therapy (ET) in metastatic breast cancer (MBC) [abstr]. Proc Am Soc Clin Oncol 2000;19:78.

19. National Institutes of Health Consensus Development Conference Statement: adjuvant therapy for breast cancer, November 1–3, 2000. J Natl Cancer Inst Monographs 2001; 30:5–15.

20. Winer EP, Hudis C, Burstein HJ, Chlebowski RT, Ingle JN, Edge SB, Mamounas EP, Gralow J, Goldstein LJ, Pritchard KI, Braun S, Cobleigh MA, Langer AS, Perotti J, Powles TJ, Whelan TJ, Browman GP. American Society of Clinical Oncology technology assessment on the use of aromatase inhibitors as adjuvant therapy for women with hormone receptor-positive breast cancer: status report 2002. J Clin Oncol 2002; 20: 3317–3327.

21. Benz CC, Scott, GK, Sarup JC, Johnson RM, Tripathy D, Coronado E, Shepard HM, Osborne CK. Estrogen-dependent, tamoxifen-resistant tumorigenic growth of MCF-7 cells transfected with HER2/neu. Breast Cancer Res Treat 1992; 24:85–95.

22. Ellis MJ, Coop A, Singh B, Mauriac L, Llombert-Cussac A, Janicke F, Miller WR, Evans DB, Dugan, M, Brady C, Quebe-Fehling E, Borgs M. Letrozole is a more effective neoadjuvant endocrine therapy than tamoxifen for ErbB1- and/or ErbB2-positive, estrogen receptor-positive primary breast cancer: evidence from a phase III randomized trial. J Clin Oncol 2001;19:3808–3816.

23. Kurokawa H, Lenferink AEG, Simpson JF, Pisacane PI, Sliwkowski MX, Forbes JT, Arteaga CL. Inhibition of HER2/neu (ErbB2) and mitogen-activated protein kinases

enhances tamoxifen action against HER2-overexpressing, tamoxifen-resistant breast cancer cells. Cancer Res 2000; 5887–5894.

24. Massarweh S, Shou J, Mohsin SK, Ge M, Wakeling AE, Osborne CK, and Schiff R. Inhibition of epidermal growth factor/HER2 receptor signaling using ZD1839 (Iressa) restores tamoxifen sensitivity and delays resistance to estrogen deprivation in HER2-overexpressing breast tumors [abstr]. Proc Am Soc Clin Oncol 2002; 21:33a.

25. Kunisue H, Kurebayashi J, Otsuki T, Tang CK, Kurosumi M, Yamamoto S, Tanaka K, Doihara H, Shimizu N, Sonoo H. Anti-HER2 antibody enhances the growth inhibitory effect of anti-estrogen on breast cancer cells expressing both oestrogen receptors and HER2. Br J Cancer 2000; 82:46–51.

26. Schiff R, Massarweh S, Shou J, Osborne CK. Breast cancer endocrine resistance: how growth factor signaling and estrogen receptor coregulators modulate response. Clin Cancer Res. 2003; 9:447s–454s.

27. Kurokawa H, Arteaga CL. ErbB (HER) receptors can abrogate antiestrogen action in human breast cancer by multiple signaling mechanisms. Clin Cancer Res 2003; 9:511s–515s.

28. Johnston SRD, Head J, Pancholi S, Detre S, Martin L-A, Smith IE, Dowsett M. Integration of signal transduction inhibitors with endocrine therapy: an approach to overcoming hormone resistance in breast cancer. Clin Cancer Res 2003; 9:524s–532s.

29. Collins P, Webb C. Estrogen hits the surface. Nat Med 1999; 5:1130–1131.

30. Kousteni S, Han L, Chen J-R, Ålmeida M, Plotkin LI, Bellido T, Manolagas SC. Kinase-mediated regulation of common transcription factors accounts for the bone-protective effects of sex steroids. J Clin Invest 2003; 111:1651–1664.

31. McDonnell DP, Norris JD. Connections and regulation of the human estrogen receptor. Science 2002; 296:1642–1644.

32. Lonard DM, Smith CL. Molecular perspectives on selective estrogen receptor modulators (SERMs): progress in understanding their tissue-specific agonist and antagonist actions. Steroids 2002; 67:15–24.

33. Stoica GE, Franke TF, Wellstein A, Morgan E, Czubayko F, List H-J,Reiter R, Martin MB, Stoica A. Heregulin-β1 regulates the estrogen receptor-αgene expression and activity via the ErbB2/PI3-K/Akt pathway. Oncogene 2003; 22:2073–2087.

34. Labriola L, Salatino M, Proietti CJ, Pecci A, Coso OA, Kornblihtt AR, Charreau EH, Elizalde PV. Heregulin induces transcriptional activation of the progesterone receptor by a mechanism that requires functional ErbB2 and mitogen-activated protein kinase activation in breast cancer cells. Mol Cell Biol 2003; 23:1095–1111.

35. Treeck O, Diedrich K, Ortmann O. The activation of an extracellular signal-regulated kinase by oestradiol interferes with the effects of trastuzumab on HER2 signalling in endometrial adenocarcinoma cell lines. Eur J Cancer 2003; 39:1302–1309.

36. Bishop PC, Myers T, Robey R, Fry DW, Liu ET, Blagosklonny MV, Bates SE. Differential sensitivity of cancer cells to inhibitors of the epidermal growth factor receptor family. Oncogene 2002; 21:119–127.

37. Lai H, Lin L, Nadji M, Lai S, Trapido E, Meng L. Mutations in the p53 tumor suppressor gene and early onset breast cancer. Cancer Biol & Ther 2002; 1:31–36.

38. Olivier M, Hainaut P. TP53 mutation patterns in breast cancers: searching for clues of environmental carcinogenesis. Cancer Biol 2001;11:353–360.

39. Liu ET. Molecular oncodiagnostics: where we are and where we need to go. J Clin Oncol 2003; 21:2052–2055.

40. Sorlie T, Perou CM, Tibshirani R, Aas T, Geisler S, Johnson H, Hastie T, Eisen MB, van de Rijn M, Jeffrey SS, Thorsen T, Quist H, Matese JC, Brown PO, Botstein D, Lonning PE, Borresen-Dale A-L. Gene expression patterns of breast carcinomas distinguish tumor subclasses with clinical implications. Proc Natl Acad Sci (USA) 2001; 98:10869–10874.

41. Gruvberger S, Ringner M, Chen Y, Panavally S, Saal LH, Borg A, Ferno M, Peterson C, Meltzer PS. Estrogen receptor status in breast cancer is associated with remarkably distinct gene expression patterns. Cancer Res 2001; 61:5979–5984.

42. Schafer JM, Lee ES, O'Regan RM, Yao K, Jordan VC. Rapid development of tamoxifen-stimulated mutant p53 breast tumors (T47D) in athymic mice. Clin Cancer Res 2000; 4373–4380.

16

Beyond Antihormones in the Targeted Therapy of Breast Cancer

Robert I. Nicholson, Iain Hutcheson, Janice Knowlden, David Britton, Maureen Harper, Nicola Jordan, Steven Hiscox, Denise Barrow, and Julia Gee

Welsh School of Pharmacy
Cardiff University
Cardiff, Wales

I. OVERVIEW

Estrogen-receptor (ER) signaling plays a central role in the pathogenesis of breast cancer. However, recent research has identified other signal elements within the breast cancer phenotype that have a potential to influence ER signaling. Targeting of such elements might more effectively limit the activity of estrogens in breast cancer development, and perhaps enhance the effects of antihormonal therapies. The clinical result would be to enhance antitumor activity of antihormones and provide novel, effective treatments for both de novo and acquired resistant states that might improve patient survival. This chapter examines the relationship between growth-factor-signaling pathways and antihormone failure in tumor models of breast cancer, and suggests a possible strategy for using signal transduction inhibitors to improve the actions of antihormones and block the aggressive disease progression that often accompanies the development of endocrine-resistant states.

II. INTRODUCTION

Current conceptions regarding the role of endocrine response pathways in the pathogenesis of breast cancer continue to recognize the central importance of estrogen and ER signaling. It would be naïve, however, to consider this signaling pathway in isolation. Research findings have identified many other signal elements within the breast cancer phenotype that could influence—and be influenced by—ER signaling, and thus have the potential not only to alter the sensitivity of developing breast cancer cells to estrogens, but also have the potential, when aberrantly expressed, to adversely influence therapeutic responses to antihormonal drugs. Targeting of such elements might, therefore, more effectively limit the actions of estrogens in terms of breast cancer development, and also at presentation could enhance the quality and duration of response to antihormonal drugs, thereby providing novel, effective treatments for both de novo and acquired resistant states that improve patient survival.

III. ANTIHORMONE FAILURE: EPIDERMAL GROWTH FACTOR RECEPTOR AND HER-2 SIGNALING

Figure 1 shows the relationship between antihormone failure, and epidermal growth factor receptor (EFGR) and HER-2 signaling. The tamoxifen-resistant variant shown on the right was derived from wild-type (wt) MCF-7 cells through prolonged exposure to 4-hydroxytamoxifen. Although the parental cells on the left show only modest levels of EGFR and HER-2, there is a substantial increase in the expression of these erbB family members as tamoxifen resistance develops. Immunostaining is visibly situated on the tumor cells' plasma membranes.

Most importantly, such a cobblestone appearance (Fig. 1, right) in clinical breast cancer specimens is often associated not only with loss of ER but also with emergence of other aggressive features of the disease. In this light, it is noteworthy that the increases in EGFR and HER-2 in tamoxifen-resistant variants promote about a two-fold increase both in basal growth rates and in cell motility. There is also about a four-fold increase in the invasiveness of the cells as demonstrated by Matrigel penetration (1, 2).

It seems unlikely that the increased levels of growth factor receptors present in the tamoxifen-resistant cells are merely bystanders in the process of the development of resistance. Immunoprecipitation studies indicate that the erbB receptors are heterodimerized and display an increased basal level of activation. This serves to recruit multiple signal transduction cascades involved in the regulation of cell proliferation and survival, including ras, raf, MAPK, PI3K/AKT, and PKC isoforms, each of which is substantially activated in the tamoxifen-resistant cells (3, 4). Sustained induction of such proliferation and survival signals by growth

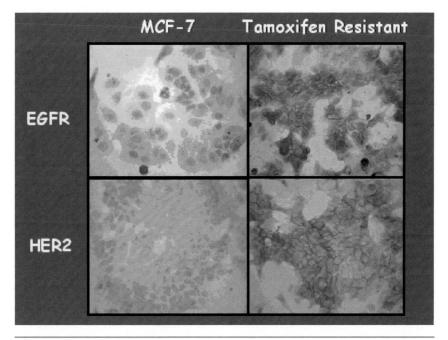

Figure 1 Relationship between EGFR and HER-2 signaling, and anti-estrogen failure. Tamoxifen-resistant variant (right) derived from wt MCF-7 cells (left) through prolonged exposure to 4-hydroxytamoxifen. (From Ref. 7)

factors ultimately serves to override the growth-inhibitory effects of antihormones and drives endocrine-resistant growth.

A.   ER Phosphorylation

An obvious and complicating issue is how this interfaces with the ER. Several growth-factor-induced protein kinases, including MAPK and AKT, are also able to target and phosphorylate key regulatory sites on the ER protein. This crosstalk enables the activity of the ER as a nuclear transcription factor, even driving some of the estrogen-like properties of antihormonal drugs. Compared to parental cells, tamoxifen-resistant cells show a substantial increase in the basal phosphorylation of the ER on serine 118 and 167 (Fig. 2), which are target sites for EGFR/HER-2-induced MAPK/AKT. This leads to an increase in the expression of several EGFR ligands and establishes a new self-propagating autocrine growth-regulatory loop that efficiently drives tamoxifen-resistant cell growth (5, 6).

In this model, the resistant growth originates from the growth-factor pathway rather than directly from the ER protein. If ER signaling is blocked with the pure

p-ser118

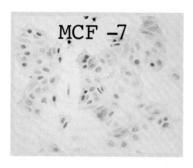 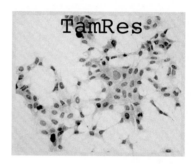

p-ser167

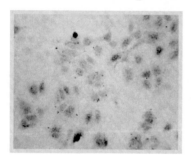 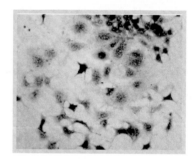

Figure 2 Tamoxifen-resistant cells show a substantial increase in the basal phosphorylation of the ER on serine 118 (top) and serine 167 (bottom), target sites for EGFR/HER-2-induced MAPK and AKT.

anti-estrogen fulvestrant, add-back experiments in which cells are exposed to exogenous TGFa not only fully activate EGFR, HER-2, ERK MAPK, and akt signaling, but also support substantial tumor cell growth in the presence of the normally growth-inhibitory drug (6). Strengthening of the EGFR pathway is thus able to entirely circumvent the catastrophic effects of this antihormone on the ER protein in such cells.

B. IGF-1R

Recent data supporting this autocrine model of tamoxifen resistance indicate significantly elevated levels of total and activated IGF-1R, which appear to contribute to EGFR-driven growth responses. Challenge of the tamoxifen resistant cells with IGF-II results, not only in the predicted increase in IGF-1R phosphorylation, but also in a reproducible increase in EGFR activation. These events can be reduced in parallel by preincubation of the cells with an IGF-1R selective inhibitor, AG1024 (2, 7).

Significantly, a neutralizing antibody to IGF-II reduces both basal IGF-1R phosphorylation and EGFR phosphorylation in a dose-dependent manner, consistent with the concept that IGF-1R signaling may contribute to EGFR-driven responses. These interactions, however, appear unidirectional insofar as challenge with EGF, which results in a massive phosphorylation of EGFR, does not activate IGF-1R. Furthermore, blockade with Iressa® is without inhibitory effect on p-IGF-1R (2, 7).

IV. ANTIGROWTH FACTOR THERAPIES

These tumor-model data provide good evidence that growth-factor signaling, notably EGFR, HER-2, and IGF-1R, make a significant contribution to the development of antihormone resistance. Is it possible, then, to negate these effects using antigrowth factor therapies and treat antihormone resistance with its potentially more aggressive phenotype? The answer is certainly "yes," bearing in mind that increases in EGFR signaling, for example, result not only in changes in endocrine response but also in increases in the motility and invasiveness of cells.

At an effective dose, Iressa decreases phosphorylation of EGFR and inhibits the growth of tamoxifen resistant breast cancer cells (3, 5). The decrease in phosphorylation of EGFR is accompanied by a decrease in tumour-cell motility and invasiveness, confirming the importance of EGFR to the aggressive phenotype (1). Herceptin® (humanized monoclonal a/b to HER-2) produces the same end result, indicating the importance of the HER-2 receptor, and AG1024 can similarly be used to inhibit cell growth, at least in part because of the contribution of IGF-1R to EGFR signaling. However, all these inhibitory actions in tamoxifen-resistant cells are only temporary; acquired resistant variants to Iressa, Herceptin, and AG1024 emerge within 2–6 months. In the case of Iressa, the resistance does not arise because of a failure of Iressa to continuously suppress phosphorylation of EGFR. Rather, it appears to result from a raised level of IGF-1R signaling onto downstream molecules such as AKT, PKC, delta, and ER (8).

Interestingly, the increases in p-AKT and PKC delta are progressive from wt cells, to tamoxifen-resistant cells, to dually tamoxifen-resistant and Iressa-resistant cells. Iressa-resistant cells also develop co-resistance to Herceptin, probably as a consequence of increases in IGF-1R signaling. Furthermore, cells with combined resistance show an increase in their level of invasiveness—a nearly two-fold increase compared to cells resistant to tamoxifen alone (8). Thus, although antigrowth-factor therapies are successful at inhibiting antihormone-resistant cells, they are in turn subject to resistant mechanisms that can also generate an increasingly invasive phenotype.

V. STRATEGIES TO PREVENT RESISTANCE

The emergence of dually resistant breast cancer cells has implications for the sequencing of therapies, including administration of antihormonal drugs and now signal transduction inhibitors. This last section discusses strategies designed to delay or prevent the development of such resistance by combining the primary treatment with drugs that anticipate and abrogate the recruited resistance mechanism.

Figure 3 (a–c) shows the typical results of treatment of endocrine-sensitive breast cancer cells using tamoxifen. The increase in EGFR signaling is apparent as early as 5 weeks, although at this time it is insufficient to drive resistant growth. The subsequent emergence of resistance occurs by week 12, when EGFR levels are further upregulated and the EGFR-signaling pathway is prominent. In one experimental model, Iressa is combined with tamoxifen in anticipation of the cells using EGFR for the resistant growth that develops on anti-estrogen challenge. Figure 4 compares graphically the results of therapy with tamoxifen and/or Iressa vs. control on cell growth; the typical appearance of combined tamoxifen-Iressa treatment after 5 weeks is shown in Figure 3d. Iressa has very little effect initially because of low levels of EGFR signaling. Tamoxifen shows the expected inhibitory effect in this 5-week period, while the combination of tamoxifen and Iressa is the most effective treatment (9).

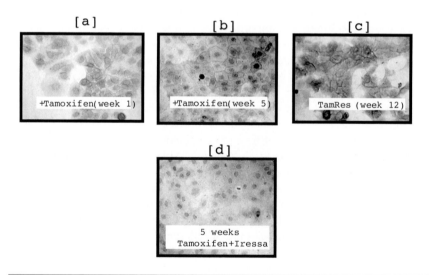

Figure 3 Results of treatment of endocrine-sensitive breast cancer cells on EGFr expression using tamoxifen at weeks 1, 5, and 12 (a–c), and results at week 5 when Iressa is combined with tamoxifen (d). (From Ref. 9)

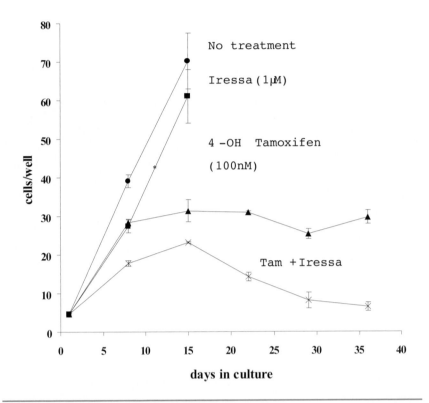

Figure 4 Results of treatment using Iressa, tamoxifen, tamoxifen plus Iressa, and control (no treatment) on cell growth rates during the first 5-week period. (From Ref 9. Copyright 2003 The Endocrine Society.)

Excitingly, if continued out to the time frame in which tamoxifen resistance normally develops, the combination of agents prevents the evolution of resistance and also results in a total cell loss (Fig. 5). Iressa blocks the antihormone-induced increases in EGFR in endocrine-sensitive cells, with co-treatment further depleting the activity of MAPK and AKT. The end result is a reduction in proliferation and a higher level of apoptosis within the cells (9).

As already indicated, Iressa and AG1024 are growth inhibitory to tamoxifen resistant cells, but in each instance resistance develops. Applying the logic of combining Iressa and tamoxifen, what would be the effect of adding AG1024 in anticipation of the cells adopting IGF-1R for resistant growth? As shown in Figure 6, our preliminary studies indicate that co-treatment with AG1024 prevents the evolution of Iressa resistance, with its more aggressive phenotype, and increases cell loss. The combination appears very much more effective than the use of either agent alone.

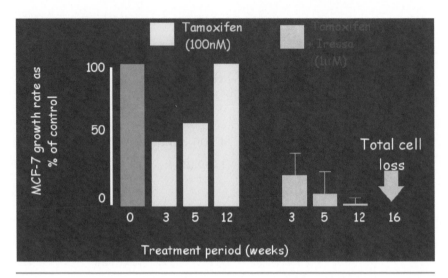

Figure 5 Effects of treatment with tamoxifen (left) and tamoxifen plus Iressa (right) on cell growth rates during a 12-week treatment period. (From Ref. 9)

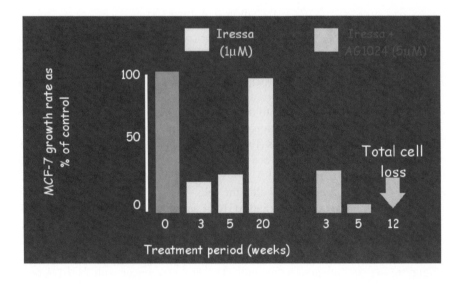

Figure 6 Effects of treatment with Iressa (left) and Iressa plus AG1024 (right) on cell growth rates during a 12-week treatment period.

VI. SUMMARY

Alterations in growth-factor signal elements have a considerable potential to influence cellular and growth responses, not only to antihormones, but to antigrowth factors as well. Evidence of this is beginning to appear in trials of antigrowth factors, which do not work in all patients and in whom acquired resistance clearly develops. Changes in growth-factor-signaling pathways appear to allow cells to survive initial drug treatment, ultimately driving resistant growth together with aggressive invasive behavior. Research evidence to date suggests a strategy for developing treatment options to combat both endocrine and antigrowth factor resistance, possibly resulting in greater efficacy for signal transduction inhibitors through their combination with endocrine therapy. This would probably apply not only to the pathways discussed here—EGFR, IGF-1R, and HER-2—but would also be applicable to inhibitors of downstream signaling. Hopefully this line of inquiry will improve breast cancer survival rates.

REFERENCES

1. Hiscox SE, Barrow D, Dutkowski C, Wakeling AE, Nicholson RI. Tamoxifen resistance in breast cancer cells is accompanied by an enhanced motile and invasive phenotype: inhibition by gefitinib (Iressa', ZD1839). Submitted.
2. Nicholson RI, Hutcheson IR, Knowlden JM, Jones HE, Harper ME, Jordan N, Hiscox SE, Barrow D, Gee JMW. Non-endocrine pathways and endocrine resistance: observations with anti-oestrogens and signal transduction inhibitors in combination. Clin Cancer Res 2004; 10:346S–354S.
3. Knowlden JM, Hutcheson IR, Jones HE, Madden TA, Gee JMW, Harper ME, Barrow D, Wakeling AE, Nicholson RI. Elevated levels of EGFR/c-erbB2 heterodimers mediate an autocrine growth regulatory pathway in tamoxifen resistant MCF-7 cells. Endocrinology 2003; 144:1032–1044.
4. Nicholson RI, Gee JMW. Oestrogen and growth factor cross-talk and endocrine insensitivity and acquired resistance in breast cancer [review]. Br J Cancer 2000; 82:501-513.
5. Nicholson RI, Hutcheson IR, Harper ME, Knowlden JM, Barrow D, McClellend RA, Jones HE, Wakeling AE, Gee JMW. Modulation of EGFR endocrine resistant, ER positive breast cancer. Endocr Relat Cancer 2001; 8:175–182.
6. Hutcheson IR, Knowlden JM, Madden TA, Barrow D, Gee JMW, Wakeling AE, Nicholson RI. Oestrogen receptor-mediated modulation of the EGFR/MAPK pathway in tamoxifen resistant MCF-7 cells. Breast Cancer Res Treat 2003. In press.
7. Knowlden JM, Hutcheson IR, Barrow D, Nicholson RI. IGF-1R and EGFR cross-talk in tamoxifen resistant MCF-7 breast cancer cells [abstr]. San Antonio Breast Cancer Symposium, San Antonio, TX, Dec 3–6, 2003.
8. Jones HE, Goddard L, Gee JMW, Hiscox SE, Rubini M, Barrow D, Knowlden JM, Williams S, Wakeling AE, Nicholson RI. Insulin-like growth factor-1-receptor signaling

and acquired resistance to gefitinib (ZD1839, Iressa™) in human breast and prostate cancer cells. Submitted.

9. Gee JMW, Harper ME, Hutcheson IR, Madden TA, Barrow D, Knowlden JM, McClellend RA, Jordan N, Wakeling AE, Nicholson RI. The anti-EGFR agent gefitinib (ZD1839, Iressa™) improves anti-hormone response and prevents development of resistance in breast cancer in vitro. Endocrinology 2003;144. In press.

17

Novel Therapeutics

Adrian L. Harris
Churchill Hospital
Oxford, England

I. OVERVIEW

Many novel therapeutic anticancer agents specifically targeting key aspects of cancer growth and progression are under development. One key element of tumor progression is angiogenesis. Many complex molecular and cellular mechanisms govern tumor angiogenesis, including vascular endothelial growth factor (VEGF). Expression of VEGF in breast cancer tumors has been shown to correlate with poor prognosis. However, a recent Phase III trial with an anti-VEGF monoclonal antibody (bevacizumab) has not demonstrated a survival benefit when bevacizumab was added to chemotherapy in breast cancer patients. However, VEGF is only one element of the angiogenic pathway and it is possible that blocking the pathway further upstream would be more effective. Another confounding factor is the heterogeneity of angiogenesis and VEGF expression in breast tumors. It is likely that targeting those tumors with an angiogenic phenotype would confer more benefit. Bevacizumab has shown promising results in clear cell renal cancer, a tumor type known to be associated with high levels of VEGF.

II. INTRODUCTION

Clinical trials on many of the novel cancer drugs developed in recent years have failed to reproduce the potential shown by animal models. For endocrine treatments, measurable pharmacodynamic markers exist, for example, estrogen levels in the blood and other tumor markers. For newer therapies, where the pathway of action has not been fully mapped out, these measurable markers of efficacy are not necessarily available.

The characteristics of cancer can be classified into six areas: 1) self-sufficiency in growth signals, 2) insensitivity to antigrowth signals, 3) tissue invasion and metastasis, 4) limitless replicative potential, 5) sustained angiogenesis, and 6) evasion of apoptosis (1). An important question in breast cancer biology is whether estrogen is involved in all these pathological processes or whether other estrogen-independent pathways are responsible for tumor growth and metastasis.

Key elements of these six pathways represent attractive targets for novel therapeutics. Indeed, many agents acting on these targets are currently in development. New targets include key gene products involved in growth signaling (e.g., EGFr, HER-2, bcr-abl, kit, aurora kinases), cell cycle progression (including chk1, chk2, cdk1, cdk2, cdk4), apoptosis (bcl2, survivin, trail, MDM2 p53), invasion proteolysis, and angiogenesis. Other novel agents, such as histone deacetylase inhibitors, proteasome inhibitors, and hsp60 blockers, do not fit into the concept of six main areas quite so well. Other important novel therapeutic targets are DNA repair inhibitors, immunotherapy, and gene therapy. However, the most successful drugs besides endocrine therapy are antimetabolites and drugs that block proliferation.

There are several novel anticancer agents involving many pathways under development. One area that has been the focus of recent research is prevention of tumor angiogenesis.

III. TUMOR ANGIOGENESIS

Tumor angiogenesis is essential for growth, invasion, and metastasis of a tumor; thus it represents an attractive target for cancer therapeutics (2). Moreover, in breast cancer, angiogenesis is switched on early, before invasion, and occurs extensively in ductal carcinoma in situ (DCIS). One of the most important angiogenic factors is VEGF. The actions of VEGF include endothelial cell mitogenesis and migration, remodeling of the extracellular matrix via induction of proteinases, increased vascular permeability and vasodilation, and inhibition of endothelial cell apoptosis. VEGF has three endothelial cell surface receptors: VEGF-R1 (Flt-1), VEGF-R2 (KDR/Flk-1), and VEGF-R3 (FLT-4) (Fig. 1). Overexpression of VEGF in animal models has been shown to confer resistance to chemotherapy, radiotherapy, and immunosuppression. Moreover, higher levels of VEGF in breast cancer correlate with a worse prognosis.

VEGF inhibitors have been in development for at least 5 to 6 years. Initially, drugs were developed that blocked the VEGF-R2 (VEGF kinase 2), which is a multidomain receptor with at least three ligands (VEGF-A, VEGF-C, VEGF-D).

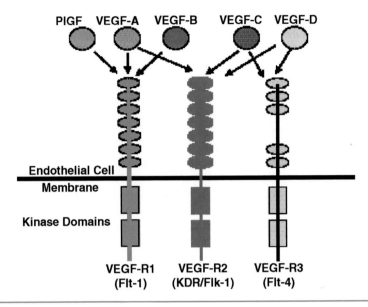

Figure 1 VEGF family and receptors.

Recently, bevacizumab (Avastin™), an antibody to VEGF-A has shown a survival advantage in metastatic colon cancer when combined with chemotherapy (3). However, inhibiting VEGF-A alone will not block VEGF-C or D, which are also ligands of VEGF-R2.

It was originally thought that VEGF-R2 was the most important endothelial cell receptor in cancer; however, recent data have shown that VEGF-R1 may also be important (4). Moreover, VEGF-R3 is normally present in embryonic endothelial cells and is switched off in normal adult cells, but switched on in tumor endothelial cells (5). Therefore, inhibitors of just one receptor or ligand may not be effective at preventing tumor angiogenesis. Nevertheless, despite recent disappointments in the field of VEGF kinase inhibitors, bevacizumab has shown encouraging results in advanced metastatic renal cancer (6). It is possible that the correct targets are not yet being blocked. Several other compounds that inhibit the VEGF pathway are under development, including a ribozyme—a VEGF-R1 inhibitor—and SU11248—a broad spectrum tyrosine kinase inhibitor that inhibits VEGF-R2, platelet-derived growth-factor receptor (PDGFr), c-kit, and fetal liver tyrosine kinase 3 (7, 8).

A. Influence of Hypoxia on Angiogenesis

Microenvironmental alterations are a key feature of tumors. Hypoxia is present in many solid tumors and generally occurs over 100 μm away from functional blood vessels (9). Hypoxia, as well as being a marker of malignant growth, is associated with rapid growth, metastasis and poor response to treatment (10, 11). In hypoxia, VEGF is induced and in situ hybridization can demonstrate VEGF expression in breast cancer sections around the hypoxic zone.

Hypoxia exerts direct effects on pathways involved in tumor development and expansion, including angiogenesis, apoptosis, glycolysis, and cell cycle regulation (9). Over the past 2 years, there have been great advances in the understanding of this pathway. A key enzyme in this process is proline hydroxylase, which hydroxylates the transcription factor hypoxia-inducible factor (HIF)-1α in the presence of oxygen. Hydroxylated HIF-1α is then a substrate for the von Hippel Lindau (VHL) gene product, a ubiquitin ligase, which targets it for destruction in the proteasome. However, in conditions of hypoxia, there is less hydroxylation of HIF-1α and, instead of proteolysis, HIF-1α translocates to the nucleus and heterodimerizes with an aryl hydrocarbon nuclear translocator. The heterodimers then bind to specific hypoxia response elements, thereby activating specific genes (12). Key genes activated in response to hypoxia include GLUT1 (involved in glucose transport), VEGF (angiogenesis), and LDH A (glycolysis, which is essential for tumor survival under hypoxic conditions) (9). Therefore, many of the cardinal signs of cancer are regulated by hypoxia.

In total, 15 angiogenic factors or pathways are regulated by hypoxia. These factors include endothelin 1 and 2, adrenomedullin, plasminogen activator inhibitor 1, histone deacetylase and platelet-derived growth factor (PDGF).

A probable endogenous marker of tumor hypoxia is the enzyme carbonic anhydrase 9 (CA9), a transmembrane glycoprotein with an extracellular enzymatic site. CA9 is responsible for reversible conversion of carbonic acid to carbon dioxide and water. This enzyme has a low expression in normal tissue but is induced by hypoxia (13). Staining breast cancer sections with monoclonal antibodies against CA9 showed a very strong pattern approximately 100 μm from the blood vessel, which is exactly the diffusion distance of oxygen and is related to radiation resistance in these areas.

CA9 has been shown to be a strong prognostic indicator in breast cancer. Patients without CA9 expression had a significant survival advantage over those who had CA9 expression ($p = 0.001$) (14). However, is CA9 just a marker of hypoxia or does it play a fundamental role in cellular survival under conditions of hypoxia? In experiments on breast cancer cell lines, RNA inhibitor (RNAI) treatment to switch off hypoxia-inducible CA9 shows that RNAI slows the growth of cells in low-density culture, although cell growth eventually reached the same density as control samples. Moreover, in dense cultures, cells never reached the same density as the control cells. If these cultures are then subjected to clonogenic survival assays under conditions of hypoxia, then 50% of remaining clones died. Thus, CA9 is clearly involved in a hypoxia survival pathway. Furthermore, hydrogen ions can enter cells six times more rapidly if CA9 is switched on than if it is switched off, thus CA9 may exert its biological effect through regulation of microenvironmental pH (13).

B. Selecting the Correct Therapeutic Target

Angiogenesis is, however, a complex process and is regulated by many different pro- and anti-angiogenic factors, which has led to difficulties in determining the most effective target to halt tumor angiogenesis. In addition to the microenviron-mental influence on angiogenesis, many other factors induce angiogenesis (Fig. 2). For example, oncogenes such as ras and EGFr switch on VEGF and angiogenesis. Hypoxia synergizes with these pathways to activate HIF-1α, producing hypoxia-inducible angiogenic factors including VEGF, PDGFα, and adrenomedullin. The angiogenic enzyme thymidine phosphorylase can also induce production of angiogenic factors such as IL-8, VEGF, and metalloproteases. Cell adhesion molecules upregulated in tumor endothelial cells also enhance angiogenesis. Tissue factor and endoglin additionally have proangiogenic effects. Tyrosine kinase receptors for VEGF and other pathways are also involved in the complex process of tumor angiogenesis. Pathways involved in the inhibition of angiogenesis are also lost. Cytoskeletal changes in the tumor endothelial cells also promote growth of tumor endothelial cells. Macrophages are additionally recruited, which are essential for tumor growth. The tumor produces IL6, among other cytokines, which stimulate the bone marrow to produce platelets. The platelets then aggregate in the tumor and release VEGF.

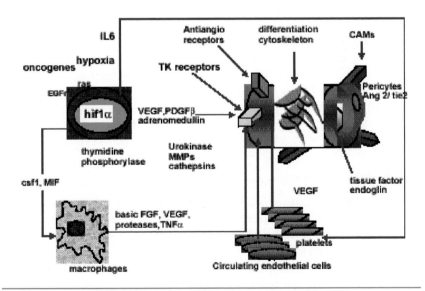

Figure 2 Angiogenesis pathways.

The tumor also produces factors that stimulate circulating endothelial cells to form the vasculature of the tumor. Given these manifold pathways involved in angiogenesis, what is the most suitable therapeutic target for attenuating tumor angiogenesis?

The size and stage of a tumor are important considerations when designing new therapeutic targets. The effect of some of the most widely studied antiangiogenic agents was investigated in animal tumor models of differing sizes/stages (15). These agents were BB94 (a metalloprotease inhibitor), AGM1470 (a fumagillin analogue), endostatin, angiostatin, and endostatin and angiostatin combined. The results showed that these drugs are effective at different stages. In the early lesion, endostatin and angiostatin were most effective at reducing tumor burden; however, this combination is less effective in the invasive stage. Similarly, the metalloprotease inhibitor was not very effective in the early lesion or in the invasive stage, but was more effective in small tumors.

The problems facing the development of anti-angi/ogenesis therapy are identical to those facing all novel therapies that target new molecules. Namely, there are multiple complex mechanisms involved in angiogenesis. New understanding of the biology of these processes is occurring in parallel to new drug developments. Moreover, angiogenesis mechanisms may be different in the primary and secondary tumors. Furthermore, not all metastases have an angiogenic phenotype. The size of the tumor is also critical to the effectiveness of chemotherapy and probably endocrine therapy.

There is a large degree of heterogeneity in the extent of tumor angiogenesis and VEGF expression in breast cancer tumors. Greater numbers of blood vessels and higher microvessel density in tumor correlate with poorer prognosis. The location of receptor-bound VEGF in sections of tumors was determined using a specific antibody (16). It could be assumed that vessels staining positively for VEGF are the active blood vessels that have been stimulated to grow. Indeed, receptor-bound VEGF is associated with a significantly poorer prognosis ($p < 0.001$). Thus, treating patients with anti-VEGF therapy is clearly potentially of value in patients who are positive for VEGF. However, treating patients negative for VEGF with anti-VEGF therapy is likely to be less effective.

C. Angiogenesis in Metastases

When blood vessels in lung metastases from breast cancer patients were stained using CD31 antibody, two distinct patterns were seen in these sections (Fig. 3) (17). The first was a typical pattern of angiogenesis, with increased blood vessels in a chaotic pattern around the tumor cells. The second pattern was of alveolar blood vessels with tumor cells within them. Although there was only a small number of patients studied, it was apparent that those patients with the typical angiogenic phenotype had a very poor 5-year survival rate after resection of the lung metastases,

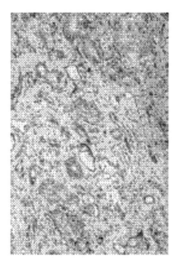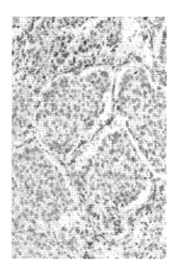

Figure 3   Staining of blood vessels in lung metastases with CD31 antibody. The section on the left shows a typical angiogenic phenotype in a lung metastasis of breast cancer; the section on the right shows a nonangiogenic phenotype, with alveolar blood vessels staining for CD31.

whereas the patients with the nonangiogenic phenotype survived more than 5 years after resection. The latter group of patients most likely did not have an angiogenic phenotype as yet and thus tumor cells were colonizing pre-existing blood vessels. The patients with the typically angiogenic phenotype generally developed more secondaries, even after resection of the lung metastases.

When liver secondaries from breast cancer patients were examined, it was found that of the 32 samples, 30 were pathologically determined to be nonangiogenic and two had an angiogenic phenotype. All the nonangiogenic metastases were negative for the hypoxia marker CA9, whereas both of the angiogenic samples were positive for CA9. In 46 samples of liver secondaries from colon cancer patients, 25 were pathologically nonangiogenic and 20 of these were negative for CA9. Of the 21 angiogenic tumor samples, 13 had an activated hypoxia pathway (i.e., were CA9 positive).

The results of these small studies might suggest that inhibition of angiogenesis would be less effective in breast cancer liver metastases than for colon cancer liver metastases, because more of the colon cancer secondaries had an angiogeneic phenotype compared with the breast cancer secondaries. This may in some way explain the lack of efficacy of bevacizumab in breast cancer. While response rates to monotherapy in Phase II trials have been promising, a Phase III trial with bevacizumab and the chemotherapeutic agent capecitabine failed to increase the survival time in comparison with chemotherapy alone (18). However, it is not clear how many breast cancer cases actually use VEGF as a main angiogenic pathway, as VEGF expression in breast cancer is very heterogeneous. Bevacizumab has, however, shown promising results in renal cancer. There was a highly significant dose response to bevacizumab treatment—the higher the dose, the better the response (6). This is possibly because all cases of clear-cell renal cancer have a VHL mutation. Because VHL is a key regulator of HIF-1α and mutated VHL can no longer degrade HIF-1α, large amounts of VEGF accumulate.

Although there is a clear biological interaction with bevacizumab in renal cancer (progression-free survival difference between the control and high-dose anti-VEGF was $p = 0.0011$), there may be more benefit in blocking HIF-1α itself, because 15 other angiogenic pathways are regulated by the HIF-1α pathway. Blocking the angiogenesis pathway further upstream, i.e., blocking HIF-1α, is the focus of current research.

IV. CONCLUSIONS

Genetic changes or well-defined biochemical changes that drive tumor progression are key targets for novel therapeutics. Care should be taken so that molecularly targeted drugs are used on tumors that are actually utilizing the relevant pathway. Thus, it is important to know the molecular pathways in subpopulations of patients to determine whether a particular novel agent is likely to have a beneficial effect.

Although many targets inhibit angiogenesis, is it necessary to inhibit one key target or multiple pathways? Improved trial design is needed to determine how the target is inhibited, by use of imaging, biopsies, and pharmacodynamic endpoints. Moreover, combination of novel targeted agents with conventional agents such as radiation, chemotherapy, hormone therapy, and immunotherapy is generally more effective in preclinical models. Thus, in clinical practice, where the situation is even more complex, combination of novel therapeutics with conventional treatments is likely to be more effective than monotherapy.

In summary, we are only just beginning to understand the complexity of angiogenesis and hence how to develop this area properly.

REFERENCES

1. Hanahan D, Weinberg RA. The hallmarks of cancer. Cell 2000; 100:57–70.
2. Folkman J. What is the evidence that tumors are angiogenesis dependent? J Natl Cancer Inst 1990; 82:4–6.
3. Kabbinavar F, Hurwitz HI, Fehrenbacher L, Meropol NJ, Novotny WF, Lieberman G, Griffing S, Bergsland E. Phase II, randomized trial comparing bevacizumab plus fluorouracil (FU)/leucovorin (LV) with FU/LV alone in patients with metastatic colorectal cancer. J Clin Oncol 2003; 21:60–65.

4. Luttun A, Tjwa M, Moons L, Wu Y, Angelillo-Scherrer A, Liao F, Nagy JA, Hooper A, Priller J, DeKlerck B, Compernolle V, Daci E, Bohlen P, Dewerchin M, Herbert JM, Fava R, Matthys P, Carmeliet G, Collen D, Dvorak HF, Hicklin DJ, Carmeliet P. Revascularization of ischemic tissues by PlGF treatment, and inhibition of tumor angiogenesis, arthritis and atherosclerosis by anti-Flt1. Nat Med 2002; 8:831–840.

5. Neuchrist C, Erovic BM, Handisurya A, Fischer MB, Steiner GE, Hollemann D, Gedlicka C, Saaristo A, Burian M. Vascular endothelial growth factor C and vascular endothelial growth factor receptor 3 expression in squamous cell carcinomas of the head and neck. Head Neck 2003; 25:464–474.

6. Yang JC, Haworth L, Sherry RM, Hwu P, Schwartzentruber DJ, Topalian SL, Steinberg SM, Chen HX, Rosenberg SA. A randomized trial of bevacizumab, an anti-vascular endothelial growth factor antibody, for metastatic renal cancer. N Engl J Med 2003; 349:427–434.

7. Weng DE, Usman N. Angiozyme: a novel angiogenesis inhibitor. Curr Oncol Rep 2001; 3:141–146.

8. Schueneman AJ, Himmelfarb E, Geng L, Tan J, Donnelly E, Mendel D, McMahon G, Hallahan DE. SU11248 maintenance therapy prevents tumor regrowth after fractionated irradiation of murine tumor models. Cancer Res 2003; 63:4009–4016.

9. Knowles HJ, Harris AL. Hypoxia and oxidative stress in breast cancer. Hypoxia and tumourigenesis. Breast Cancer Res 2001; 3:318–322.

10. Höckel M, Schlenger K, Aral B, Mitze M, Schaffer U, Vaupel P. Association between tumor hypoxia and malignant progression in advanced cancer of the uterine cervix. Cancer Res 1996; 56:4509–4515.

11. Brizel DM, Scully SP, Harrelson JM, Layfield LJ, Bean JM, Prosnitz LR, Dewhirst MW. Tumor oxygenation predicts for the likelihood of distant metastases in human soft tissue carcinoma. Cancer Res 1996; 56:941–943.

12. Harris AL. von Hippel-Liddau syndrome: target for anti-vascular endotherlial growth factor (VEGF) receptor therapy. Oncologist 2000; 5(suppl 1):32–36.

13. Wykoff CC, Beasley NJP, Watson PH, Turner KJ, Pastorek J, Sibtain A, Wilson GD, Turley H, Talks KL, Maxwell PH, Pugh CW, Ratcliffe PJ, Harris AL. Hypoxia-inducible expression of tumor-associated carbonic anhydrases. Cancer Res 2000; 60:7075–7083.

14. Chia SK, Wykoff CC, Watson PH, Han C, Leek RD, Pastorek J, Gatter KC, Ratcliffe P, Harris AL. Prognostic significance of novel hypoxia-regulated marker, carbonic anhydrase IX, in invasive breast carcinoma. J Clin Oncol 2001; 19:3660–3668.

15. Bergers G, Javaherian K, Lo KM, Folkman J, Hanahan D. Effects of angiogenesis inhibitors on multistage carcinogenesis in mice. Science 1999; 284:808–812.

16. Koukourakis MI, Giatromanolaki A, Thorpe PE, Brekken RA, Sivridis E, Kakolyris S, Georgoulias V, Gatter KC, Harris AL. Vascular endothelial growth factor/KDR activated microvessel density versus CD31 standard microvessel density in non-small cell lung cancer. Cancer Res 2000; 60:3088–3095.

17. Pezzella F, Manzotti M, DeBacco A, Viale G, Nicholson AG, Price R, Ratcliffe C, Pastorino U, Gatter KC, Harris AL, Altman DG, Pilotti S, Veronesi U. Evidence for novel non-angiogenic pathway in breast cancer metastasis. Lancet 2000; 355:1787–1788.

18. Abstracts of the 25th Annual San Antonio Breast Cancer Symposium. San Antonio, TX, Dec 11–14, 2002. Breast Cancer Res Treat 2002; 76(suppl 1):S29–180.

18

Surrogate Biomarkers and Neoadjuvant Endocrine Therapy

Matthew J. Ellis
Washington University
St. Louis, Missouri, U.S.A.

I. INTRODUCTION

Endocrine treatment with a third generation aromatase inhibitor (AI) is an effective neoadjuvant regimen for strongly hormone receptor-positive primary breast cancer in postmenopausal women, as shown by a recent trial of letrozole versus tamoxifen. However, although AI responses are frequently sufficient to improve surgical outcomes, the rate of pathologically complete response is less than 5%. Alternative clinical or biomarker surrogates for drug efficacy must, therefore, be identified. Currently the most investigated biomarker is Ki67. This cell cycle regulated protein usually falls dramatically with neoadjuvant endocrine treatment. The finding that Ki67 is suppressed more by letrozole than tamoxifen (1) correlates well with the clinical advantages of a third-generation AI in the neoadjuvant, adjuvant, and advanced disease settings (2) and supports a role for Ki67 as a surrogate endpoint in Phase III neoadjuvant studies addressing strategies to enhance adjuvant AI efficacy. Less certain is the value of changes in Ki67 (ΔKi67) as an endocrine therapy sensitivity test that could be used to plan adjuvant treatment. It will take much larger studies than those currently planned to validate ΔKi67 for this use. It seems likely that additional surrogates, such as those obtained through gene expression profiling, will be necessary to reach the

269

level of certainty required to individualize adjuvant therapy based on a clinical or biomarker response to neoadjuvant AI treatment.

II. DEFINING THE QUESTIONS REGARDING SURROGATE BIOMARKERS FROM NEOADJUVANT THERAPIES

From the clinical perspective, there are at least two very distinct motivations for conducting neoadjuvant studies in breast cancer: 1) to identify promising systemic therapies for further testing in larger scale adjuvant trials, and 2) to identify individuals with primary tumors that are resistant to standard treatment modalities. Different clinical trial design considerations, measurement parameters, and statistical techniques are required to address these two issues. When comparing drug regimens, a number of different biochemical, histological, and clinical endpoints can be used in an analytical approach that focuses on group rather than individual outcomes—i.e., is there evidence that overall tumor regression rates, induction of cell death, or inhibition of proliferation are more frequent on one arm of the study than the other? In contrast, studies that attempt to capitalize on the potential of neoadjuvant therapy to predict the effectiveness of standard adjuvant therapy must focus on individual outcomes. In other words, does tumor regression, reduction in tumor proliferation, or increase in cell death in response to neoadjuvant endocrine therapy translate into a higher individual chance of long-term remission in comparison to patients whose tumors responded poorly? In this latter instance, surrogate endpoints must: 1) be closely correlated with long-term outcomes; 2) be subject to a low degree of measurement error; and 3) be analyzable as a discontinuous variable (high or low risk) to simplify decision making regarding the treatment approaches. Currently, there are no robust surrogate endpoints or biomarkers that meet these essential parameters in the context of neoadjuvant endocrine therapy. Thus, large prospective trials must be conducted if we are to test a strategy of neoadjuvant endocrine therapy for the purposes of sensitivity testing in a definitive way. An alternative approach is to define new baseline biomarkers for endocrine responsiveness in the neoadjuvant setting (as they relate to response), and then test them in retrospective series of patients treated long term for adjuvant therapy with the same class of endocrine agent.

III. PATHOLOGICAL COMPLETE RESPONSE AS A SURROGATE ENDPOINT: STRENGTHS AND WEAKNESSES

Pathological complete response of primary breast cancer in response to neoadjuvant chemotherapy is a validated surrogate endpoint for long-term outcomes with a number of clear advantages. First, pathological assessments are already routinely applied. Second, measurement error, while present, is presumably at a relatively low level. Third, pCR is a binary outcome (pCR: yes or no?) so that simple statistics based on contingency tables and chi-square statistics are appropriate, and clinical algorithms can be developed. Finally, pCR is not based on a change from baseline measurement but is simply assessed on a post-treatment specimen. When surrogate analysis requires two data points (before and after therapy), difficulties with measurement error and establishing cut points (when is the change significant in terms of prognosis?) become a critical concern. Not taking into account the size of the original tumor does create some issues with pCR because pCR occurs more frequently with small tumors than large tumors. Therefore, the association of pCR with better long-term outcomes must be, in part, related to the prognostic associations with tumor size. The published estimates for the rate of pCR in response to neoadjuvant endocrine therapy are less than 5% (3). Although strategies to increase pCR in response to endocrine therapy must be explored (treating smaller tumors, extending the period of neoadjuvant therapy, or adding a second agent), other surrogates for drug effect and long-term outcomes need to be studied. Arguably, this is also the case with chemotherapy because patients who experience pCR still suffer systemic relapses, just with reduced frequency. Perhaps the problem of relapse, despite the occurrence of a pCR, is largely why we have yet to see the application of pCR as an interim endpoint in a clinical trial where treatment is randomized, to further chemotherapy versus not according to the presence of pCR after a standard chemotherapy regimen.

IV. ALTERNATIVES TO PCR FOR NEOADJUVANT ENDOCRINE STUDIES

The clinical findings from the randomized neoadjuvant trial comparing letrozole versus tamoxifen established that clinical response, radiological response, and rates of breast-conserving surgery are all valuable endpoints in comparing the relative efficacy of two endocrine approaches for the treatment of early stage breast cancer (Table 1). The letrozole 024 results mirror the conclusion from the >9000-patient ATAC trial that a third generation aromatase inhibitor (AI) would be more effective adjuvant endocrine therapy than tamoxifen (4). It is, therefore, of considerable interest that the letrozole 024 study predicted the outcome of the ATAC study with a much smaller sample size (328) and with only 4 months of follow up. These findings establish the concept that a positive result from a neoadjuvant study could, in the future, be viewed as essential preliminary data for the activation of any future adjuvant endocrine therapy study. In terms of tissue-based surrogate endpoints, Ki67 analysis has been conducted on paired specimens from the letrozole 024 study. This cell cycle regulated protein usually shows a dramatic fall with endocrine treatment of ER+ primary breast cancers and was, therefore, chosen as an additional surrogate with which to compare letrozole and tamoxifen. The statistical analysis of Ki67 changes presents

Table 1 Clinical Results Summary for "On-Study Biopsy" Confirmed ER+ and/or PR+ Cases from a Randomized Neoadjuvant Endocrine-Therapy Trial that Compared Tamoxifen and Letrozole

	Letrozole	Tamoxifen	p value[a]
Confirmed (ER+/PR+)	124 (100%)	126 (100%)	
Overall tumor response (CR + PR)			
Clinical	74 (60%)	52 (41%)	0.004
Ultrasound	48 (39%)	37 (29%)	0.119
Mammography	47 (37%)	25 (20%)	0.002
Breast-conserving surgery	60 (48%)	45 (36%)	0.036
Clinical disease progression	10 (8%)	15 (12%)	0.303

[a] Stratified Mantel-Haenszel chi-squared test.
Source: Ref. 6.

some challenges because the raw data are not normally distributed. The data are, therefore, presented using the median, range, and geometric mean before and after therapy. Nonparametric tests are then applied, in particular the Wilcoxon signed rank test, for assessing treatment induced changes within treatment groups. The Mann Whitney two-sample test is also applied to compare the overall degree of change for letrozole versus tamoxifen. However, a disadvantage of the Mann Whitney test is that it has less statistical power when compared to a parametric test (based on the mean and standard deviation of a normally distributed population). Also, there is no method to adjust the data for differences between the two groups in terms of baseline values. An alternative approach is to take the natural log of the Ki67 value to simulate a normal distribution and then apply analysis of covariance (ANCOVA) (5). ANCOVA is a type of regression analysis in which the slopes of the two lines generated by plotting the before- and after-treatment values on the two treatment arms are compared. Using these methodologies, it was established that the fall in Ki67 was more profound with letrozole than tamoxifen (Fig. 1). This result establishes Ki67 analysis as an additional useful surrogate endpoint for the assessment of endocrine agents in neoadjuvant trials. This conclusion was underscored by comparing the relative effects of tamoxifen and letrozole within subsets defined by HER-1 (epidermal growth factor receptor) and HER-2 (erbB2) as a combined category of HER-1- and/or HER-2+ versus both negative. In the assessment of the clinical data it had been established that within the group of patients with ER+ and HER-1/2+ disease, letrozole was dramatically more effective than tamoxifen (6). The Ki67 analysis correlated with this finding because the treatment-induced reduction in Ki67 was greater on the letrozole arm in both subsets (Fig. 1). These data suggest that Ki67 can also be used to assist in

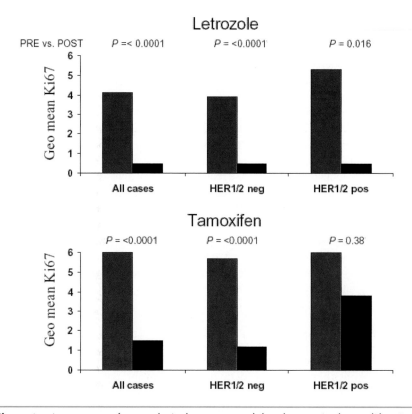

Figure 1 A summary of an analysis that compared the changes in the proliferation related biomarker Ki67 between letrozole and tamoxifen. The fall in Ki67 was greater with letrozole therapy regardless of HER-1 and HER-2 status.

the exploration of relationships between signal transduction pathways and therapeutic effects of different classes of endocrine agent.

V. GLOBAL GENE EXPRESSION PROFILING: A NEW SURROGATE FOR THE EFFICACY OF ENDOCRINE AGENTS IN THE NEOADJUVANT SETTING

Neoadjuvant endocrine therapy trials tend not to demonstrate close correlation between changes in Ki67 and clinical and radiological response (7). In fact, analysis of the letrozole 024 trial found no difference in the degree of change in Ki67 between tumors responding to letrozole and those tumors recorded to exhibit stable or progressive disease. This finding suggests that tumor regression is prevented by the inability of letrozole to trigger therapeutic events such as cell death or perhaps vascular collapse, rather than a failure to inhibit tumor proliferation. One approach to improve our understanding of the nature of tumor responsiveness to estrogen deprivation is to conduct global gene expression profiling on tumor biopsy samples taken before and after the initiation endocrine therapy. Limited information is available from a responding case of an ongoing study in which a baseline expression array was compared with analysis of a sample taken at 1 month after the initiation of letrozole therapy (8). Genes showing the greatest decrease include members of a proliferation cluster, topoisomerase (DNA) II alpha (170kD), ribonucleotide reductase M2 polypeptide, 5-methyltetrahydrofolate-homocysteine methyltransferase reductase and cell division cycle 2 G1 to S and G2 to M), an invasion cluster [matrix metalloproteinase 1 (interstitial collagenase), carboxypeptidase B1 (tissue), CD36 antigen (collagen type I receptor, thrombospondin receptor), and protein regulator of cytokinesis 1], and the apoptosis suppression cluster [baculoviral IAP repeat-containing 5 (survivin), and nucleolar protein 3 apoptosis repressor w/CARD domain]. When we have a sufficient number of cases it will be of great interest to compare these changes between responding and nonresponding cases.

VI.   CONCLUSIONS

There is increasing evidence that the neoadjuvant setting provides an effective means to obtain preliminary data on the adjuvant potential of endocrine approaches to treatment. The next trial to provide data to test this hypothesis is the IMPACT trial. This neoadjuvant study was designed to mimic the three

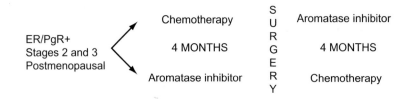

Followed by aromatase inhibitor for 5 years

Figure 2   A proposal for a clinical trial to explore the impact of neoadjuvant endocrine therapy on survival from ER+ breast cancer. This trial would have sufficient power to investigate the relationships between clinical and biomarker responses to endocrine therapy and long-term outcomes. $n =$ approx 1,000, based on the hypothesis that neoadjuvant endocrine therapy is associated with a survival advantage.

arms of the ATAC trial. Clearly, if neoadjuvant anastrozole proves to be more effective than tamoxifen in this trial, and the combination is no better than the tamoxifen-alone arm, this investigation will provide further strong evidence for the predictive value of neoadjuvant endocrine studies. The hypothesis raised by the marked advantage for letrozole in ER+ HER-1/2+ patients also deserves to be further investigated, both in adjuvant and neoadjuvant settings. In contrast to the general enthusiasm regarding neoadjuvant endocrine therapy as a biomarker discovery platform, or as a way to test new biological agents, there are no current studies that will investigate neoadjuvant endocrine therapy with the rigor applied to neoadjuvant chemotherapy. One approach that could be applied in the future is to randomize neoadjuvant treatment between an AI and chemotherapy followed by surgery. Those that received the AI would receive chemotherapy postoperatively. The study could be powered, analogous to NSABP B18, to demonstrate that neoadjuvant endocrine therapy improves overall survival (Fig. 2).

REFERENCES

1. Ellis MJ, Coop A, Singh B, Tao Y, Llombert-Cussac A, Janaeke F, Mauriac L, Evans DB, Quebe-Fehling E, Chaudri-Ross HA, Miller WR. Letrozole inhibits tumor proliferation more effectively than tamoxifen independent of HER1/2 expression status. Cancer Res 2003. In press.
2. Smith IE, Dowsett M. Aromatase inhibitors in breast cancer. N Engl J Med 2003; 348:2431–2442.
3. Eiermann W, Paepke S, Appfelstaedt J, Llombart-Cussac A, Eremin J, Vinholes J, Mauriac L, Ellis M, Lassus M, Chaudri-Ross HA, Dugan M, Borgs M. Preoperative treatment of postmenopausal breast cancer patients with letrozole: a randomized double-blind multicenter study. Ann Oncol 2001; 12:1527–1532.
4. Anastrozole alone or in combination with tamoxifen versus tamoxifen alone for adjuvant treatment of postmenopausal women with early breast cancer. First results of the ATAC randomised trial. Lancet 2002; 359:2131–2139.
5. Vickers AJ, Altman DG. Statistics notes: Analysing controlled trials with baseline and follow up measurements. Br Med J 2001; 323:1123–1124.
6. Ellis MJ, Coop A, Singh B, Mauriac L, Llombert-Cussac A, Janicke F, Miller WR, Evans DB, Dugan M, Brady C, Quebe-Fehling E, Borgs M. Letrozole is more effective neoadjuvant endocrine therapy than tamoxifen for ErbB-1- and/or ErbB-2-positive, estrogen receptor-positive primary breast cancer: evidence from a phase III randomized trial. J Clin Oncol 2001; 19:3808–3816.
7. Miller WR, Dixon JM, Macfarlane L, Cameron D, Anderson TJ. Pathological features of breast cancer response following neoadjuvant treatment with either letrozole or tamoxifen. Eur J Cancer 2003; 39:462–468.
8. Ellis MJ, Rosen E, Dressman H, Marks J. Neoadjuvant comparisons of aromatase inhibitors and tamoxifen: pretreatment determinants of response and on-treatment effect. J Steroid Biochem Mol Biol 2003. In press.

19

Aromatase Localization in Human Breast Cancer with Development of New Antibodies

Hironobu Sasano,[1] D. P. Edwards,[2] T. J. Anderson,[3] S. G. Silverberg,[4]
Dean B. Evans,[5] Richard J. Santen,[6] Paul Ramage,[5] Y. Miki,[1] T. Suzuki,[1]
E. R. Simpson,[7] Ajay S. Bhatnagar,[8] and William R. Miller[9]

[1]Tohoku University School of Medicine, Sendai, Japan

[2]University of Colorado Health Sciences Center,
Denver, Colorado, U.S.A.

[3]Edinburgh University, Edinburgh, Scotland

[4]University of Maryland School of Medicine, Baltimore, Maryland, U.S.A.

[5]Novartis Pharma AG, Basel, Switzerland

[6]University of Virginia Health System, Charlottesville, Virgina, U.S.A.

[7]Prince Henry's Institute of Medical Research, Monash Medical Centre,
Clayton, Victoria, Australia

[8]WWS Group Ltd, Muttenz, Switzerland

[9]University of Edinburgh and Western General Hospital,
Edinburgh, Scotland

I. OVERVIEW

Intratumoral aromatase is a potential therapeutic target for the treatment of post-menopausal estrogen-dependent breast cancers. Therefore, reliable methods should be developed for routine application for the detection of intratumoral aromatase. In addition, there have been controversies about the intratumoral localization of aromatase in human breast carcinoma. Therefore, obtaining the precise intratumoral localization of aromatase in order to assess its biological significance is important. We have undertaken the following two approaches toward

277

this goal. The first approach is to separate stromal adipocytes and carcinoma or parenchymal cells, under light microscopy using laser capture microscopy (LCM). Then, mRNA was extracted from these separated fractions, and the expression of aromatase was evaluated with RT-PCR. The analysis of LCM revealed that aromatase mRNA was present in the fractions of stromal cells and adipocytes in all 15 cases examined, but aromatase mRNA was present only in 12/15 in those of carcinoma cells. These results indicated that intratumoral aromatase is present in both interstitial, or stromal, and parenchymal cells in human breast carcinoma, but intratumoral aromatase in interstitial cell types may be more predominant. The other approach is the generation of monoclonal antibodies against aromatase from a recombinant GST-aromatase fusion protein and validation of them in surgical pathology specimens of human breast carcinoma following immunohistochemical evaluation in full-term human placenta and normal cycling human ovaries. A multicenter collaborative group has been established for this purpose. Biochemical assays resulted in the selection of 23 monoclonal antibodies. These antibodies were further evaluated by immunohistochemistry (IHC) of paraffin-embedded tissue sections including normal ovary, and placenta, and a small series of ten breast carcinomas. Of the 23 mAbs, two (clone 677 and F2) were determined to specifically stain cell types known to express aromatase in normal tissues. In breast carcinomas, staining of malignant epithelium, adipose tissue, and normal/benign and stromal compartments was detected. Then, IHC was performed and independently evaluated by three pathologists (H.S., T.A., and S.G.S.), each using the same evaluation criteria for staining intensity and proportion of immunopositive cells. With these two mAbs, interpathologist and intralaboratory variations were small in comparison with differences that could be detected between tissue specimens and antibodies.

II. INTRODUCTION

Estrogens are considered to play important roles in the development and progression of hormone-dependent human breast cancer. The overexpression of aromatase appears to play an important role in estrogen-related development and progression of some human breast cancers (1–4). Aromatase-inhibitor (AI) therapy is one of the endocrine treatments available to breast cancer patients. Therefore, predicting which patients will respond prior to initiation of therapy has become important. Some studies have demonstrated a positive correlation between intratumoral aromatase activity and response to treatment with various AIs (3, 4). Immunohistochemical analysis of intratumoral aromatase can provide information about an overall activity or expression of aromatase in human breast carcinoma. For this purpose, a precise, sensitive, and quantifiable immunohistochemical method for detecting aromatase in archival materials or formalin-fixed and paraffin-embedded tissue has been explored. However, no anti-aromatase antibodies have been specifically designed for this purpose.

Existing antibodies directed against aromatase are available. However, they are in dwindling supply and the results from studies using them have been controversial in terms of tumor aromatase localization (5–9). Several studies reported the predominance of aromatase localization in stromal or interstitial cells including adipocytes in human breast carcinoma specimens (5–7), whereas other studies reported its predominance in parenchymal or carcinoma cells (8, 9). Precise localization of aromatase and identification of cell types expressing aromatase in human breast carcinoma tissue would be helpful in elucidating the biological significance of intratumoral aromatase. Therefore, an international collaborative study group was formulated in order to develop antibodies that can be used to assess aromatase expression in fixed breast cancer tissue and test whether these measurements are predictive of responsiveness to AIs. In addition, the development of laser capture microdissection (LCM) with RT-PCR has made it possible to evaluate gene expression in particular types of cells in the tissues. Results of LCM may be less influenced by the modes of tissue preparation even compared to mRNA in situ hybridization, another method of evaluating mRNA localization in tissue specimens. Therefore, in this study, we isolated fractions of stromal or interstitial cells, parenchymal or carcinoma cells, and adipocytes under light microscopy and evaluated aromatase mRNA expression separately in these cell fractions in order to obtain the precise distribution of intratumoral aromatase.

III. GENERATION OF AROMATASE MONOCLONAL ANTIBODIES

The strategy for screening hybridomas was to assay the initial fusion wells by enzyme-linked immunosorbent assay (ELISA) against purified GST-aromatase used as antigen and with free glutathione-S-transferase GST. Only positives for GST-aromatase and negatives for the GST moiety of the antigen were selected. ELISA positives were further screened by Western blot against purified GST-aromatase, GST-aromatase in crude extracts of Sf9 cells and free GST. Hybridoma products that gave a specific reaction for GST-aromatase by Western blot with little or no cross-reaction with other proteins in crude cell extracts were submitted to screening by IHC of normal ovary and placenta. The criteria for specific IHC detection of aromatase in placenta were staining exclusively in the plasma membrane of syncytiotrophoblasts of chorionic villi and in the ovary by staining in granulosa cells of ovarian follicles. Hybridomas that passed this screening criteria were subcloned, isotyped, and the mAb products were purified and used for subsequent characterizations.

From the cell fusions of mice injected with unfixed antigen, 60 hybridomas were positive by ELISA, 11 of these reacted specifically by Western blot with aromatase, and 4 of the Western blot positives gave specific staining of placenta and ovary by IHC (clones 636, 677, 1157, and 1255). From the cell fusions with

Table 1 Summary of Monoclonal Antibodies Selected

Clone	Mouse Isotype	Antigen
677/H7	IgG2a	Unfixed GST-aromatase
1255/H6	IgG1	Unfixed GST-aromatase
Grp10/F2	IgG1	Fixed GST-aromatase
Grp15/F11	IgG1	Fixed GST-aromatase

fixed antigen there were 105 ELISA positives, 22 of these were positive by Western blot criteria and 5 of the Western blot positives gave specific staining of placenta and ovary by IHC. Purified mAbs were used for further characterization of all nine of the hybridomas selected from the two cell fusions by the above screening strategy. By IHC of ten cases of human invasive ductal breast carcinoma, four of the nine mAbs were determined to be optimal in terms of specific cytoplasmic staining of epithelial cancer cells and minimal background staining, i.e., no staining in nucleus or acellular areas. The four mAbs selected by this screening strategy are listed in Table 1, along with antibody subtypes for each.

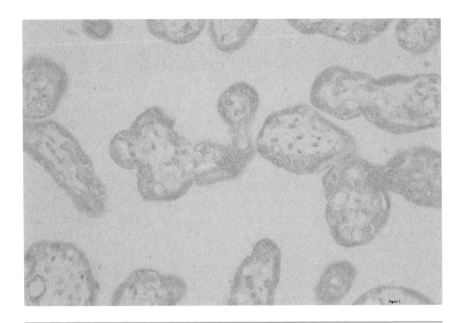

Figure 1 Immunohistochemistry of aromatase in full term human placenta using monoclonal antibody #677. Aromatase immunoreactivity was detected in syncytiotrophoblasts of chorionic villi.

Western blot screening results demonstrated that each mAb reacted with the 82–85kDa GST-aromatase fusion protein, but failed to react with free GST, indicating they detect an epitope in the aromatase portion of the antigen. Examples of IHC staining of term human placenta and normal cycling human ovary with one of the selected mAbs, 677, are shown in Figures 1 and 2, respectively. Immunostaining was detected in syncytiotrophoblasts of chorionic villi of placenta (Fig. 1) and predominantly in granulosa cells of ovarian follicles (Fig. 2); both are known cellular sites of aromatase expression.

IV. INDEPENDENT SCORING AND EVALUATION OF BREAST CARCINOMAS

In evaluating results of immunohistochemistry in clinical specimens, inter- and/or intrainstitutional or inter- and/or intraobserver differences can become a very serious problem in interpretation of the findings, eventually resulting in clinical management of the patients. Therefore, in our present project, three co-authors (HS, TJA, and SGS) independently performed and evaluated IHC of the same ten cases of breast carcinomas with the four selected mAbs from Table 1. In addition,

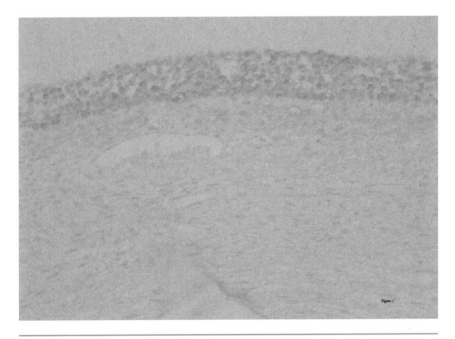

Figure 2   Immunohistochemistry of aromatase in normal cycling human ovaries using monoclonal antibody #677. Aromatase immunoreactivity was predominantly detected in membrana granulosa.

aromatase is a cytoplasmic antigen, which makes it somewhat more difficult to obtain precise assessment of immunoreactivity in clinical specimens compared to nuclear antigens, such as estrogen receptor (ER). Therefore, in our project, immunostaining was evaluated based on the following criteria: 1) the proportion of the area of the tissue sections occupied by the cells; 2) the proportion of positively stained cells; and 3) the overall staining intensity of a tissue section. These criteria were developed through simultaneous evaluation using multiheaded light microscopy. All three co-authors agreed that immunohistochemistry using mAbs 677 or F2 yielded the most satisfactory results in terms of minimal background staining, specificity, reproducibility, and interpretation of the results based on these staining criteria. With these two mAbs, immunoreactivity was detected in different compartments of breast carcinomas including parenchymal or carcinoma cells, stromal cells or fibroblasts, adipocytes, macrophages, and normal duct epithelial cells (Fig. 3). The proportion of positively stained cells varied among the ten cases. This relatively wide distribution of intratumoral aromatase indicates that the evaluation of proportion of aromatase-positive cells and amounts of aromatase in each cell types of human breast carcinoma tissues is indispensable in

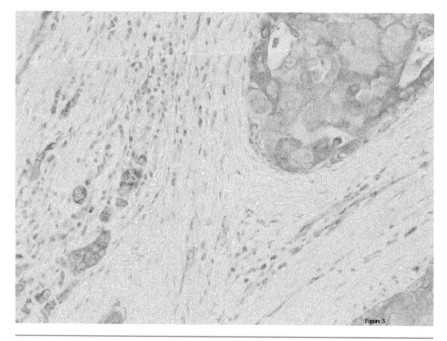

Figure 3 Immunohistochemistry of aromatase in human breast invasive ductal carcinoma. Aromatase immunoreactivity was detected in both carcinoma (parenchymal) cells and stromal cells.

Table 2 Summary of Scoring of Aromatase Immunoreactivity in Human Breast Invasive Ductal Carcinoma

1. Obtain the approximate percentage of the parenchymal or carcinoma cells in the foci of carcinoma as follows. Both cellularity and areas of carcinoma should be considered at the time of evaluation.
   0: 0%, 1: 1–25%, 2: 26–50%, 3: 51–75%, 4: 76–100%
2. Obtain the approximate percentage of aromatase-positive carcinoma as follows:
   0: 0%, 1: 1–25%, 2: 26–50%, 3: 51–75%, 4: 76–100%
3. Choose the most representative areas of aromatase positivity in carcinoma cells and grade relative immunointensity as follows:
   0: no immunoreactivity, 1: weak, 2: moderate, 3: intense
4. Evaluate relative immunointensity and proportion of stromal cells, macrophages, and other inflammatory cells and adipocytes in and /or adjacent to carcinomatous foci as follows:

   Proportion adipocytes
   0: 0%, 1: 1–25%, 2: 26–50%, 3: 51–75%, 4: 76–100%
   Normal ducts and stromal cells
   0: 0%, 1: 1–25%, 3: 26–50%, 4: more than 50%
   Intensity
   0: no immunoreactivity, 1: weak, 2: moderate, 3: intense
5. Describe the presence or absence of focal immunoractivity in the tissue sections

studying overall aromatase activity and expression in whole carcinoma tissues, especially in relation to the possible response to AIs. When correlating results of immunohistochemistry with other parameters, such as clinical outcome or response to medication, it is generally important to report the results to clinicians at least in a semiquantitative manner. Therefore, in this project, an H-score or semiquantitative scoring system for mAbs 677 and F2 was established based on staining of these ten cases of breast carcinomas (Table 2) that can be applied to future clinical correlation studies between biochemical and immunohistochemical results.

V. MICRODISSECTION/PCR

Fifteen cases of invasive ductal carcinoma of the breast were evaluated in this study. All these specimens were obtained in Tohoku University Hospital with an informed consent of the patients following an approval of Ethics Committee of Tohoku University School of Medicine, Sendai, Japan. These specimens were rapidly embedded in Optimal Cutting Temperature medium (SAKURA Co., Ltd., Tokyo, Japan) and frozen-sectioned at a thickness of 8 μm. The specimen was subsequently mounted on membrane attached glass slides (Cell Robotics,

Inc., Albuquerque, New Mexico, U.S.A.). All tissue sections were stored at $-30°C$ until analysis of LCM. These 15 sections were fixed in 100% methanol for 5 minutes and then stained with toluidine blue. Then LCM was performed using a CRI-337 (Cell Robotics) with 30–60 μm laser spot size applying default to full-strength pulse power (40–100 W) and extreme strength of the pulse width (50–00 ms). Approximately 100 cells were laser-transferred from the stroma, cancer parenchyma, and adipocytes in these 15 cases of human breast carcinoma. Total RNA was extracted from laser-transferred cells according to the RNA microisolation protocol (10, 11). Briefly, following precipitation and a 70% ethanol wash, the pellets were resuspended in 9 μl of RNase-free H_2O. Total RNA from the microdissected tissue was reverse transcribed in a reaction mixture containing 50 mM Tris acetate, pH 8.4, 75 mM potassium acetate, 8 mM magnesium acetate, 0.01 M dithiothreitol, 2 mM dNTP, 25 μM Oligo (dT)$_{12-18}$ Primer, 25 μg/μl random hexamer oligonucleotides, and SUPERSCRIPT II RNase H− Reverse Transcriptase (Life Technologies, Inc.) for 60 min at 50°C. The resulting cDNA was amplified in 25 μl of a PCR mix consisting of GeneAmp, 1xPCR Gold Buffer (PerkinElmer Life Sciences), 1.5 mM $MgCl_2$, 200 μM dNTP, and 0.125 unit of AmpliTaq Gold (PerkinElmer Life Sciences) under the following conditions: initial denaturing at 95°C for 10 min followed by 40 cycles of 1 min at 94°C, 1 min at 55°C, and 1 min at 72°C, after which PCR products were subjected to a final extension step for 7 min at 72°C. Primers used for PCR amplification were: Forward_5'-GTG AAA AAG GGG ACA AAC ATT-3', Reverse_5'-TGG AAT CGT CTC AGA AGT GT-3', Size: 215bp (1286–1500).

Following PCR for aromatase, amplified products were detected as a specific single band in stromal or interstitial cells and adipocytes adjacent to carcinoma invasion isolated by LCM, as well as in whole breast carcinoma tissues (data not shown) in all 15 cases examined (Fig. 4). Relatively low levels of aromatase mRNA were also detected in 12/15 cases of human breast carcinoma.

These findings, as well as those in internal mammary chain (IMC), demonstrated that aromatase expression was relatively widely distributed in many compartments of human breast carcinoma tissues. However, aromatase in stromal cells and/or adipocytes may be more predominant than parenchymal or carcinoma cells because of the more frequent presence of aromatase mRNA in stromal and/or adipocytes than that in carcinoma cells, and the relative abundance of aromatase mRNA in stromal and/or adipocytes components in the RT-PCR analysis of the same cycle. However, further investigation, including the more precise quantification of aromatase mRNA among these different components of breast cancer tissue, are required for clarification.

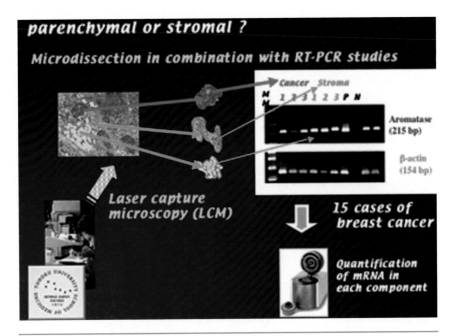

Figure 4 An example of LCM/RT-PCR: Carcinoma, stromal, or interstitial cells and adipocytes were separated by LCM as shown in this figure. RT-PCR demonstrated the presence of aromatase mRNA in all compartments of the tissue. MM represents molecular weight; P, positive control; N, negative control.

VI. SUMMARY

Monoclonal antibodies have been generated against aromatase for IMC detection of intratumoral aromatase in human breast cancer as an international collaborative study. Immunoreactivity of aromatase was widely distributed in different components of the cells types in breast cancer tissues such as cancer parenchyma, interstitial stroma, and adipocytes.

Analysis of aromatase RNA from human breast carcinoma by LCM/RT-PCR also confirmed this finding. These results indicated that an assessment of aromatase among different compartments of carcinoma tissues using a scoring system will be needed to evaluate overall aromatase expression in surgical specimens of resected breast carcinoma.

REFERENCES

1. Miller WR, Forrest APM. Oestradiol synthesis from C19 steroids by human breast cancer. Br J Cancer 1974; 33:905–911.

2. Miller WR, Hawkins RA, Forrest APM. Significance of aromatase activity in human breast cancer. Cancer Res 1982; 42:3365–3368.

3. Miller WR, O'Neil J. The importance of local synthesis of estrogen with the breast. Steroids 1987; 50:537–548.

4. Bezwoda WR, Mansoor N, Dansey R. Correlation of breast tumor aromatase activity and response to aromatase inhibition with aminoglutethimide. Oncology 1987; 44:345–349.

5. Sasano H, Nagura H, Harada N, Goukon Y, Kimura M. Immunolocalization of aromatase and other steroidogenic enzymes in human breast disorders. Hum Pathol 1994; 25:530–535.

6. Sasano H, Harada N. Intratumoral aromatase in human breast, endometrial, and ovarian malignancies. Endocr Rev 1998; 19:593–607.

7. Shenton KC, Dowsett M, Lu Q, Brodie A, Sasano H, Sacks NP, Rowlands MG. Comparison of biochemical aromatase activity with aromatase immunohistochemistry in human breast carcinomas. Breast Cancer Res Treat 1998; 49(suppl 1):S101–107; discussion S109–119.

8. Esteban JM, Warsi Z, Haniu M, Chen S. Detection of intratumoral aromatase in breast carcinomas. An immunohistochemical study with clinicopathologic correlation. Am J Pathol 1992; 940:337–343.

9. Lu Q, Nakamura J, Savinov A, Yue W, Weisz J, Dabbs DJ, Wolz G, Brodie A. Expression of aromatase protein and messenger ribonucleic acid in tumor epithelial cells and evidence of functional significance of locally produced estrogen in human breast cancers. Endocrinology 1996; 137:3061–3068.

10. Niino Y, Irie T, Takaishi M, Hosono T, Nam-ho Huh, Tachikawa T, Kuroki T. PKC_II, a new isoform of protein kinase C specifically expressed in the seminiferous tubules of mouse testis. J Biol Chem 2001; 276:36711–36717.

11. Emmert-Buck MR, Bonner RF, Smith PD, Chuaqui RF, Zhuang Z, Goldstein SR, Weiss RA, Liotta LA. Laser Capture Microdissection. Science 1996; 274:998–1001.

4

Biology and New Therapeutics

I. Craig Henderson and Manfred Kaufmann, *Chairmen*
Tuesday, July 8, 2003

I. C. Henderson: We don't really have much time left for general discussion, although we can take 5 or 10 minutes to ask some questions. I would like to start off based on several comments that Adrian [Harris] made during his presentation. This is relevant to Dr. Sasano's presentation as well. Do we really know where the target is for aromatase inhibitors? I don't think there is any question that we know what the target is. But is it really the aromatase in the breast cancer cell or in the tissue right around the breast cancer cells that is the critical aromatase? Or is it spread out throughout the body? Is total level of aromatase in the body critical?

W. Miller: Maybe I can have a go at that one. I would agree with Adrian [Harris]. I think it's very important that we have the tools to be able to identify routinely where the enzyme is. Where I might slightly disagree with Adrian is that there is literature which is quite definitive. We know in postmenopausal women that the enzyme is distributed in peripheral tissues. We can largely define those peripheral tissues. It's very difficult to find a peripheral tissue in which we don't have activity. Indeed, that's been a problem with finding the appropriate negative controls to do immunohistochemistry.

I think we can also say a little bit about the relative contribution of peripheral aromatase and local biosynthesis within breast cancer. There are two groups of studies; we performed one of these and the other was performed by Mike Reed in London. What you can do is to give patients tritiated androgen and C^{14} labeled estrogen. Then you actually extract the breast tumors and if you've got tritiated estrogen, you can make an assumption that the estrogen has come from local conversion.

At the same time, if you have got C^{14} labeled estrogen, you can calculate the relative uptake estrogen into the tumor. If you do that, what you learn is that each tumor is slightly different. There are some tumors in which it would appear that there is no local activity within the tumor. All of the estrogen can be accounted for by uptake. There are others in which it seems to be largely local biosynthesis and in most of the tumors it's a combination of both.

Both Mike [Reed] and our group have also looked at the relative contribution versus the endogenous levels and radioactive levels of estrogen within the tumor. What you can show is that if tumors not only take up estrogen but also locally synthesize it, then, in general, there tend to be higher levels of estrogen within the tumor. In certain cases, however, the levels of estrogen clearly don't totally relate to local biosynthesis and one would suspect that despite there being aromatase activity within certain tumors, peripheral synthesis and the uptake is actually more influential.

I think it's a heterogeneous situation that is typical of breast cancer across the board.

A. Harris: Your elegant work was done in maybe 10 or 20 patients. We'd like to know in some of these studies, whether 20% of the patients are high local producers because it might define your strategy and how you use the drugs.

W. Miller: I totally agree with you, Adrian. But I think the problem is that to measure tumor aromatase alone is not going to give you the answer. It's very clear that in many patients the peripheral synthesis is more inferential. Therefore, just to measure tumor aromatase will not give you the answer.

R. Santen: I think we have to mention the other pathway also. What we're really interested in is how much estrogen is present in cells in the breast. The aromatase pathway is clearly one way to produce estrogen in the breast. The other pathway is the sulfatase pathway in which estrone-sulfate is converted to free estrone. The levels of estrone sulfate in the blood are some 50- to 100-fold higher than free estrone or estradiol. The breast has a million times more sulfatase than aromatase, but its affinity for substrate is much lower than for aromatase. But clearly it's possible that some of the molecules of estradiol in the breast can be produced as a result of the sulfatase pathway.

On the other hand, you can only get estrone and its sulfate if you have aromatase. But if we really own up to what we know at this point, we're really not sure how important the sulfatase pathway is versus the aromatase pathway. We have to determine, in each individual patient, how important the contribution of local synthesis is versus the peripheral synthesis.

C. Benz: I wonder if we took an informal poll in here and, assuming that our aromatase assays were good, whether they be immunohistochemical or enzymatic, would anybody believe that tumor aromatase activity or level would be predictive of tumor responsiveness to aromatase inhibitors? From what Bill [Miller] said earlier, we might bet that, even with good reagents, a tumor aromatase assay would not be predictive.

M. Ellis: I just wanted to follow up on Dick's [Santen] comment on estrone sulfate. Mitch, I was struck looking at your data that post-aromatase inhibitor, the only estrogen you can measure with any certainty is estrone sulfate.

M. Dowsett: The measurements that we show were actually done in collaboration with Per [Lonning]. He made the estrone sulfate measurements. The starting level was 420 pmol/L. The on-treatment level with letrozole was 9 pmol/L. We had something to the extent of 98% suppression, I think, reflecting that the aromatase inhibition is complete. What Dick [Santen] did there essentially says that you only get estrone sulfate as a result of the initial aromatization.

M. Ellis: You could measure residual estrone sulfate more readily than estradiol.

M. Dowsett: True.

M. Ellis: The question being, is there enough sulfatase present in some of these tumors for that to be a mechanism for sufficient estrogen exposure to stimulate the tumor? I think we've looked at estrone sulfatase closely enough to know that.

R. Santen: There have been some extensive studies on that. Clearly homogenized tumors can convert estrone sulfate to estrone. The estimates that have been made generally suggest there is more estrogen made via sulfatase than there is via aromatase. All of those estimates are enzyme kinetics, in vitro studies, and homogenizations. Where I stand now is that we really don't know how important sulfatase is versus aromatase.

Mike Reed is really the person who has collected the most extensive data, but yes, there is enough sulfatase enzyme. It has high enough affinity. It can convert estrone-sulfate to estrone both in vivo and in vitro. In animal models, estrone sulfate will clearly stimulate breast tumors after being converted to estrone and estradiol. There is an extensive body of literature that has looked at this.

P. Lonning: But just another comment on that. You are absolutely right about the estrone sulfate in the plasma. But when you go to the tissue, the level of estrogen sulfate is lower than the level of estradiol. You can only detect something like 70% suppression. That complicates the issue if you like to look into the estrone sulfate levels in the tissue. Of course that might be because the estrone sulfate is rapidly metabolized to estradiol. But we don't know.

H. Sasano: I would like to comment about the possible value of intratumoral aromatase. I think it is true that there is no correlation between estrogen-receptor-alpha expression and intratumoral aromatase. So, if you only look at intratumoral aromatase without looking at estrogen-receptor-alpha status, this probably cannot be a predictive factor. If you have both estrogen-receptor-alpha positive and abundant intratumoral aromatase, this could be a predictive factor. Of course, you have to think of estrogen sulfatase and sulfo transferase and 17beta-hydroxy-steroid dehydrogenase. But I think the basic idea of looking at the intratumoral aromatase in combination with estrogen-receptor-alpha is the best method available at this juncture. So, only intratumoral aromatase by itself cannot predict it unless one studies it along with estrogen-receptor-alpha expression in the tumor cells.

C. Benz: When we talk about estrone sulfate levels, we should also be considering circulating DHEA sulfate levels which are even higher and are converted to DHEA by the same sulfatase that acts on estrone sulfate. In addition to being converted to the aromatase substrate androstenedione, DHEA can also get converted to ADIOL by 17beta-HSD, and while ADIOL is structurally an androgen, it can bind with high affinity to the estrogen receptor and thus represents a potentially important estrogenic stimulus produced independent of the aromatase pathway.

M. Dowsett: I had a couple of points to make to Chris Benz, which are connected. I think it might get back to the growth factor receptor aspect of this particular session. You showed the inverse relationship, Chris, between estrogen receptor and HER-2 in these age relationships. First, does age actually disrupt the relationship between estrogen receptor and HER-2, or does the estrogen receptor/HER-2 inverse relationship persist with age? estrogen receptor goes up with age, HER-2 goes down with age, but does the inverse relationship between estrogen receptor and HER-2 persist if you look at that?

C. Benz: Within age groups, yes, it does.

M. Dowsett: We recently looked at about 2,000 tumors from an ongoing clinical trial in this country called TACT, and looked at the various different correlates with HER-2 expression. Age was one, along with estrogen receptor, nodal status, size, and grade. Actually, age was a univariate predictor of HER-2. But when you added the others in, it dropped completely out.

C. Benz: The complication here is that by dichotomizing between estrogen-receptor-plus and estrogen-receptor-negative tumors, we oversimplify. We have molecular mechanisms by which both the estrogen receptor can down-regulate the erbB system and vice versa. I don't think we fully understand these mechanisms, but I really think they are quite important and somehow impact upon endocrine sensitivity.

M. Dowsett: I needed to take that one step further. The fact that we get very few high estrogen-receptor-positive, high HER-2+, they almost don't exist, yet the cells which you derived from the MCF7 cells had a 45-fold amplification of the gene, the MCF7/HER2-18, yes? So what is your take-home message on the relevance to that cell line, to de novo resistance? It looks like that's in the one percentile.

C. Benz: I think it is an unusual situation relative to being a clinical model. I think we have to take that as a caveat. Likewise, many of us work with the MCF7 cell line as if it's supposed to represent all estrogen-receptor-positive breast cancers. I think that's a bit hazardous as well.

One thing that I did overlook when we were first characterizing that cell line was the phenomenon that Rakesh Kumar picked up on with his identification of the variant corepressor, MTA1s (metastatic-associated protein 1, splice variant). He showed that much of the estrogen receptor in the MCF/HER-2-18 subline is largely in the cytosol and actually co-localizing with the MTA1s protein. In fact, as I recall our early studies, when I did quantitative assays of the estrogen receptor in that cell line, they were very comparable to the original cell lines, somewhat reduced but still very highly overexpressed. When we did immunohistochemical assays, my interpretation was clouded by the fact that I saw cytoplasmic estrogen receptor and discounted it because that was ten years ago and we don't score cytoplasmic estrogen receptor. I think this observation needs to be revisited.

P. Lonning: I'm just jumping to another issue because I think you said something very important, Adrian, about the targeting. If you look away from the aromatase and take some of the other examples you mentioned like, for example, the cyclins, that's very important. If we think about two tumors, one could have a normal cyclin CDK4. The other one is amplified, really amplified for cyclin D. If you give a CDK4 inhibitor to these two tumors, in one case you're more or less trying to inhibit a normal physiological process of the cell cycle. In the other case, you are trying to correct perhaps some of the driving pathology in the cells. It may be that it could work in both cases, but [it] is quite likely that the response could be very different. I think it's extremely important when we put these drugs into trials to really explore the biology of each tumor to know the background in which setting we're using the drugs.

C. K. Osborne: Getting at the issue of the lower estrogen receptor and the HER-2, even in your data when you looked at Chris' [Benz] data, and you looked at the error bars, there were quite a few high estrogen receptors in the HER-2+ group. Yes, the MCF7 may be a little bit unusual, but let me talk about a couple of things that I think would suggest that low estrogen receptor is not the only explanation for resistance in the HER-2+ group.

First of all, as we've published, with Craig Allred, the biggest difference between response, as defined by disease-free survival, is no estrogen receptor versus very low estrogen receptor. That's the biggest separation. So, very low estrogen receptor responds quite well to tamoxifen. Then you get a little bit better response as you get more estrogen receptor. The biggest difference is between less than 1% and greater than 1% up to 10%. That's the biggest difference in tamoxifen benefit. So having a little less estrogen receptor in an HER-2 positive tumor should not make a major difference.

Low estrogen receptor responds very well. Secondly, in our study of HER-2 overexpression and AIB1 overexpression, yes, the estrogen receptor was a little bit less than the HER-2+ group, but in a multivariate analysis it didn't come out at all being significant.

Finally, another study that Chris Benz has on one of his slides that we published, Richard Elledge was the first author, showed that HER-2 wasn't a very significant factor in predicting response to tamoxifen in metastatic disease. You showed a certain borderline significance. We've reanalyzed that data doing FISH and including EGFR, a receptor we often don't look at in these settings. Now using FISH, HER-2 is significant and it's significant regardless of quantitative estrogen receptor again, but when you include it in a model, with EGFR, then EGFR overwhelms everything. It's dramatic. The hazard ratio for high EGFR was approximately 4.1. It overwhelmed quantitative estrogen receptor, HER-2, or any other parameter. It may be that EGFR, although not commonly overexpressed in breast cancer, may turn out to be a key player that we should routinely measure.

C. Benz: Was that independent, Kent?

C. K. Osborne: Independent. I don't think that low estrogen receptor per se explains all or maybe even very much of the resistance. But, in the analysis, EGFR was independent of estrogen receptor and HER-2 in predicting less responsiveness to tamoxifen.

M. Ellis: In the result of the randomized trial of letrozole versus tamoxifen, when we're looking at estrogen receptor, HER-1, and HER-2, we specifically excluded any case that had estrogen receptor level lower than 10%. So, we're looking at cases with estrogen receptor levels in the conventionally positive range. In that situation, the HER-1 and- 2 expressers did not have lower average levels of estrogen receptor compared to the non expressers. But we excluded those marginal cases because the eligibility criteria for the trial required 10% or more. Those were considered to be, in a biomarker sense, ineligible cases.

C. Benz: Matt, in that same analysis, wasn't it true that letrozole seemed to be more effective in the low Allred scoring estrogen receptor positive cases than tamoxifen?

M. Ellis: Right. There are relatively few of those and almost all were HER-2 − and HER-1 − as it turned out.

I.C. Henderson: Let's stop the session here and go on. We'll turn it over to Adrian [Harris] and Kent [Osborne] for wrap up and additional discussion.

Final Discussion and Wrap-up

Adrian L Harris and C. Kent Osborne, *Chairmen*

Tuesday, July 8, 2003

C. K. Osborne: Maybe I can start and paint a broad picture from an historic view—thinking about where we were when I was an intern, 31 years ago, to where we are today, then look back at the progress, and, finally, look toward where we need to go. When I was an intern, we were just starting to use chemotherapy single agents and hormone therapy was king at that time. The hormone therapies were hypophysectomy, adrenalectomy, and high-dose estrogens and other steroid hormones.

The big argument I remember at that time was transfrontal hypophysectomy versus transnasal hypophysectomy. When you consider the side effects—there was a 17% incidence of cerebrospinal fluid leak after hypophysectomy. This was difficult therapy. You can imagine the other side effects that people had in those days with bilateral adrenalectomy and hypophysectomy.

Obviously we've come a long way. I think one of the problems is that endocrine therapy, at least in the United States, lost its "king" status for awhile. I think it was lost because the effectiveness of combination chemotherapy became apparent in the 1970s and it wasn't until the late 1970s that we had endocrine therapies that were less toxic, the first one being tamoxifen. In addition, there was a lot of enthusiasm with the curability of Hodgkin's disease and lymphomas to move toward chemotherapy in other types of cancer.

I'm not sure I ever left the idea that endocrine therapy was king, but certainly a lot of people in the United States and, I suspect, in other countries did. Today, there's no question that endocrine therapy is dominant for the right tumor, and I hope that we all agree that endocrine-receptor-negative

(ER–) tumors do not benefit from any endocrine therapy and that patients with such tumors should not be included in any future study of endocrine therapy. That goes for endocrine receptor (ER) unknown as well.

I hope that is settled. Too many of the studies that we've had are simply confounded and complicated by the inclusion of people who don't respond and can't respond to the therapy. There should be no ER-unknown patients in studies anymore. Excluding ER– and unknown patients will help a great deal in understanding the effectiveness of these newer therapies.

M. Dowsett: I don't want to forget this small group of ER−/PR+. We always see them as being in effect ER+. The people that aren't aware of that message may well just rely on the estrogen-receptor-negative status. Essentially nowadays in the elderly group, or perhaps overall, we see 80% of our patients ER+, leaving only 20% ER−. A considerable proportion of those are PGR+ perhaps—15% of that residual 20%—and we don't want to lose those from our treatment.

C. K. Osborne: It's true. But they are so infrequent that [it's] hard to be really sure how well they respond. We just published an article in the *JCO*: 14,000 women from our tumor bank, looking at the value of progesterone receptor (PR), in addition to ER in predicting response to tamoxifen adjuvant therapy. All the assays were done in two experienced labs. We clearly showed that ER+/PR+ patients, in contrast to what the meta-analysis shows, benefit more from tamoxifen than ER+/PR− patients. But even in that large data set, there were so few ER−/PR+, at least defined by our criteria, that we couldn't show conclusively that they actually did benefit from tamoxifen adjuvant therapy.

It's an uncommon group. I don't know what the right answer is. In metastatic disease we showed a long time ago that they do seem to benefit. I'm just not certain in the adjuvant setting.

M. Dowsett: In our study, we collected the NATO and CRC samples together. We ended up with 813 samples. These were old samples. Clearly, I can't tell you for sure that they have no fixation artifacts. What I can tell you is that all the relationships which we would expect—inverse relationships between ER and HER-2, relationships between ER and PR, the epidermal growth factor receptor (EGFR) relationships—they were all present and as significant as we'd expect.

In that setting there were between 3% and 5% of those samples which were ER−/PR+. They actually did better than any of the other groups. The confidence intervals were really wide, of course, but they certainly benefited from the tamoxifen. The point is that they did better than the ER+ PR+ group. What it sort of provokes in my mind was that, within the NATO trial, an accidental and disproportionate number of ER−/PR+ did well, driving forward the idea that ER− patients overall got some benefit. This is sort of an accident of history that has driven us forward, particularly in this country, to continue to support that view. I would certainly not say that ER−/PR− group could get any benefit whatsoever. Those data do encourage me to think that ER−/PR+ do benefit.

M. Dixon: I'm with Kent [Osborne] on this one. We do get rapid fixation on our tissues. We see a negligible number of patients who are ER−/PR+. I think Mitch's [Dowsett] series is an historic data set. Fixation techniques have changed over time. Our experience with modern fixatives rapidly applied to tissues is that the number of patients that are ER−/PR+ is incredibly small.

C. K. Osborne: For the fallback position I think you're right. I think the fact that PR is there probably indicates that ER must be there, maybe at very low levels or maybe a false negative. For the moment, they probably ought to be treated with hormone therapy.

N. Wolmark: In the days of cytosolic receptor analyses, we saw ER−/PR+ in about 6%. They behaved like ER+ patients.

C. K. Osborne: All of the data in this 14,000-patient study, which I mentioned, were ligand-binding assay. We saw it in about 5% of the patients. Even there we couldn't dissect out a clear benefit. It was just such a small number.

I think we've come a long way. We now have better endocrine therapies that are more tolerable. There is no question in ER+ postmenopausal women that adjuvant endocrine therapy is two or three times better than chemotherapy in terms of reducing the risk of recurrence.

We heard a lot today about new agents. Steve Johnston reviewed the data on the newer SERMs. I have to agree with him. It's disappointing. I don't see any new SERMs on the horizon that are going to replace tamoxifen. Maybe there is one out there. I think there are two or three on his slide, the GW compound, lasofoxifene, and maybe one other that are still under investigation.

Maybe they will be useful in prevention similar to raloxifene with less uterotropic action. But I don't see any being non-crossresistant with tamoxifen, for instance. I don't see any that are waiting in the wings to replace tamoxifen. I think tamoxifen or toremifene is it for the foreseeable future.

Also I think we need to get over this idea that tamoxifen is dead. Yes, the aromatase inhibitors look a little bit better. Maybe they will replace it if they haven't already in advanced disease as first-line therapy. Every time we have a new endocrine therapy that has a different mechanism of action, it [has] always found a place in the sequential use of the treatment of the disease.

Yes, maybe one drug will now be put to the front, but that doesn't mean that the other one will not be used later in sequence.

Furthermore, with the new molecular biology and new understanding about how ER works, it may well be that with the combination of a growth factor inhibitor plus tamoxifen that the bone-sparing effects of tamoxifen will be preserved, which may be by a different mechanism. But the combination may render tamoxifen as active or even more so than aromatase inhibitors if preclinical data are confirmed. I think we still need to keep an open mind about tamoxifen and not just throw it away and quit studying it.

We heard a little bit about the SERDs, and those are very interesting drugs. I worked on fulvestrant in its preclinical development. I think the problem with this drug is we don't know the optimal way to use it yet. I think the dose that we have now is too low. It's also very expensive. If I were the company I would definitely spend some dollars trying to figure out the optimal dose of fulvestrant before I initiated a lot of other clinical trials.

Obviously, the aromatase inhibitors were a major topic of today's and yesterday's discussions. I think they do represent an advance. I think it's an interesting conceptual advance, too. What it's telling us is you get a greater level of anti-estrogenicity, if you will, in the tumors by lowering the ligand for the receptor than you do by blocking the receptor with a SERM. I think the reason is because the little bit of agonist activity of SERMs prevents them from being as effective at lowering the ligand concentration in the tumor to very low levels. That's important in thinking about how these various drugs work.

Again, it points out the fact that SERMs are not active antagonists. They are only antagonists in the presence of a more effective agonist, like estrogen. By themselves, they're weak agonists. They do not inhibit gene expression by themselves but do act as antagonists in the presence of estrogen.

I think, though, we have a lot to learn about aromatase inhibitors. I'm still a little bit concerned about some of the long-term toxicities. We've got 15 or 16 million patient years of exposure to tamoxifen. We probably know more about that drug than we know about any drug that we use to treat any disease today, when you think about it, with 75,000 women on randomized controlled trials. Estrogen replacement therapy used to be the most-used treatment. We never had a randomized trial other than the 75-patient study done in the '70s to show that it relieved hot flashes, until now.

We know an awful lot about tamoxifen. One of the questions I wanted to ask the aromatase mavens here is: The brain has significant levels of aromatase; it must be there for a reason. Is long-term inhibition of that going to be good or is it going to be bad? The dementia problem now reported with estrogen may be related to microinfarcts from its vascular effects rather than an effect on the brain itself. I wondered if somebody could talk about that.

I'm also concerned about the long-term cardiovascular effects and obviously bone. I wonder if maybe Mitch [Dowsett] could comment. Do we know what aromatase does in the brain? Is there a concern about inhibiting it for a long period of time?

M. Dowsett: I don't know of any studies that define what the aromatase is doing in the brain. I think you're right. It remains a concern that the aromatase inhibitors in a preventive context could be detrimental to this. What I would say is that within IBIS-II, there is a cognitive function subprotocol, which is being designed by Leslie Fallowfield and her group, that will be a detailed assessment of this. I don't know of any answers at the present time.

N. Wolmark: That would be the best setting to test it in because we're becoming more and more aware of chemo brain. It's probably a multifactorial issue if you use advanced disease as a measurement for it.

A. Bhatnagar: We have to step back at least in time before we begin to try to answer the question regarding the significance of aromatase in the brain of postmenopausal women. The biological reason for aromatase in the brain, both in premenopausal women and in men, is that it produces the feedback signal for the gonadotropins. We've shown that very well in men now, that when you inhibit aromatase in adult men, luteinizing hormone (LH) signal goes up. The LH signal drives the testes to make more testosterone and it does that very, very effectively. Estrogens in men are actually the feedback signal.

In premenopausal women, estrogens are also the feedback signal in the brain in terms of cyclicity and in terms of the premenopausal status. It may be that what we're dealing with in the postmenopausal brain is an aromatase that is a remnant from the premenopausal situation. It may not really have very much primary significance in terms of its being there. If there were a reason for aromatase to disappear when it's not being used anymore, maybe we wouldn't see aromatase in the brains of postmenopausal women. It certainly is there for the premenopausal women to ensure reproduction, to ensure procreation of the species, and the normal endocrine functions of a premenopausal woman.

R. Santen: I think we have to be very careful about this. There is aromatase in many parts of the brain. There is ER-alpha as well as ER-beta. Dr. Toran-Allerand at Columbia University has conducted several studies using cultured neuronal cells and has shown major direct effects of estrogen produced via aromatase on neuronal cells. Fred Naftolin of Yale University also has shown morphologic effects in the brain 20 minutes after estrogen administration.

I think this is one of the issues very much like the issue of hormone replacement therapy. If we're going to expose a large number of women to an agent that could potentially do something, I think it's incumbent on us to begin to look at the endpoints carefully so that we will know in 10 years whether these aspects will be correct or not.

I think the other aspect, as Kent [Osborne] mentioned, is the whole cardiovascular area. A variety of basic biologic data suggests that estrogen exerts important effects on the cardiovascular system. These effects are mediated at least partially by the nongenomic receptors on the endothelial cells. A number of pathways such as the nitrous oxide pathway can mediate these effects. Clearly the Women's Health Initiative Study showed that estrogen can exacerbate heart disease. One could predict that aromatase inhibitors might have the opposite effect.

I think it's really quite important that when we expose a large number of women to these agents, and particularly in the preventive setting, we must look very closely at these parameters in addition to some that we really haven't thought about at this point.

P. Goss: Just to comment on this. I don't think anybody planning aromatase inhibitor trials is not cognizant of these potential side effects. For instance, in our own planning for our aromatase inhibitor trial, we've spent many, many months consulting with all the quality-of-life experts, including the investigators involved in prevention and adjuvant trials such as IBIS-II, Leslie Fallowfield and Ian Tannock. To date, we don't think there are any gross cognitive dysfunctions in the trials that have been conducted. As far as possible, we are going to look at this in the MA17 study.

What we need is very careful tools to examine executive function, higher cognitive function, subtle changes, which are important but difficult to measure. [As] in IBIS-II, with Leslie's [Fallowfield] tools, we are developing similar very careful cognitive function substudies, to look not just at mini-mental-status level of cognitive change, but at very subtle cognitive dysfunction over prolonged periods of time.

C. K. Osborne: Another area that we discussed briefly, which I think is an exciting strategy, is that of neoadjuvant endocrine therapy. I can't understand why American clinicians and some European clinicians are so reluctant to try that. Maybe you get a little higher collagen receptor (CR) rate from chemotherapy and a little more rapid reduction of the tumor, but you've got to look at the survival of the patient. In a postmenopausal woman, endocrine therapy eradicates micrometastases much more frequently than chemotherapy and it results in superior survival.

I think this is an area in which we can also learn a lot about biology that may give us markers predicting who should get tamoxifen adjuvant therapy or an aromatase inhibitor after surgery. It's attractive to me for a variety of reasons. There ought to be more studies of neoadjuvant endocrine therapy, not only as a tool to learn about biology but also to see if it is more efficacious in some way.

M. Dowsett: One clear issue that Matt [Ellis] brought up, which we didn't get much time to really speak about, was the surrogate marker issue. It regarded whether or not these short-term changes might actually predict long-term outcome. In particular, I think you said, Matt, that we don't have indications that the changes in Ki67 actually predict for adjuvant usage.

M. Ellis: Not for aromatase inhibitors; I know there is a little data coming out for tamoxifen now from the Edinburgh group.

M. Dowsett: I think that's sort of key issue here. We concentrated on the early changes—the 2-week changes—which I'd see as sort of intermediate predictive markers. We're just getting the data now from the IMPACT trial, which would allow us to determine whether or not the change in Ki67 at 2 weeks for anastrozole, tamoxifen, and the combination, if done earlier, would have predicted the outcome of the ATAC trial.

I think that will be an important result, [and] I'd be quite keen to get your response to that.

M. Ellis: I think it is. But drug development is a different motivation for doing a neoadjuvant study. Individual prediction of drug sensitivity is a different question, which is what I was trying to get at in my talk. What I think the letrozole versus tamoxifen neoadjuvant trial showed, and I think probably what IMPACT will show, is that in terms of drug development decisions, our current intermediate endpoints are rather good.

Asking drug development questions in the neoadjuvant setting, that's what is appealing to me. For example, we have plans to do an exemestane versus exemestane/celecoxib neoadjuvant study because there is a big neoadjuvant study testing this question.

Neoadjuvant studies are a way to avoid tripping over ourselves. The many opportunities with new biologic agents are going to be a challenge and the question will be which combination is the best to take forward into a very large, adjuvant study. Therefore, I'm quite hopeful in the same way you are that a neoadjuvant approach is the answer here. I am a little less hopeful in terms of using neoadjuvant endocrine therapy as a way to predict the long-term effectiveness of adjuvant endocrine therapy on an individual basis because a very large study will be necessary.

M. Dowsett: I agree entirely. Perhaps there is a slight middle way on this, if you like, which we're beginning to use. One thing that has become clear is that the 2-week change that you get in proliferation is quite closely associated with the change that you see at 3 months in these neoadjuvant studies. We've got a trial, which should start in September, that is designed around that observation. That is, all patients started on an aromatase inhibitor would get a 2-week biopsy.

Then 50% are randomized to an additional agent and 50% stay on an aromatase inhibitor. What we'll be trying to see is whether this group with the aromatase inhibitor stays relatively high and has an unchanging Ki67 on its own, whether the addition of this new agent would actually lead to antiproliferative response in that group. It's still looking at groups rather than individuals.

C. K. Osborne: I have just two more comments before Adrian (Harris) can take over and talk about today's activities. That is, we had a couple of talks on endocrine therapy in premenopausal women. One of the things that struck me is that while we know quite a bit about adjuvant endocrine therapy in postmenopausal women, we have a lot to learn in premenopausal women. I suppose some of the reasons for that is the misconception about the endocrine responsiveness of premenopausal women that existed for a decade until we finally concluded that if you administered it for 5 years, tamoxifen was just as effective as in older women. Maybe that's one reason.

Another reason is that pharmaceutical companies don't like to study their new hormonal type drugs in premenopausal women. It is about marketing issues. They tend to focus on post-, where there are more patients who are much easier to study. Now we've got to sort things out in the younger woman. I think we have a lot to learn. We don't even know for sure about combination endocrine/chemotherapy, which patients should get ovarian ablation and which should not. What is the role of aromatase inhibitors along with ovarian ablation? LHRH plus tamoxifen seems better than LHRH alone, but is it better than just tamoxifen? There are a lot of issues there that I think we need to study more carefully regarding endocrine therapy in the premenopausal woman and try and get over this mental block that these patients are chemotherapy patients, which I think still exists in a lot of places.

J. Ingle: In the discussion after the premenopausal session the other day, we talked about the portfolio of studies in premenopausal adjuvant that will be beginning. I think this has taken years to get people together. I guess Ajay [Bhatnagar] maybe wasn't aware at least of what North American Intergroup and IBCSG and BIG will be doing. We'll be looking at three studies to address some of the major questions. I think they have to be publicized for more support.

C. K. Osborne: Lastly, we've heard a lot of talk today and yesterday about selecting the proper patient by evidence that the target is there. I'm really concerned about that. We have already three targets that we know are valuable clinically, HER-2, ER, and PR. Yet, we have not established standards to measure those, despite the fact that ER has been around for a long time and HER-2 for 12 or 15 years.

This is a pathology test that would seem to be the responsibility of the leadership in pathology to standardize and quality control to make sure that patients are treated correctly.

There are patients at risk of dying because they're being mistreated on the basis of false receptor assays. Prognostic and predictive markers are only going to become more and more important as we go into the era of molecular medicine.

H. Sasano: I think from the standpoint of the pathologists, in ideal situations, everything should be centralized in one or several laboratories. However, for instance, in cases [in] Japan, it is practically impossible because of billing or other problems. Scientifically, if it is going to be centralized in one lab, this would be fine, but it may be difficult in a real environment. Therefore, continuous education to those involved in the laboratories is very important like USCAP or ASCP or other relevant meetings. That is probably the most practical way. However, I would like to emphasize that the centralization is key for the standardization.

N. Wolmark: There are other ways to get quality control. B-31, our initial analysis of the immunohistochemistry for HER-2/neu, was disconcerting. By limiting analyses to larger labs, by insisting that FISH be done for the "plus" cases, you can certainly increase accuracy, but it's a major effort. There are ways to improve accuracy, but they are extremely time consuming and expensive, and we're not in the business of quality control.

H. Sasano: Also I'd like to add one thing. [As] Mike [Dixon] mentions, the fixation, durations of the fixation, and the time from taking out the specimen to fixation is also very important in quality control. I think that this also should be emphasized from the pathologists to surgeons or the other clinicians.

I. C. Henderson: You touched on chemotherapy in premenopausal women. You touched on it in [the] neoadjuvant situation. It seems to me that we should go a little bit beyond that. The overviews have always come up with the conclusion that chemotherapy and endocrine therapy are additive in all situations. It seems to me that there are sufficient data from individual trials, and maybe the most remarkable of those is the International Breast Cancer Study Group, to say that they probably are not additive in all situations.

A priority going forward, particularly in the United States where almost everybody gets both, is that there seem to be a number of situations where they really are not additive. In fact, it may be the opposite direction.

We worry about the effects of 5 years of an aromatase inhibitor on cognitive function as a theoretical construct in our studies. I think the questions of the effects of chemotherapy and quality of life are much more clear-cut and are an issue that certainly, in North America, require much more attention going forward in trying to define that group which may be a substantial percentage of receptor-positive patients, where there really isn't any advantage of adding chemotherapy, given the quality of endocrine therapies we have today.

M. Ellis: Perhaps in a couple [of] years time we'll be able to report on some progress in that area. Together with CTEP, NCI, and the Breast Intergroup, there are moves toward a trial that would take patients who had ER+ tumors that were node negative, and then run a prognostic cluster, and separate patients into three groups. These would include a prognostic group in which the outcome on endocrine therapy is thought to be excellent and the calculated benefit from chemotherapy is insignificant. There would be a gray area group where they would randomize to chemo versus not. Then a third area with poor prognosis ER+ disease, perhaps that luminal subtype B that was discussed earlier, who will get chemotherapy. Using molecular markers to rationalize who gets chemotherapy is something that we'll be trying to do over the next 5 to 10 years.

A. Harris: One of the things I thought particularly interesting this morning was other potential roles of estrogen that Dick Santen put forward, as to whether it has direct genotoxicity, as shown in this elegant work he has done.

What I would like [more] see is to work with the animal model, not at the very high estrogen level he used, but using levels mimicking the human estrogen level, which are much lower. I don't know what you think about that, how way out the estrogen levels are compared to the levels you might find in patients?

R. Santen: That's a very critical point. With the model, we can actually clamp the levels of estradiol at any desired levels. Our current studies are lowering the dosage to determine minimally effective doses. The problem, of course, may be the issue of magnitude of dose versus duration of exposure. The higher the dose, the shorter the time of exposure needed. This is a model of carcinogenesis, so it may be difficult to observe the animals long enough to really focus on dose sufficiently, carefully, but it's an excellent point.

A. Harris: How much estrogen-receptor inhibition do we need and how much depletion do we need to get maximal effect? It looks as if, when you get escape from effects of Zoladex®, you actually need to eliminate every trace of estrogen. Is more suppression sufficient to stop resistance emerging? It is relevant to the design of the trials we have heard about in terms of how early and how much depletion you need in terms of DCIS or ADH if you want to prevent tumors. Then an issue would be whether patients could tolerate severe depletion.

R. Santen: I could comment briefly that the model would suggest that it's stoichiometric. The higher level of estrogen, the greater number of mutations that would ultimately be produced. The effect of estrogen on self-proliferation ought to be dose-response related also. The concept could clearly accommodate a partial suppression with a partial reduction.

A. Harris: What Mitch [Dowsett] is putting forth is to give hormone replacement on the suppressant estradiol levels—trying it as a more global health viewpoint. You're talking about women that have no cancer, who have a moderate risk of cancer. One of the things that is missing is folate as has been shown to be potentially valuable. That's folate deficiency seems to be related to the risk of alcohol and breast cancer. You try to talk about giving universal tablets to people. In fact, you're missing other elements of epidemiology that could be fed in to the global pill for women's health. I don't know if you have any comments on that, Mitch.

M. Dowsett: That's a cracking idea.

J. Ingle: The point about alcohol and breast cancer risk—a small amount of folate would help.

P. Lonning: Adrian, the reason why we like to put in folate is because you expect an increase of homocysteine levels and cardiovascular risk, for example. In the 027 placebo-controlled study, we're actually determining homocysteine levels, which is the best surrogate parameter for functional folate status. We will reveal that with respect to exemestane.

A. Harris: Then the mechanism of the evolution of the ER– tumors, and whether they actually come from receptor-positive tumors is obviously quite important, as to what stage of breast cancer evolution you give these aromatase inhibitors—whether you actually are going to prevent the evolution of the ER– tumors. Would anyone like to comment on that, that ER– tumors may develop from a stem cell from a separate pathway or do you think they come from the ER+ tumors?

R. Santen: I quite honestly don't think you'll get a consensus on that. It has been suggested that ER+ tumors later become ER– tumors. I personally don't believe there is any direct data to prove either way, whether there are two pathways or one pathway. I think we'll have to learn that in time. My sense is that a number of people feel that most of the tumors start as ER+ and go to ER−. We will clearly have to get the data to demonstrate that.

P. Lonning: Probably one of the interesting things will be the basal cell tumors. It could be interesting to look into the gene profiling of DCIS to see whether some of these early stage tumors also reveal the basal cell gene expression profile. There can be the question whether these are derived by different pathways.

C. Benz: There is also the substantial preclinical evidence indicating that when you give known carcinogens to animals that then develop ER− mammary cancers that you can also interrupt this ER− carcinogenic pathway by doing ovariectomies or even administering anti-estrogens to these animals. So, you don't need to invoke conversion of an ER+ to an ER− breast cancer cell to appreciate that there are essential paracrine interactions between ER+ and ER− mammary cells driving normal glandular development that may also be preserved and then lost somewhere between primary tumor growth and metastatic progression.

A. Harris: I think the evolution of resistance and the different pathways that three speakers are talking [about], as well as the new data on the membrane ER pathways, are particularly exciting. I wonder whether you can assess the membrane pathway on tumor samples yet? It may be possible to follow the evolution of resistance.

C. K. Osborne: I think it would be very difficult with the tools we have right now to assess that in any quantitative fashion. People are just beginning to even see it. As Craig [Allred] has often told me, pathologists have optimized their estrogen receptor assay by immunohistochemistry to nuclear staining. By doing so, we may have inadvertently gotten rid of an important component, thinking it was background. I think that we need to start looking at that again.

C. Allred: Certainly these are just anecdotal observations, but at least given the general level of sensitivity of the types of detection systems we're using in immunochemistry now, observing ER-alpha anywhere but the nucleus is a pretty rare thing, at least in substantial levels. So there might be a pony there, but I would be surprised.

Having said that, I'm working with DAKO to help them develop a kit for ER and PR akin to what they've done for HER-2 in the Hercept test. They're trying to apply a new generation of detection systems that are at least ten-fold more sensitive than anything that we've been using. I'm not disclosing any secrets or anything; you can actually buy the detection system independently now. It's just the application to ER that I think is interesting.

Just in the very early pilot studies that we're doing trying to titer sensitivity in that, we're seeing ER everywhere, in every kind of cell. This may get muddier before it gets more clear.

A. Harris: I think it is exciting that the different pathways—the ER in the membrane and tyrosine kinases—are proving valid targets for overcoming resistance. But each presenter has found different pathways depending on how they set up their model. I think that is showing the complexity of trying to devise clinical trials. The point I was making in my talk before is profiling. You need to profile people in advance for these pathways. For example, Iressa plus tamoxifen in hormone resistance, analyzing IGF1 receptor, HER-2, and other pathways on the samples should be done, even though you do not stratify patients by those in advance. I think it's really important that some of the methodology problems are overcome to allow this type of analysis serially.

M. Dowsett: The data which I showed at ASCO this year in collaboration with Kent's [Osborne] group indicated a discordance between primary tumors and recurrent tumors and the expression of the two common factors, HER-2 and ER. There were also clearly quite substantial changes in the P38 MAP kinase. This provokes all sorts of different thoughts. For example, the rather strange results we get sometimes from metastatic-disease studies. It suggests this may well be due to discordance in the phenotype of primary and metastatic disease.

I'd be interested in the clinicians' responses to what proportion of patients with metastatic disease one could reasonably expect to get a one or more sample of a metastatic lesion to do these tests with. We don't just want skin lesions. Can you respond to that, Kent?

C. K. Osborne: If we could prove that it was really important to get it, you could get it on a lot of them. I have biopsied lungs and livers back in the 1970s for ER assay. We don't do that now because ER is relatively stable and we'll just go ahead and treat if the primary tumor is ER+. I think though, we're coming to a point, maybe in the near future, that we're not going to be able to rely on the primary tumor to give accurate information on a particular signaling pathway years after chemotherapy and so forth. We're going to have to, if I'm right, start biopsying people with recurrent disease on a regular basis just before the treatment, and that may require a biopsy of the liver or lung. But we are going to have to assess their molecular profile in order to determine what treatment to use.

We've just spent a lot of time in preparation for the clinical trials that I listed on our slide. Trying to develop assays that we think will somewhat accurately assess molecules like IGF receptor, MAP kinase, AKT, P38 and others may be important. I think we're there on most of those. We can apply those now particularly to the neoadjuvant setting, which I think is a very valuable setting to begin to explore how these things affect response to various endocrine therapies, with or without growth factor inhibitors and so forth.

It's going to turn out to be a very complex story. If you look at primary disease, endocrine therapy is curative in some patients with microscopic metastases. When you look at metastatic disease, at best what we can achieve is control of the disease for a relatively short period of time from the patient's point of view. There is a big difference in the tumor, not just sheer numbers of tumor cells, but a large difference in the biology of the tumor, between the primary setting and the metastatic setting.

Maybe in the primary setting, the tumor is reliant on one or two pathways as its major driving force. After additional progression in the metastatic disease setting, there may be multiple pathways operative. I hope that we don't abandon therapies, particularly these growth factor inhibitors and angiogenesis inhibitors, by studying only metastatic disease. It's amazing to me in the colon cancer metastatic studies that inhibiting one of the many angiogenesis factors has any effect at all. I'm terribly surprised about that.

I think we're going to have to change our whole paradigm in studying these new agents. We're going to have to bite the bullet and study them earlier. I would predict, based on our model, if you give an EGF receptor tyrosine kinase inhibitor alone to a group of breast cancer patients that it wouldn't work. But if you use it in the right setting, perhaps along with endocrine therapy, it will. I think the days of treating everybody with one therapy and hoping that it works are gone. We're really going to have to use our brains as well as sophisticated molecular tests to select the patients.

I. C. Henderson: Taking your comment one step further, and I think this applied to some of the things that Adrian [Harris] said as well. Perhaps we don't have to give up this idea that we always start and evaluate each new intervention separately. It's clear from a lot of things that have been said that we're probably not going to maximize, particularly reduction, or affect things that affect signal-transduction pathways, just by affecting one.

We may need to affect two or three or four, maybe try to go for a maximum effect and then back off, rather than the more traditional approach where, in truth, each one of them may have only a marginal effect. Without huge trials we're not going to detect that. We're not going to be able to get proof of principle. Maybe we need to jump forward with multiple interventions and then sort out later which ones are the critical ones.

C. K. Osborne: I think you're absolutely right, but you're going to have to convince the FDA in the United States and drug companies to work together. The FDA will have to allow multiple new drugs to be used in the same patients. Right now I don't think they permit it, even though that makes the most sense.

J. Klijn: There are two major problems. The acceptance of two experimental drugs in one trial. But furthermore, you need frequently the cooperation of more than one pharmaceutical company.

R. Santen: I'd just like to make one last comment. We've been focusing on a number of things in this session, but I think if we look ahead 10 years, we'd like to prevent breast cancer. We have the tools now to potentially accomplish this. Risk is a component of the series of questions that we have. If we were to prioritize now how we as a group could make the biggest impact on breast cancer, my sense would be that we would identify the patients at highest risk of breast cancer and begin to apply the tools that we have now. I think that with prevention strategies we will have many fewer problems with development of resistance, problems with genetic mutations in other pathways, and so on.

I sit here thinking that we now have the ability to really prevent breast cancer. That's what we ought to be focusing on. We do have the tools to do it.

P. Goss: Just to endorse what you're saying, Dick, there was a very excellent paper published by Polyak and her colleagues from Harvard toward the end of last year where they biopsied breast tissue at all stages from normal epithelium through to advanced metastatic cancer. They did detailed analysis of all the tissues.

Really the conclusion of their paper was that between groups of specimens from patients, you only had genetic consensus up to the level of atypical ductal hyperplasia. Even when you got to DCIS, there was genetic chaos and multiple pathways between different individuals. So I agree with Dick [Santen]. Staring at us in the face is an opportunity for simple prevention technique with the potential for a large preventive effect, by intervening early in the pathway. I think to identify the right patient and to use these tools is going to have the most important public health impact on the disease. To me, that's where the aromatase inhibitors are really important.

J. Klijn: Just a problem is the cost–benefit ratio in metastatic disease, indeed, you cannot cure.

But in prevention you are overtreating a lot of women. So how to find a compromise?

P. Goss: We've got to refine our selection criteria for women at high risk, as we've said.

A. Bhatnagar: I think we've come to the end of the second day now. I'm just going to say a couple of words. I think I said what I had to say at the beginning of the meeting. The one thing that I did not say, which I'd like to say now, is that I think if you look at all the people around the table, the ones who are here and also the few who unfortunately had to leave, the one thing that is most valuable to all of us around the table is our time. I sincerely hope that for all the people that were here, you felt that the expenditure of these two days of time was, for you personally, something that was a positive benefit.

I can tell you that the reader of the proceedings that come out of the Gleneagles meeting now will certainly have a lot of ideas, a lot of new thoughts, hypotheses to chew on. I think that this contribution to the open literature in the area of endocrine therapy of breast cancer will again be a positive contribution. I want to thank all of you for the 2 days that we've had. A lot of stimulating discussion.

I want to thank our co-chairs, Jim Ingle and Mitch Dowsett, and all the discussion leaders, the speakers, and the discussants themselves, because as I said before, the essence of this meeting is discussion, controversy, and more discussion. So thanks once again to all of you, and I hope we will see you again at this meeting in 2 years, at the latest.

Index

Index

Index

Index